NURSES' HANDBOOK OF
HEALTH
ASSESSMENT

Sixth Edition

Janet R. Weber, EdD, RN
Professor
Department of Nursing
Southeast Missouri State University
Cape Girardeau, Missouri

Wolters Kluwer | Lippincott Williams & Wilkins
Health

Philadelphia · Baltimore · New York · London
Buenos Aires · Hong Kong · Sydney · Tokyo

Senior Acquisitions Editor: Elizabeth Nieginski
Development Editor: Renee Gagliardi/Katherine Burland
Editorial Assistant: Kristin Sheppard
Senior Production Editor: Mary Kinsella
Director of Nursing Production: Helen Ewan
Senior Managing Editor / Production: Erika Kors
Art Director, Illustration: Brett MacNaughton
Interior Designer: Joan Wendt
Senior Manufacturing Manager: William Alberti
Manufacturing Coordinator: Karin Duffield
Indexer: Gaye Tarallo
Compositor: Circle Graphics
Printer: R. R. Donnelley, Shenzhen, China

6th Edition

9 8 7 6 5 4 3 2 1

Library of Congress Cataloging-in-Publication Data

Nurses' handbook of health assessment / [edited by] Janet R. Weber. — 6th ed.
   p. ; cm.
 Includes bibliographical references and index.
 ISBN-13: 978-0-7817-6632-6 (alk. paper)
 ISBN-10: 0-7817-6632-X (alk. paper)
 1. Nursing assessment—Handbooks, manuals, etc. I. Weber, Janet.
 [DNLM: 1. Nursing Assessment—methods—Handbooks. 2. Medical History
Taking—methods—Handbooks. 3. Physical Examination—methods—Handbooks.   WY
49 N97296 2008]
   RT48.N863 2008
   616.07'5—dc22   2006100108

DISCLAIMER

LWW.com

To my loving husband, Bill,
for all your wise encouragement,
patience, and confidence

To my son, Joe, for teaching me to live more
fully by relaxing and taking risks

To my son, Wesley, for your endless,
energizing humor and wise insights

To my mom for photocopying
and tending to details

To my colleagues, Jane and Ann,
for all your contributions that hold
this guide together

To all my students who teach me
how to teach

To all the nurses who inspire me to
continue to write

Contributors

Jill Cash, MSN, FNP, RN-CS
Family Nurse Practitioner
Carbondale Family Medicine
Carbondale, Illinois
Instructor, Graduate Family Nurse Practitioner Program
Southern Illinois University
Edwardsville, Illinois

Jane Kelley, PhD, RN
Professor of Nursing
School of Nursing University of Mississippi Medical Center
Jackson, Mississippi

Suha Ballout, MSN, RN
Masters Candidate
American University of Beirut Medical Center
Beirut, Lebanon

Ann Sprengel, EdD, RN
Professor of Nursing
Southeast Missouri State University
Cape Girardeau, Missouri

Cathy Young, DNS, APRN, BC
Sexual Assault Nurse Examiner and Forensic Examiner
Paragould, Arkansas

Preface

PURPOSE

The sixth edition of the *Nurses' Handbook of Health Assessment* continues to provide students and practicing nurses with an up-to-date reference and guide to assist with interviewing clients and performing a physical assessment.

This guide will remind the student or nurse of questions to ask, examinations to make, and procedures to carry out when assessing the client. In addition, it clearly identifies normal versus abnormal findings and supplies examples of precise descriptive language that will make documentation easy and accurate.

KEY FEATURES AND NEW CHAPTERS

Key features of this handbook include full-color anatomy and physiology images, illustrations of normal and abnormal physiologic findings, highlighted risk factors, the three-column format of assessment procedures, and the spiral binding that allows the handbook to stay open on any flat surface.

The sixth edition includes two new chapters important for every encounter with all types of clients: Chapter 5, "Pain Assessment: The Fifth Vital Sign," and Chapter 22, "Assessment of Families Using Violence."

ORGANIZATION

The handbook has 22 chapters. The first three provide an overview of the nursing assessment process and its rationale.

Chapter 1 explains the purpose of a nursing health history. *Chapter 2* contains guidelines needed to elicit subjective data for a complete nursing health history, and begins with questions for a client profile and developmental history followed by health history questions organized according to Gordon's 11 functional health patterns (Gordon, 1994). The reader is referred to specific physical assessment chapters for related objective data as appropriate. A list of associated nursing diagnoses that may be identified by client response follows each section. The nursing diagnoses are based on the currently accepted North American Nursing Diagnosis Association (NANDA) taxonomy of diagnostic categories. The functional health patterns format focuses the health history within the independent domain of professional nursing. *Chapter 3* consists of guidelines for performing the physical assessment.

Chapters 4 through *19* present assessment procedures in an easy to understand format. Each chapter contains the following:

- Focus questions specific to the body system being assessed
- Illustrations of relevant anatomy or physiologic processes
- Equipment needed for the examination
- Physical assessment procedure
- Pediatric variations
- Geriatric variations
- Cultural variations
- Selected and related collaborative problems
- Teaching tips

Chapters 20, 21, and *22* are a guide to special assessments:

- Assessment of the Childbearing Woman
- Assessment of Newborns and Infants
- Assessment of Families Using Violence

COLLECTION OF STANDARD ASSESSMENT TOOLS

Appendices at the end of the text bring together in one convenient place the many reference tools needed for health assessment. These include nursing assessment forms, developmental norms, growth charts, immunization schedules, sample of an adult health history and physical assessment, a family assessment, breast and skin self-examination guides, blood pressure classification and management guide, nursing diagnoses, and collaborative problems. New appendices to this edition include testicular self-examination guidelines and a convenient Spanish translation guide for nursing health history and physical examination.

Janet R. Weber, EdD, RN

Contents

THE NURSING HEALTH HISTORY

DEFINITION AND PURPOSE

A nursing health history can be defined as the systematic collection of subjective data (stated by the client) and objective data (observed by the nurse) used to determine a client's functional health pattern status (Table 1–1). The nurse collects physiologic, psychological, sociocultural, developmental, and spiritual client data. These data assist the nurse in identifying nursing diagnoses and/or collaborative problems.

Nursing diagnoses may fall into one of three categories: actual, risk, or wellness (Table 1–2). An "actual" nursing diagnosis is a human response to health conditions/life processes that currently exists in an individual, family, or community that can be validated by the defining characteristics of that diagnostic category. A "risk" diagnosis describes human responses of an individual, family, or community and is supported by risk factors that contribute to increased vulnerability. A "wellness" nursing diagnosis describes human responses about an individual, family, or community that have a readiness for enhancement (NANDA, 2005–2006).

Wellness diagnoses may be described as opportunities for enhancement of a healthy state (Kelley, Avant, & Frisch, 1995). There are occasions when clients are ready to improve an already healthy level of function. When such an opportunity exists, the nurse can support the client's movement toward greater health and wellness by identifying "opportunities for enhancement."

Carpenito-Moyet (2006) defines collaborative problems as certain "physiological complications that nurses monitor to detect their onset or changes in status. Nurses manage collaborative problems using both physician-prescribed and nursing-prescribed interventions to minimize the complications of the events." The definitive treatment for a nursing diagnosis is developed by the nurse; the definitive treatment for a collaborative problem is developed by both the nurse and the physician. Not all physiologic complications are collaborative problems. If the nurse can prevent the complication or provide the primary treatment, then the problem may very well be a nursing diagnosis. For example, nurses can prevent and treat pressure ulcers. The NANDA nursing diagnosis to use, therefore, is Risk for Impaired Skin Integrity. See Table 1–2 for an example of these three categories

TABLE 1–1	COMPARING SUBJECTIVE AND OBJECTIVE DATA	

	Subjective	Objective
Description	Data elicited and verified by the client	Data directly or indirectly observed through measurement
Sources	Client Family and significant others Client record Other health care professionals	Observations and physical assessment findings of the nurse or other health care professionals Documentation of assessments made in client record Observations made by the client's family or significant others
Methods used to obtain data	Client interview	Observation and physical examination
Skills needed to obtain data	Interview and therapeutic communication skills Caring ability and empathy Listening skills	Inspection Palpation Percussion Auscultation
Examples	"I have a headache." "It frightens me." "I am not hungry."	Respirations 16 per minute BP 180/100, apical pulse 80 and irregular X-ray film reveals fractured pelvis

and directions for stating each type of diagnosis. Nursing diagnoses, risk nursing diagnoses, wellness nursing diagnoses, and collaborative problems are listed in Appendices 14 and 15.

Collaborative problems are equivalent in importance to nursing diagnoses but represent the interdependent or collaborative role of nursing, whereas nursing diagnoses represent the independent role of the nurse (Carpenito-Moyet, 2006). Figure 1–1 illustrates the decision-making process involved in distinguishing a nursing diagnosis from a collaborative health problem. The nurse can use this model to decide

TABLE 1–2	COMPARISON OF WELLNESS, RISK, AND ACTUAL NURSING DIAGNOSES		
	Wellness Diagnoses	Risk Diagnoses	Actual Nursing Diagnoses
Client status	Human responses to levels of wellness that have a readiness for enhancement (NANDA, 2005–2006)	Human responses that may develop in a vulnerable individual, family, or community (NANDA, 2005–2006)	Human responses to health conditions/life processes that exist (NANDA, 2005–2006)
Format for stating	"Readiness for Enhanced . . ."	"Risk for . . ."	"Nursing diagnoses and related to clause"
Examples	Readiness for Enhanced Body Image Readiness for Enhanced Family Processes Readiness for Enhanced Effective Breast-feeding Readiness for Enhanced Skin Integrity	Risk for Disturbed Body Image Risk for Interrupted Family Processes Risk for Ineffective Breast-feeding Risk for Impaired Skin Integrity	Disturbed Body Image related to wound on hand that is not healing Dysfunctional Family Processes: Alcoholism Ineffective Breast-feeding related to poor mother–infant attachment Impaired Skin Integrity related to immobility

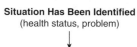

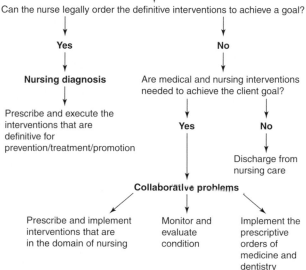

FIGURE 1-1 Differentiation of nursing diagnoses from collaborative problems. (Carpenito-Moyet, L. J. [2006]. *Nursing diagnoses: Application to clinical practice* [11th ed.]. Philadelphia: Lippincott Williams & Wilkins, p. 23. © 1990 Lynda Juall Carpenito.)

whether the identified problem can be treated independently as a nursing diagnosis, or whether the nurse will monitor and use both medical and nursing interventions to treat or prevent the problem. If collaborative medical and nursing interventions are not needed, the problem is discharged from nursing care and referred to medicine and/or dentistry. The difference between a medical diagnosis, collaborative problem, and nursing diagnosis is explained in Table 1–3. Guidelines for formulating nursing diagnoses and collaborative problems can be found in Table 1–4.

A nursing health history usually precedes the physical assessment and guides the nurse as to which body systems must be assessed. It also assists the nurse in establishing a nurse–client relationship, and allows client participation in identifying problems and goals. The primary source of data is the client; valuable information may also be obtained from the family, other health team members, and the client record.

TABLE 1-3 EXAMPLES OF MEDICAL DIAGNOSES, COLLABORATIVE PROBLEMS, AND NURSING DIAGNOSES

Medical Diagnoses	Collaborative Problems	Nursing Diagnoses
Fractured jaw	Potential complication: aspiration	Altered Oral Mucous Membrane related to difficulty with hygiene secondary to fixation devices Acute Pain related to tissue trauma
Diabetes mellitus	Potential complication: hyperglycemia	Impaired Skin Integrity related to poor circulation to lower extremities Deficient Knowledge (effects of exercise on need for insulin)
Pneumonia	Potential complication: hypoglycemia Potential complication: hypoxemia	Ineffective Airway Clearance related to presence of excessive mucus production Deficient Fluid Volume related to poor fluid intake

TABLE 1-4 COMPARISON OF NURSING DIAGNOSES AND COLLABORATIVE PROBLEMS

Identifying Criteria of a Nursing Diagnosis	Identifying Criteria of a Collaborative Problem
1. The client problem is physiologic, psychosocial, or spiritual.	1. The client problem is a physiologic complication.
2. The nurse monitors and treats.	2. The nurse monitors for signs and symptoms of the complication and notifies the physician if a change occurs. (In some cases the nurse may initiate interventions.)
3. The nurse independently orders and implements the primary nursing interventions.	3. The physician orders the primary treatment, and the nurse collaborates to implement additional treatments that are licensed to be implemented and monitors for responses to and effectiveness of treatments.

Format and Follow-up for Nursing Diagnoses	Format and Follow-up for Collaborative Problems
1. Use diagnostic category + "related to" + etiology.	1. Use "Potential complication: _____."
2. Write specific client goals.	2. Write nursing goals.
3. Write specific nursing orders (interventions), including assessments, teaching, counseling, referrals, and direct client care.	3. Write which parameters the nurse must monitor, including how often. Indicate when the physician should be notified. Identify nursing interventions to prevent the complication and those to be initiated if a change occurs.

NURSING MODEL VERSUS MEDICAL MODEL

Several models of nursing may be used to guide the nurse in data collection. Marjory Gordon's Functional Health Pattern assessment framework (1994) is particularly useful, however, in collecting health data to formulate nursing diagnoses. Gordon has defined 11 functional health patterns that provide for a holistic client database. A pattern is a sequence of related behaviors that assists the nurse in collecting and categorizing data. These 11 functional health patterns can be used for nursing assessment in any practice areas for clients of all ages and in the assessment of families and communities. For the purpose of this handbook, assessment is focused on the individual. However, guideline questions for families organized according to functional health patterns are included in Appendix 10. The NANDA list of accepted nursing diagnoses has been grouped according to the appropriate functional health patterns. These diagnoses are listed at the end of each functional health pattern section in Chapter 2. Box 1–1 presents a brief overview of the subjective and objective assessment focus data needed for each functional health pattern.*

Using a functional health pattern framework assists the nurse with collecting data necessary to identify and validate nursing diagnoses. This approach eliminates repetition of medical data already obtained by physicians and other members of the health care team. The medical systems model (biographical data, chief complaint, present health history, past medical history, family history, psychosocial history, and review of systems) is more useful for the physician in making medical diagnoses. Clients often complain that the same information is requested by both nurses and physicians. A nursing history based on functional health patterns, however, will help eliminate this problem by assisting the nurse to assess client responses associated with nursing diagnoses and collaborative problems.

It is important for the nurse to assess each functional health pattern with clients because alterations in health can affect functioning in any of these areas, and alterations in functional health patterns can, in turn, affect health. See Appendix 1 for a sample nursing assessment form based on functional health patterns.

GUIDELINES FOR OBTAINING A NURSING HEALTH HISTORY

Phases of the Nursing Interview

Professional interpersonal and interviewing skills are necessary to obtain a valid nursing health history. The nursing interview is a com-

---

*Adapted from Gordon, M. (1994). *Nursing diagnosis: Process and application* (3rd ed.). St. Louis: Mosby–Year Book.

BOX 1–1 • Subjective and Objective Assessment Focus for Functional Health Patterns

1. Health Perception–Health Management Pattern
   Subjective data: Perception of health status and health practices used by client to maintain health
   Objective data: Appearance, grooming, posture, expression, vital signs, height, weight

2. Nutritional–Metabolic Pattern
   Subjective data: Dietary habits, including food and fluid intake
   Objective data: General physical survey, including examination of skin, mouth, abdomen, and cranial nerves (CN) V, IX, X, and XII

3. Elimination Pattern
   Subjective data: Regularity and control of bowel and bladder habits
   Objective data: Skin examination, rectal examination

4. Activity–Exercise Pattern
   Subjective data: Activities of daily living that require energy expenditure
   Objective data: Examination of musculoskeletal system, including gait, posture, range of motion (ROM) of joints, muscle tone, and strength; cardiovascular examination; peripheral vascular examination; thoracic examination

5. Sexuality–Reproduction Pattern
   Subjective data: Sexual identity, activities, and relationships; expression of sexuality and level of satisfaction with sexual patterns; reproduction patterns
   Objective data: Genitalia examination, breast examination

6. Sleep–Rest Pattern
   Subjective data: Perception of effectiveness of sleep and rest habits
   Objective data: Appearance and attention span

7. Cognitive–Perceptual Pattern
   For the purposes of this handbook, the cognitive–perceptual pattern has been divided into two parts: (1) the sensory–perceptual pattern, to include the senses of hearing, vision, smell, taste, and touch, and (2) the cognitive pattern, to include knowledge, thought perception, and language.
   a. Sensory–Perceptual Pattern
      Subjective data: Perception of ability to hear, see, smell, taste, and feel (including light touch, pain, and vibratory sensation)

> ### BOX 1-1 • (continued)
>
>   **Objective data:** Visual and hearing examinations, pain perception, cranial nerve examination; testing for taste, smell, and touch
>   b. Cognitive Pattern
>   **Subjective data:** Perception of messages, decision making, thought processes
>   **Objective data:** Mental status examination
>
> 8. Role–Relationship Pattern
>   **Subjective data:** Perception of and level of satisfaction with family, work, and social roles
>   **Objective data:** Communication with significant others, visits from significant others and family, family genogram
>
> 9. Self-perception–Self-concept Pattern
>   **Subjective data:** Perception of self-worth, personal identity, feelings
>   **Objective data:** Body posture, movement, eye contact, voice and speech pattern, emotions, moods, and thought content
>
> 10. Coping–Stress Tolerance Pattern
>   **Subjective data:** Perception of stressful life events and ability to cope
>   **Objective data:** Behavior, thought processes
>
> 11. Value–Belief Pattern
>   **Subjective data:** Perception of what is good, correct, proper, and meaningful; philosophical beliefs; values and beliefs that guide choices
>   **Objective data:** Presence of religious articles, religious actions and routines, and visits from clergy

munication process that focuses on the client's developmental, psychological, physiologic, sociocultural, and spiritual responses that can be treated with nursing and collaborative interventions. The nursing interview has three basic phases, explained below by describing the roles of the nurse and the client during each phase.

Introductory Phase

Introduce yourself and describe your role (ie, RN, student, etc.). Address the client with surname. Next, explain the purpose of the interview to the client (ie, to collect data, to understand the client's needs, and to plan nursing care). Explain the purpose of note taking, confidentiality, and the type of questions to be asked. Provide comfort, privacy, and confidentiality.

Working Phase

Facilitate the client's comments about major biographical data, reason for seeking health care, and functional health pattern responses. Use critical thinking skills to listen for and observe cues, and to interpret and validate information received from the client. Collaborate with the client to identify problems and goals. The approach used for facilitation may be either free flowing or more structured with specific questions, depending on available time and type of data needed.

Summary and Closure Phase

Summarize information obtained during the working phase and validate problems and goals with the client. You may begin to discuss possible plans to resolve the problems (nursing diagnoses and collaborative problems). Allow the client time to express feelings, concerns, and questions.

Specific Communication Techniques

Specific communication techniques are used to facilitate the interview. Following are specific guidelines for phrasing statements and questions to promote an effective and productive interview.

Types of Questions to Use

- Use open-ended questions to elicit the client's feelings and perceptions. These questions begin with "What," "How," or "Which," and require more than a one-word response.
- Use closed-ended questions to obtain facts and zero in on specific information. The client can respond with one or two words. These questions begin with "Is," "Are," "Will," "When," or "Did," and help avoid rambling by the client.
- Use a laundry list (scrambled words) approach to obtain specific answers. For example, "Is the pain severe, dull, sharp, mild, cutting, piercing?" "Does the pain occur once every year, day, month, hour?" This reduces the likelihood of the client's perceiving and providing an expected answer.
- Explore all data that deviate from normal with the following questions: "What alleviates or aggravates the problem?" "How long has it occurred?" "How severe is it?" "Does it radiate?" "When does it occur?" "Is its onset gradual or sudden?"

Types of Statements to Use

- Rephrase or repeat your perception of the client's response to reflect or clarify information shared. For example, "You feel you have a serious illness?"
- Encourage verbalization of client by saying "Um hum," "Yes," or "I agree," or nodding.
- Describe what you observe in the client. For example, "It seems you have difficulty on the right side."

Additional Helpful Hints

- Accept the client; display a nonjudgmental attitude.
- Use silence to help the client and yourself reflect and reorganize thoughts
- Provide the client with information during the interview as questions and concerns arise.

Communication Styles to Avoid

- Excessive or insufficient eye contact (varies with cultures).
- Doing other things while taking the history, and being mentally distant or physically far away from client (more than 2–3 feet).
- Biased or leading questions—for example, "You don't feel bad, do you?"
- Relying on memory to recall all the information or recording all the details.
- Rushing the client.
- Reading questions from the history form, distracting attention from the client.

Specific Age Variations

When interviewing the pediatric client from birth to early adolescence (through age 14 years), information from the history should be validated for reliability with the responsible significant other (eg, parent, grandparent).

Use the following guidelines when interviewing the geriatric patient:

- Use a gentle, genuine approach.
- Use simple, straightforward questions in lay terms. Let the client set the pace of the conversation. Be patient and listen well. Allow ample time.
- Introduce yourself, but remember that an older client may soon forget your name—you may have to write it for the client later in the interview.
- Use direct eye contact and sit at client's eye level. Establish and maintain privacy (especially important).
- Assess hearing acuity; with loss, speak slowly, face the client, and speak on the side on which hearing is more adequate. Speak louder only if you confirm client has a hearing deficit. Turn off any background noises.
- *Remember:* Age affects and often slows all body systems within an individual to varying degrees.
- Wear a name tag and provide written notes for the client to refer to in the future.

Emotional Variations

- *Angry client:* Approach in a calm, reassuring, in-control manner. Allow ventilation of client's feelings. Avoid arguing and provide personal space.

- *Anxious client:* Approach with simple, organized information. Explain your role and purpose.
- *Manipulative client:* Provide structure and set limits.
- *Depressed client:* Express interest and understanding in a neutral manner.
- *Sensitive issues* (eg, sexuality, dying, spirituality): Be aware of your own thoughts and feelings. These factors may affect the client's health and need to be discussed with someone. Such personal, sensitive topics may be referred when you do not feel comfortable discussing these topics.

Cultural Variations

Ethnic variations in communication and self-disclosure styles may seriously affect the information obtained. Be aware of possible variations in the communication styles of yourself and client. If misunderstanding or difficulty in communicating is evident, seek help from a "culture broker" who is skilled at cross-cultural communication. Frequently noted ethnic variations include:

- Reluctance to reveal personal information to strangers for various culturally based reasons.
- Variation in willingness to express emotional distress or pain openly.
- Variation in ability to receive information and/or listen.
- Variation in meaning conveyed by use of language (eg, by non-native speakers, by use of slang).
- Variation in use and meaning of nonverbal communication: eye contact, stance, gestures, demeanor (eg, eye contact may be perceived as rude, aggressive, or immodest by some cultures, but lack of eye contact may be perceived as evasive, insecure, or inattentive by other cultures; slightly bowed stance may indicate respect in some groups; size of personal space affects one's comfortable interpersonal distance; touch may be perceived as comforting or threatening).
- Variation in disease/illness perception; culture-specific syndromes or disorders are accepted by some groups (eg, *susto* in Latin America). *Susto* (fright or emotional shock) is perceived to cause general malaise, insomnia, irritability, depression, nightmares, and wasting away (dePaula, Laganá, & Gonzalez-Ramirez, 1996, p. 217).
- Variation in past, present, or future time orientation (eg, United States dominant culture is future-oriented; other cultures vary).
- Variation in family decision-making process: person other than client or client's parent may be the major decision maker re: appointments, treatments, or follow-up care for client.

Assessing Non–English-Speaking Clients

- Use a bilingual interpreter familiar with the client's culture and with health care, when possible (eg, a nurse culture broker).

- Consider the relationship of the interpreter to the client. If the interpreter is a child or of a different sex, age, or social status, interpretation may be impaired.
- Not all clients can read. Basic care terms can be communicated best by pictures.

COMPONENTS OF THE NURSING HEALTH HISTORY

HEALTH HISTORY BY FUNCTIONAL HEALTH PATTERN

Following are the components of a nursing health history incorporating a functional health pattern approach (Gordon, 1994). Prior to data collection for each functional health pattern, a client profile and developmental history are obtained.

1. Client Profile
2. Developmental History
3. Health Perception–Health Management Pattern
4. Nutritional–Metabolic Pattern
5. Elimination Pattern
6. Activity–Exercise Pattern
7. Sexuality–Reproduction Pattern
8. Sleep–Rest Pattern
9. Sensory–Perceptual Pattern
10. Cognitive Pattern
11. Role–Relationship Pattern
12. Self-Perception–Self-Concept Pattern
13. Coping–Stress Tolerance Pattern
14. Value–Belief Pattern

The purpose of each nursing health history component is explained, followed by guideline statements and questions to elicit subjective data from the client. Guideline questions should be preceded by open-ended statements to encourage the client to verbalize freely. Then ask specific questions to obtain specific information. It is important to remember that not every question will apply to every client. Use common sense and professional judgment to determine which questions are a priority and appropriate for each individual client.

Certain factors such as comfort level, anxiety level, age, and current health status must be considered as they influence the client's ability to participate fully in the interview. When appropriate, an objective data outline follows the subjective data questions and refers the examiner to the section where the specific examination technique, normal findings, and deviations from normal are located. At the end of each section is a list of corresponding nursing diagnostic categories for that specific nursing health history component. This list is divided into wellness, risk, and actual (problem) nursing diagnoses. Although clients can be at risk for most problem diagnoses, only NANDA-approved and a few selected other risk diagnoses are listed. Appendix 1 provides a documentation form for collection of subjective and objective data for each of the functional health patterns.

CLIENT PROFILE

Purpose

The purpose of the client profile is to determine biographical client data and to obtain an overview of past and present medical diagnoses and treatment that may alter a client's response. This section also helps the interviewer elicit collaborative health problems.

Subjective Data: Guideline Questions

Biographical Data

What is your name?
Tell me about your background.
When were you born?
What is your ethnic origin?
How old are you?
What level of education have you completed?
Have you ever served in the military?
Do you have a religious preference? Specify.
Where do you live?
What form of transportation do you use?
Where is the closest health care facility to you that you would go to if ill or in an emergency?

Reason for Seeking Health Care and Current Understanding of Health

Use the following mnemonic—**COLDSPA**—to explore any abnormal signs, symptoms, or problems the client reports:
Character: Describe the sign or symptom.
Onset: When did it begin?
Location: Where is it? Does it radiate?
Duration: How long does it last? Does it recur?
Severity: How bad is it?
Pattern: What makes it better? What makes it worse?
Associated factors: What other symptoms occur with it?
Explain your major reason for seeking health care.
What has the doctor told you regarding your health?
Do you understand your medical diagnosis? Explain.

Treatments/Medications

Describe the treatments and medications you have received.
How has your illness been treated in the past?

What is being planned for your treatment now?
Do you understand the purpose of your treatment?
Have you been satisfied with past treatments? Explain.
What prescribed medications are you taking?
What over-the-counter medications are you taking?
Do you have any difficulties with these medications?
How do they make you feel?
What is the purpose of these medications?

Past Illnesses/Hospitalizations

Tell me about any past illnesses/surgeries you have had.
Have you had other illnesses in the past? Specify.
How were the past illnesses treated?
Have you been in hospital before? Where? For what purpose?
How did you feel about your past hospital stays?
How can we help to improve this hospital stay for you?
Have you received any home health care? Explain.
How satisfied were you with this care?

Allergies

Are you allergic to any drugs, foods, or other environmental
    substances (eg, dust, molds, pollens, latex)?
Describe the reaction you have when exposed to the allergen.
What do you do for your allergies?

DEVELOPMENTAL HISTORY

Purpose

The purpose of the developmental history is to determine the physical, cognitive, and psychosocial development of the client to assess any developmental delays. Subjective data obtained from assessment of the functional health patterns (Role–Relationship, Cognitive, Value–Belief, and Coping–Stress Tolerance) will assist you in determining cognitive and psychosocial development. Appendix 2 provides a comparison developmental table for the child. Psychosocial development of the adult and aging adult is provided in Appendix 4. Objective data obtained from the physical examination regarding height, weight, and musculoskeletal function provide a basis for determining physical development (see Developmental Information, Appendix 2, and growth charts, Appendix 5).

Subjective Data: Guideline Questions

Describe any physical handicaps you have.
Tell me about your health and growth as a child.
Tell me about your accomplishments in life.
What are your lifelong goals?
Has your illness interfered with these goals?

Objective Data

Appendices 3, 6, and 7 provide normal information and developmental norms based on age to provide a baseline by which to compare your client's physical, psychosocial, and cognitive development.

Does this client have obvious developmental lags that need further assessment?

Does this client's illness interfere with the ability to accomplish the necessary developmental, physical, psychosocial, and cognitive tasks required at each age level for normal development?

Does this client have any physical, psychosocial, or cognitive developmental lags that aggravate his or her illness or inhibit self-care?

HEALTH PERCEPTION–HEALTH MANAGEMENT PATTERN

Purpose

The purpose of assessing the client's health perception–health management pattern is to determine how the client perceives and maintains his or her health. Compliance with current and past nursing and medical recommendations is assessed. The client's ability to perceive the relationship between activities of daily living and health is also determined.

Subjective Data: Guideline Questions

Client's Perception of Health

Describe your health.
How would you rate your health on a scale of 1 to 10 (10 is excellent) now, 5 years ago, and 5 years ahead?

Client's Perception of Illness

Describe your illness or current health problem.
How has this affected your normal daily activities?
How do you feel your current daily activities have affected your health?
What do you believe caused your illness?
What course do you predict your illness will take?
How do you believe your illness should be treated?
Do you have or anticipate any difficulties in caring for yourself or others at home? If yes, explain.

Health Management and Habits

Tell me what you do when you have a health problem.
When do you seek nursing or medical advice?
How often do you go for professional exams (dental, Pap smears, breast, blood pressure)?

What activities do you believe keep you healthy? Contribute to illness?

Do you perform self-exams (blood pressure, breast, testicular)?

When were your last immunizations? Are they up to date? (See Immunization Schedule, Appendix 5.)

Do you use alcohol, tobacco, drugs, caffeine? Describe the amount and length of time used.

Are you exposed to pollutants or toxins? Describe.

Compliance with Prescribed Medications and Treatments

Have you been able to take your prescribed medications? If not, what caused your inability to do so?

Have you been able to follow through with your prescribed nursing and medical treatment (eg, diet, exercise)? If not, what caused your inability to do so?

Objective Data

Refer to Chapter 4, General Physical Survey.

Associated Nursing Diagnostic Categories to Consider

Wellness Diagnoses

Effective Therapeutic Regimen: Individual, Family, or Community Health-Seeking Behaviors

Risk Diagnoses

Risk for Adult Failure to Thrive
Risk for Altered Development
Risk for Altered Growth
Risk for Delayed Growth and Development
Risk for Delayed Surgical Recovery
Risk for Falls
Risk for Impaired Health Maintenance
Risk for Injury
Risk for Injury: Wandering
Risk for Perioperative Positioning Injury
Risk for Poisoning
Risk for Suffocation
Risk for Trauma

Actual Diagnoses

Delayed Growth and Development
Ineffective Health Maintenance
Energy Field Disturbance
Ineffective Therapeutic Regimen Management: Community
Ineffective Therapeutic Regimen Management: Family

Ineffective Therapeutic Regimen Management: Individual Noncompliance (Specify)

NUTRITIONAL–METABOLIC PATTERN

Purpose

The purpose of assessing the client's nutritional–metabolic pattern is to determine the client's dietary habits and metabolic needs. The conditions of hair, skin, nails, teeth, and mucous membranes are assessed.

Subjective Data: Guideline Questions

Dietary and Fluid Intake

Describe the type and amount of food you eat at breakfast, lunch, and supper on an average day.
Do you attempt to follow any certain type of diet? Explain.
What time do you usually eat your meals?
Do you find it difficult to eat meals on time? Explain.
What types of snacks do you eat? How often?
Do you take any vitamin supplements? Describe.
Do you take herbal supplements? Describe.
Do you consider your diet high in fat? Sugar? Salt?
Do you find it difficult to tolerate certain foods? Specify.
What kind of fluids do you usually drink? How much per day?
Do you have difficulty chewing or swallowing food?
When was your last dental exam? What were the results?
Do you ever experience a sore throat, sore tongue, or sore gums? Describe.
Do you ever experience nausea and vomiting? Describe.
Do you ever experience abdominal pains? Describe.
Do you use antacids? How often? What kind?

Condition of Skin

Describe the condition of your skin.
Describe your bathing routine.
Do you use sunscreens, lotions, oils? Describe.
How well and how quickly does your skin heal?
Do you have any skin lesions? Describe.
Do you have excessively oily or dry skin?
Do you have any itching? What do you do for relief?

Condition of Hair and Nails

Describe the condition of your hair and nails.
Do you use artificial nails? How often? How long? Have you ever had problems with these nails?
Do you have excessively oily or dry hair?
Have you had difficulty with scalp itching or sores?

Do you use any special hair or scalp care products
(ie, permanents, coloring, straighteners)?
Have you noticed any changes in your nails? Color? Cracking?
Shape? Lines?

Metabolism

What would you consider to be your ideal weight?
Have you had any recent weight gains or losses? Describe.
Have you used any measures to gain or lose weight? Describe.
Do you have any intolerances to heat or cold?
Have you noted any changes in your eating or drinking habits?
Explain.
Have you noticed any voice changes?
Have you had difficulty with nervousness?

Objective Data

Assess the client's temperature, pulse, respirations, and height and
weight. Refer to Chapter 7, Skin, Hair, and Nail Assessment; Chapter 8,
Head and Neck Assessment; and Chapter 11, Mouth, Throat, Nose, and
Sinus Assessment

Associated Nursing Diagnostic
Categories to Consider

Wellness Diagnoses

Readiness for Enhanced Effective Breast-feeding
Readiness for Enhanced Nutritional Metabolic Pattern
Readiness for Enhanced Skin Integrity

Risk Diagnoses

Imbalanced Nutrition: Risk for Less Than Body Requirements
Imbalanced Nutrition: Risk for More Than Body Requirements
Risk for Delayed Surgical Recovery
Risk for Imbalanced Body Temperature
  Hypothermia
  Hyperthermia
Risk for Aspiration
Risk for Deficient Fluid Volume
Risk for Impaired Skin Integrity
Risk for Infection
Risk for Latex Allergy

Actual Diagnoses

Impaired Dentition
Imbalanced Nutrition: Less Than Body Requirements
Imbalanced Nutrition: More Than Body Requirements
Impaired Oral Mucous Membrane
Ineffective Protection

Decreased Intracranial Adaptive Capacity
Deficient Fluid Volume
Excess Fluid Volume
Impaired Skin Integrity
Impaired Swallowing
Impaired Tissue Integrity
Ineffective Breast-feeding
Ineffective Infant Feeding Pattern
Ineffective Thermoregulation
Interrupted Breast-feeding
Latex Allergy

ELIMINATION PATTERN

Purpose

The purpose of assessing the client's elimination pattern is to determine the adequacy of function of the client's bowel and bladder for elimination. The client's bowel and urinary routines and habits are assessed. In addition, any bowel or urinary problems and use of urinary or bowel elimination devices are examined.

Subjective Data: Guideline Questions

Bowel Habits

Describe your bowel pattern. Have there been any recent changes?
How frequent are your bowel movements?
What is the color and consistency of your stools?
Do you use laxatives? What kind and how often do you use them?
Do you use enemas? How often and what kind?
Do you use suppositories? How often and what kind?
Do you have any discomfort with your bowel movements? Describe.
Have you ever had bowel surgery? What type? Ileostomy? Colostomy?

Bladder Habits

Describe your urinary habits.
How frequently do you urinate (when and number of times)?
What is the amount and color of your urine?
Do you have any of the following problems with urinating:
    Pain?
    Blood in urine?
    Difficulty starting a stream?
    Incontinence?
    Voiding frequently at night?
    Voiding frequently during day?
    Bladder infections?
Have you ever had bladder surgery? Describe.
Have you ever had a urinary catheter? Describe. When?
    How long?

Objective Data

Refer to Chapter 16, Abdominal Assessment, and the External Rectal Area Assessment section in Chapter 17.

Associated Nursing Diagnostic Categories to Consider

Wellness Diagnoses

Readiness for Enhanced Bowel Elimination
Readiness for Enhanced Urinary Elimination

Risk Diagnoses

Risk for Impaired Urinary Elimination
Risk for Constipation

Actual Diagnoses

Bowel Incontinence
Diarrhea
Perceived Constipation
Risk for Constipation
Impaired Urinary Elimination
Functional Urinary Incontinence
Reflex Urinary Incontinence
Stress Urinary Incontinence
Total Urinary Incontinence
Urge Urinary Incontinence
Urinary Retention

ACTIVITY–EXERCISE PATTERN

Purpose

The purpose of assessing the client's activity–exercise pattern is to determine the client's activities of daily living, including routines of exercise, leisure, and recreation. This includes activities necessary for personal hygiene, cooking, shopping, eating, maintaining the home, and working. An assessment is made of any factors that affect or interfere with the client's routine activities of daily living. Activities are evaluated in reference to the client's perception of their significance in his or her life.

Subjective Data: Guideline Questions

Activities of Daily Living

Describe your activities on a normal day (including hygiene activities, cooking activities, shopping activities, eating activities, house and yard activities, other self-care activities).
How satisfied are you with these activities?
Do you have difficulty with any of these self-care activities? Explain.

Does anyone help you with these activities? How?

Do you use any special devices to help you with your activities?

Does your current physical health affect any of these activities (eg, dyspnea, shortness of breath, palpitations, chest pain, pain, stiffness, weakness)? Explain.

Leisure Activities

Describe the leisure activities you enjoy.

Has your health affected your ability to enjoy your leisure? Explain.

Do you have time for leisure activities?

Describe any hobbies you have.

Exercise Routine

Describe those activities that you believe give you exercise.

How often are you able to do this type of exercise?

Has your health interfered with your exercise routine?

Occupational Activities

Describe what you do to make a living.

How satisfied are you with this job?

Do you believe it has affected your health? If yes, how?

How has your health affected your ability to work?

Objective Data

Refer to Chapter 12, Thoracic and Lung Assessment; Chapter 14, Heart Assessment; Chapter 15, Peripheral Vascular Assessment; and Chapter 18, Musculoskeletal Assessment.

Associated Nursing Diagnostic Categories to Consider

Wellness Diagnoses

Readiness for Enhanced Tissue Perfusion

Readiness for Enhanced Activity–Exercise Pattern

Readiness for Enhanced Breathing Pattern

Readiness for Enhanced Cardiac Output

Readiness for Enhanced Effective Diversional Activity Pattern

Readiness for Enhanced Home Maintenance Management

Readiness for Enhanced Self-Care Activities

Readiness for Enhanced Organized Infant Behavior

Risk Diagnoses

Risk for Impaired Respiratory Function

Risk for Disorganized Infant Behavior

Risk for Disuse Syndrome

Risk for Perioperative Positioning Injury

Risk for Peripheral Neurovascular Dysfunction

Actual Diagnoses

Activity Intolerance
Ineffective Tissue Perfusion (specify type: Cerebral,
   Cardiopulmonary, Renal, Gastrointestinal, Peripheral)
Decreased Intracranial Adaptive Capacity
Decreased Cardiac Output
Disorganized Infant Behavior
Disuse Syndrome
Deficient Diversional Activity
Dysfunctional Ventilatory Weaning Response
Impaired Bed Mobility
Impaired Gas Exchange
Impaired Home Maintenance
Impaired Physical Mobility
Impaired Walking
Impaired Wheelchair Mobility
Impaired Transfer Ability
Inability to Sustain Spontaneous Ventilation
Self-Care Deficit (specify type: Feeding, Bathing/Hygiene,
   Dressing/Grooming, Toileting)
Ineffective Airway Clearance
Ineffective Breathing Pattern

SEXUALITY–REPRODUCTION PATTERN

Purpose

The purpose of assessing the client's sexuality–reproduction pattern
is to determine the client's fulfillment of sexual needs and perceived
level of satisfaction. The reproductive pattern and developmental level
of the client are determined, and perceived problems related to sexual activities, relationships, or self-concept are elicited. The physical
and psychological effects of the client's current health status on his or
her sexuality or sexual expression are examined.

Subjective Data: Guideline Questions

Female

• Menstrual history
  How old were you when you began menstruating?
  On what date did your last cycle begin?
  How many days does your cycle normally last?
  How many days elapse from the beginning of one cycle until the
     beginning of another?
  Have you noticed any change in your menstrual cycle?
  Have you noticed any bleeding between your menstrual cycles?
  Do you experience episodes of flushing, chillings, or intolerance
     to temperature changes?

Describe any mood changes or discomfort before, during, or
after your cycle.

What was the date of your last Pap smear? Results?

- Obstetric history

How many times have you been pregnant?

Describe the outcome of each of your pregnancies.

If you have children, what are the ages and sex of each?

Describe your feelings with each pregnancy.

Explain any health problems or concerns you had with each
pregnancy.

If pregnant now:

Was this a planned or unexpected pregnancy?

Describe your feelings about this pregnancy.

What changes in your lifestyle do you anticipate with this
pregnancy?

Describe any difficulties or discomfort you have had with this
pregnancy.

How can I help you meet your needs during this pregnancy?

Male or Female

- Contraception

What do you or your partner do to prevent pregnancy?

How acceptable is this method to both of you?

Does this means of birth control affect your enjoyment of
sexual relations?

Describe any discomfort or undesirable effects this method
produces.

Have you had any difficulty with fertility? Explain.

Has infertility affected your relationship with your partner? Explain.

- Perception of sexual activities

Describe your sexual feelings. How comfortable are you with
your feelings of femininity/masculinity?

Describe your level of satisfaction from your sexual relationship(s)
on scale of 1 to 10 (with 10 being very satisfying).

Explain any changes in your sexual relationship(s) that you
would like to make.

Describe any pain or discomfort you have during intercourse.

Have you (has your partner) experienced any difficulty achieving an
orgasm or maintaining an erection? If so, how has this affected
your relationship?

- Concerns related to illness

How has your illness affected your sexual relationship(s)?

How comfortable are you discussing sexual problems with your
partner?

From whom would you seek help for sexual concerns?

- Special problems

Do you have or have you ever had a sexually transmitted
disease? Describe.

What method do you use to prevent contracting a sexually transmitted disease?
Describe any pain, burning, or discomfort you have while voiding.
Describe any discharge or unusual odor you have from your penis/vagina.
• History of sexual abuse
Describe the time and place the incident occurred.
Explain the type of sexual contact that occurred.
Describe the person who assaulted you.
Identify any witnesses present.
Describe your feelings about this incident.
Have you had any difficulty sleeping, eating, or working since the incident occurred?

Objective Data

Refer to Chapter 13, Breast Assessment; Chapter 16, Abdominal Assessment; and Chapter 17, Genitourinary Assessment.

Associated Nursing Diagnostic Categories to Consider

Wellness Diagnosis

Readiness for Enhanced Sexuality Patterns

Risk Diagnosis

Risk for Ineffective Sexuality Pattern

Actual Diagnoses

Ineffective Sexuality Pattern
Sexual Dysfunction

SLEEP–REST PATTERN

Purpose

The purpose of assessing the client's sleep–rest pattern is to determine the client's perception of the quality of his or her sleep, relaxation, and energy levels. Methods used to promote relaxation and sleep are also assessed.

Subjective Data: Guideline Questions

Sleep Habits

Describe your usual sleeping time and habits (ie, reading, warm milk, medications, etc.) at home.
How long does it take you to fall asleep?
If you awaken, how long does it take you to fall asleep again?
Do you use anything to help you fall asleep (ie, medication, reading, eating)?
How would you rate the quality of your sleep?

Special Problems

Do you ever experience difficulty with falling asleep? Remaining asleep?

Do you ever feel fatigued after a sleep period?

Has your current health altered your normal sleep habits? Explain.

Do you feel your sleep habits have contributed to your current illness? Explain.

Sleep Aids

What helps you fall asleep?
  Medications?
  Reading?
  Relaxation technique?
  Watching TV?
  Listening to music?

Objective Data

Observe Appearance

Pale
Puffy eyes with dark circles

Observe Behavior

Yawning
Dozing during day
Irritability
Short attention span

Associated Nursing Diagnostic Categories to Consider

Wellness Diagnosis

Readiness for Enhanced Sleep

Risk Diagnoses

Risk for Sleep Deprivation
Risk for Disturbed Sleep Pattern

Actual Diagnoses

Disturbed Sleep Pattern
Sleep Deprivation

SENSORY–PERCEPTUAL PATTERN

Purpose

The purpose of assessing the client's sensory–perceptual pattern is to determine the functioning status of the five senses: vision, hearing, touch (including pain perception), taste, and smell. Devices and methods used to assist the client with deficits in any of these five senses are assessed.

Subjective Data: Guideline Questions

Perception of Senses

Describe your ability to see, hear, feel, taste, and smell.
Describe any difficulty you have with your vision, hearing, ability to feel (eg, touch, pain, heat, cold), taste (salty, sweet, bitter, sour), or smell.

Pain Assessment (See Chapter 5 for detailed pain assessment.)

Describe any pain you have now.
What brings it on? What relieves it?
When does it occur? How often? How long does it last?
What else do you feel when you have this pain?
Show me on this drawing (of a figure) where you have pain.
Rate your pain on a scale of 1 to 10, with 10 being the most severe pain. (Have a child use the Oucher Scale, with faces ranging from frowning to crying.)
How has your pain affected your activities of daily living?

Special Aids

What devices (eg, glasses, contact lenses, hearing aids) or methods do you use to help you with any of these problems?
Describe any medications you take to help you with these problems.

Objective Data

Refer to the section on Nose and Sinus Assessment in Chapter 11; Chapter 9, Eye Assessment; Chapter 10, Ear Assessment; and the section on Cranial Nerve Assessment in Chapter 19.

Associated Nursing Diagnostic Categories to Consider

Wellness Diagnosis

Readiness for Enhanced Physical Comfort

Risk Diagnoses

Risk for Aspiration
Risk for Acute Pain
Risk for Autonomic Dysreflexia

Actual Diagnoses

Chronic Pain
Autonomic Dysreflexia
Acute Pain
Disturbed Sensory Perception (specify: Visual, Auditory, Kinesthetic, Gustatory, Tactile, Olfactory)
Unilateral Neglect

COGNITIVE PATTERN

Purpose

The purpose of assessing the client's cognitive pattern is to determine the client's ability to understand, communicate, remember, and make decisions.

Subjective Data: Guideline Questions

Ability to Understand

Explain what your doctor has told you about your health.
Are you satisfied with your understanding of your illness and prescribed care? Explain.
What is the best way for you to learn something new (read, watch television, etc.)?

Ability to Communicate

Can you tell me how you feel about your current state of health?
Are you able to ask questions about your treatments, medications, and so forth?
Do you ever have difficulty expressing yourself or explaining things to others? Explain.

Ability to Remember

Are you able to remember recent events and events of long ago? Explain.

Ability to Make Decisions

Describe how you feel when faced with a decision.
What assists you in making decisions?
Do you find decision making difficult, fairly easy, or variable? Describe.

Objective Data

Refer to the Mental Status Assessment section of Chapter 19.

Associated Nursing Diagnostic Categories to Consider

Wellness Diagnosis

Readiness for Enhanced Cognition

Risk Diagnosis

Risk for Disturbed Thought Processes

Actual Diagnoses

Acute Confusion
Disturbed Thought Processes
Chronic Confusion

Decisional Conflict (specify)
Impaired Environmental Interpretation Syndrome
Impaired Memory
Deficient Knowledge (specify)

ROLE–RELATIONSHIP PATTERN

Purpose

The purpose of assessing the client's role–relationship pattern is to determine the client's perceptions of responsibilities and roles in the family, at work, and in social life. The client's level of satisfaction with these is assessed. In addition, any difficulties in the client's relationships and interactions with others are examined.

Subjective Data: Guideline Questions

Perception of Major Roles and Responsibilities in Family

Describe your family.
Do you live with your family? Alone?
How does your family get along?
Who makes the major decisions in your family?
Who is the main financial supporter of your family?
How do you feel about your family?
What is your role in your family? Is this an important role?
What is your major responsibility in your family? How do you
   feel about this responsibility?
How does your family deal with problems?
Are there any major problems now?
Who is the person you feel closest to in your family? Explain.
How is your family coping with your current state of health?

Perception of Major Roles and Responsibilities at Work

Describe your occupation.
What is your major responsibility at work?
How do you feel about the people you work with?
If you could, what would you change about your work?
Are there any major problems you have at work? If yes,
   explain.

Perception of Major Social Roles and Responsibilities

Who is the most important person in your life? Explain.
Describe your neighborhood and the community in which
   you live.
How do you feel about the people in your community?
Do you participate in any social groups or neighborhood
   activities? If yes, describe.
What do you see as your contribution to society?
What would you change about your community if you could?

Objective Data

1. Outline a family genogram for your client. See Figure 2–1 for an example.
2. Observe your client's family members.
   a. How do they communicate with each other?
   b. How do they respond to the client?
   c. Do they visit, and how long do they stay with the client?

Associated Nursing Diagnostic Categories to Consider

Wellness Diagnoses

Readiness for Enhanced Caregiver Role
Readiness for Enhanced Communication
Readiness for Enhanced Grieving
Readiness for Enhanced Parenting
Readiness for Enhanced Relationships
Readiness for Enhanced Role Performance
Readiness for Enhanced Social Interaction

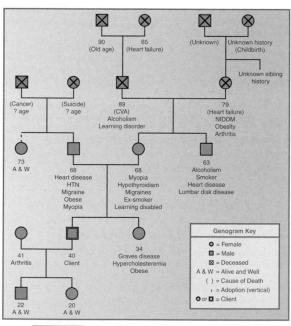

FIGURE 2–1 Genogram of a 40-year-old male client.

Risk Diagnoses

Risk for Impaired Parent/Infant/Child Attachment
Risk for Dysfunctional Grieving
Risk for Loneliness

Actual Diagnoses

Interrupted Family Processes
Dysfunctional Family Processes: Alcoholism
Impaired Parenting
Ineffective Role Performance
Anticipatory Grieving
Caregiver Role Strain
Chronic Sorrow
Dysfunctional Grieving
Impaired Social Interaction
Impaired Verbal Communication
Parental Role Conflict
Social Isolation

SELF-PERCEPTION–SELF-CONCEPT PATTERN

Purpose

The purpose of assessing the client's self-perception–self-concept pattern is to determine the client's perception of his or her identity, abilities, body image, and self-worth. The client's behavior, attitude, and emotional patterns are also assessed.

Subjective Data: Guideline Questions

Perception of Identity

Describe yourself.
Has your illness affected how you describe yourself?

Perception of Abilities and Self-Worth

What do you consider to be your strengths? Weaknesses?
How do you feel about yourself?
How does your family feel about you and your illness?

Body Image

How do you feel about your appearance?
Has this changed since your illness? Explain.
How would you change your appearance if you could?
How do you feel about other people with disabilities?

Objective Data

Refer to the procedures for observing appearance, behavior and mood in the Mental Status Assessment section of Chapter 19.

Associated Nursing Diagnostic Categories to Consider

Wellness Diagnoses

Readiness for Enhanced Self-Concept

Risk Diagnoses

Risk for Disturbed Body Image
Risk for Hopelessness
Risk for Chronic Low Self-Esteem

Actual Diagnoses

Anxiety
Death Anxiety
Disturbed Body Image
Chronic Low Self-Esteem
Fatigue
Fear
Hopelessness
Disturbed Personal Identity
Powerlessness
Disturbed Self-Esteem
Situational Low Self-Esteem

COPING–STRESS TOLERANCE PATTERN

Purpose

The purpose of assessing the client's coping–stress tolerance pattern is to determine the areas and amount of stress in a client's life and the effectiveness of coping methods used to deal with it. Availability and use of support systems such as family, friends, and religious beliefs are assessed.

Subjective Data: Guideline Questions

Perception of Stress and Problems in Life

Describe what you believe to be the most stressful situation in your life.
How has your illness affected the stress you feel? *or* How do you feel stress has affected your illness?
Has there been a personal loss or major change in your life over the last year? Explain.
What has helped you to cope with this change or loss?

Coping Methods and Support Systems

What do you usually do first when faced with a problem?
What helps you to relieve stress and tension?
To whom do you usually turn when you have a problem or feel under pressure?

How do you usually deal with problems?
Do you use medication, drugs, or alcohol to help relieve stress?
Explain.

Objective Data

Refer to the Mental Status Assessment section of Chapter 19.

Associated Nursing Diagnostic Categories to Consider

Wellness Diagnoses

Readiness for Enhanced Individual Coping
Readiness for Enhanced Family Coping
Readiness for Enhanced Community Coping
Readiness for Enhanced Spiritual Well-Being

Risk Diagnoses

Risk for Ineffective Coping (Individual, Family, or Community)
Risk for Post-Trauma Syndrome
Risk for Self-Mutilation
Risk for Spiritual Distress
Risk for Suicide
Risk for Violence (specify: Self-Directed, Other-Directed)
Risk for Relocation Stress Syndrome

Actual Diagnoses

Caregiver Role Strain
Chronic Sorrow
Impaired Adjustment
Ineffective Community Coping
Compromised Family Coping
Disabled Family Coping
Ineffective Individual Coping:
    Defensive Coping
    Ineffective Denial
Post-Trauma Syndrome
Rape–Trauma Syndrome
Relocation Stress Syndrome
Self-Mutilation

VALUE–BELIEF PATTERN

Purpose

The purpose of assessing the client's value–belief pattern is to determine the client's life values and goals, philosophical beliefs, religious beliefs, and spiritual beliefs that influence his or her choices and decisions. Conflicts between these values, goals, beliefs, and expectations that are related to health are assessed.

Subjective Data: Guideline Questions

Values, Goals, and Philosophical Beliefs

What is most important to you in life?
What do you hope to accomplish in your life?
What is the major influencing factor that helps you make decisions?
What is your major source of hope and strength in life?

Religious and Spiritual Beliefs

Do you have a religious affiliation?
Is this important to you?
Are there certain health practices or restrictions that are important
   for you to follow while you are ill or hospitalized? Explain.
Is there a significant person (eg, minister, priest) from your
   religious denomination whom you want to be contacted?
Would you like the hospital chaplain to visit?
Are there certain practices (eg, prayer, reading scripture) that are
   important to you?
Is a relationship with God an important part of your life? Explain.
Describe any other sources of strength that are important to you.
How can I help you continue with this source of spiritual
   strength while you are ill in the hospital?

Objective Data

Observe religious practices:
   Presence of religious articles in room (eg, Bible, cards, medals,
      statues)
   Visits from clergy
   Religious actions of client: prayer, visit to chapel, request for
      clergy, watching of religious TV programs or listening to
      religious radio stations
Observe client's behavior for signs of spiritual distress:
   Anxiety
   Anger
   Depression
   Doubt
   Hopelessness
   Powerlessness

Associated Nursing Diagnostic Categories to Consider

Wellness Diagnosis

Readiness for Enhanced Spiritual Well-Being

Risk Diagnosis

Risk for Spiritual Distress

Actual Diagnoses

Death Anxiety
Spiritual Distress

PHYSICAL ASSESSMENT

3

PHYSICAL ASSESSMENT SKILLS

Four basic techniques are used in performing a physical assessment: *inspection, palpation, percussion,* and *auscultation*. The definition and proper technique for each of these are described below. Always use Standard Precautions as recommended by the Hospital Injection Control Practices Advisory Committee (HICPAC) and the Communicable Disease Center (COC).

Inspection

Definition

Inspection is using the senses of vision, smell, and hearing to observe the condition of various body parts, including any deviations from normal.

Technique

- Expose body parts being observed while keeping the rest of the client properly draped.
- *Always* look before touching.
- Use good lighting. Tangential sunlight is best. Be alert for the effect of bluish red-tinted or fluorescent lighting that interferes with observing bruises, cyanosis, and erythema.
- Provide a warm room for examination of the client. (Too cold or hot an environment may alter skin color and appearance.)
- Observe for color, size, location, texture, symmetry, odors, and sounds.

Palpation

Definition

Palpation is touching and feeling body parts with your hands to determine the following characteristics:

- Texture (roughness/smoothness)
- Temperature (warm/hot/cold)
- Moisture (dry/wet/moist)
- Motion (stillness/vibration)
- Consistency of structures (solid/fluid filled)

Technique

- Examiner's fingernails should be short.
- The most sensitive part of the hand should be used to detect various sensations. See Table 3–1.
- Light palpation precedes deep palpation.
- Tender areas are palpated last.
- Three different types of palpation may be used depending on the purpose of the exam. The purpose and technique for each are described in Table 3–2.

Percussion

Definition

Percussion is tapping a portion of the body to elicit tenderness or sounds that vary with the density of underlying structures. The reliability of this technique is often questioned due to variations in the specificity and sensitivity of percussion.

Technique

Two types of percussion may be used depending on purpose. These are explained in Table 3–3. Percussion notes elicited through indirect percussion vary with density of underlying structures. Five percussion notes are described in Table 3–4.

Auscultation

Definition

Auscultation is listening for various breath, heart, vasculature, and bowel sounds using a stethoscope.

Technique

Use a good stethoscope that has the following:

- Snug-fitting ear plugs
- Tubing not longer than 15 inches and internal diameter not greater than 1 inch
- Diaphragm and bell

TABLE 3–1 SENSITIVITY OF PARTS OF THE HAND	
Hand Part Used	**Type of Sensation Felt**
Fingertips	Fine discriminations, pulsations
Palmar/ulnar surface	Vibratory sensations (eg, thrills, fremitus)
Dorsal surface (back of hand)	Temperature

TABLE 3–2 TYPES OF PALPATION

Type	Purpose	Technique
Light palpation	To determine surface variations (eg, texture, tenderness, temperature, moisture, elasticity, pulsations, superficial organs, masses)	Depress skin $\frac{1}{2}$ inch to $\frac{3}{4}$ inch with finger pads.
Deep palpation	To feel internal organs and masses for size, shape, tenderness, symmetry, mobility	Depress skin $1\frac{1}{2}$ inches to 2 inches with firm, deep pressure. May use one hand on top of the other to exert firmer pressure.

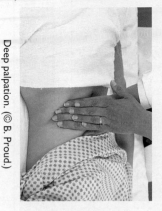

Deep palpation. (© B. Proud.)

(continued)

TABLE 3-2 TYPES OF PALPATION (Continued)

Type	Purpose	Technique
Bimanual palpation (use with caution as it may provoke internal injury) Bimanual palpation of the breast. (© B. Proud.)	To palpate breasts and deep abdominal organs	Use two hands, one on each side of body part or organs being felt. The upper hand is used to apply pressure while the lower hand is used to detect deep structures. Use one hand to push deeply on abdominal wall to move internal structure to the flank. Use the other hand to feel the structure.

TABLE 3-3 TYPES OF PERCUSSION

Type	Purpose	Technique
Direct percussion	To elicit tenderness or pain	Directly tap body part with one or two fingertips.

Direct percussion of sinuses.
(© B. Proud.)

(continued)

TABLE 3–3 TYPES OF PERCUSSION (Continued)

Type	Purpose	Technique
Indirect percussion	To elicit one of the following sounds over the chest or abdomen: tympany, resonance, hyperresonance, dullness, flatness (see Table 3–4)	Press middle finger of nondominant hand firmly on body part. Keep other fingers off body part. Strike the finger on the body part with the middle finger (with short fingernail) of the dominant hand. Flex dominant wrist (not forearm) quickly. Listen to sound. (Use quick wrist movement, as if giving an IM injection.)

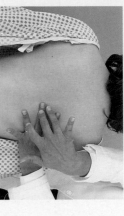

Indirect or mediate percussion of lungs.
(© B. Proud.)

TABLE 3 – 4	SOUNDS (TONES) ELICITED BY PERCUSSION				
Sound	**Intensity**	**Pitch**	**Length**	**Quality**	**Example of Origin**
Resonance (heard over part air and part solid)	Loud	Low	Long	Hollow	Normal lung
Hyperresonance (heard over mostly air)	Very loud	Low	Long	Booming	Lung with emphysema
Tympany (heard over air)	Loud	High	Moderate	Drumlike	Puffed-out cheek, gastric bubble
Dullness (heard over more solid tissue)	Medium	Medium	Moderate	Thudlike	Diaphragm, pleural effusion, liver
Flatness (heard over very dense tissue)	Soft	High	Short	Flat	Muscle, bone, sternum, thigh

The diaphragm and bell are used differently to detect various sounds, as shown in Table 3–5.

BASIC GUIDELINES FOR PHYSICAL ASSESSMENT

Obtain a nursing history and survey the client's general physical status for an overall impression prior to physical assessment. This is done to determine which specific body systems should be examined (eg, if the client complains of chest pain, a thoracic and cardiac physical exam should be performed). A complete examination of all body systems may be done only on admission; otherwise, the physical assessment may only include one or a few body systems.

Maintain privacy and proper draping.

Explain the procedure and purpose of each part of the exam to the client.

Follow a planned examination order for each body system, using the four techniques described earlier. Specific history questions related to each body part being examined may be integrated with the physical exam. (For example, when examining vision, ask the date of the client's last eye exam, if he or she has a history of blurring or double vision.)

First inspect, palpate, percuss, and then auscultate, except in the abdominal exam. To avoid alterations in bowel sounds: first auscultate and then percuss the abdomen *prior to* palpation. Use each technique to compare symmetrical sides of the body and organs.

TABLE 3–5	USES FOR DIAPHRAGM AND BELL OF STETHOSCOPE	
	Purpose	**Technique**
Diaphragm	To detect high-pitched sounds (eg, breath sounds, normal heart sounds, bowel sounds)	Press firmly on body part.
Bell	To detect low-pitched or abnormal sounds (eg, extra heart sounds, heart murmurs, carotid bruits)	Press lightly over body part.

Assess both structure *and* function of each body part and organ (eg, the appearance and condition of the ear, as well as its hearing function).

When you identify an abnormality, assess for further data on the extent of the abnormality and the client's responses to the abnormality. Is there radiation of pain to other areas? Is there an effect on eating? Bowels? Activities of daily living? (For example, with left upper quadrant abdominal pain: Is there radiation of the pain?)

Integrate client education with the physical assessment (eg, breast self-exam, testicular self-exam, foot care for the client with diabetes).

Allow time for client questions.

Remember: The most important guideline for adequate physical assessment is conscious, continuous practice of physical assessment skills.

VARIATIONS IN PHYSICAL ASSESSMENT OF THE PEDIATRIC CLIENT

The physical assessment sequence is dependent upon the development level of the client. (For a detailed discussion, see Appendix 3, Developmental Information—Age 1 Month to 18 Years.)

Establishment of rapport with the child and significant others is the most essential step in obtaining meaningful physical assessment data.

Allowing time for interaction with the child prior to beginning the examination helps to reduce fears.

In certain age groups, portions of the assessment will require physical restraint of the client with the help of another adult. Distraction and play should be intermingled throughout the examination to assist in maintaining rapport with the pediatric client.

Involving assistance from the child's significant caregiver may facilitate a more meaningful examination of the younger client. Based on the child's responses, the examiner should be prepared to alter the order of the assessment and approach to the child.

Protest or an uncooperative attitude toward the examiner is a normal finding in children from birth to early adolescence, throughout parts or even all of the assessment process. Appendix 3 describes normal behavior at various developmental levels for the pediatric client.

If restraining is needed by another health team member, allow parent to comfort child *after* the procedure.

VARIATIONS IN PHYSICAL ASSESSMENT
OF THE GERIATRIC CLIENT

Remember: Normal variations related to aging may be observed in all parts of the physical exam. To avoid fatiguing the older client, allow rest periods between parts of the physical assessment. Provide a room with a comfortable temperature setting and no drafts, close to the restroom.

Allow sufficient time for client to respond to directions and to change positions. Use silence to provide more time for the client to process thoughts and respond.

If possible, assess geriatric clients in a setting where they have an opportunity to perform normal activities of daily living to determine their optimum potential.

Conduct exam in an area with ample space to accommodate wheelchairs and other supportive devices.

GENERAL PHYSICAL SURVEY

4

Equipment Needed

- Balance beam scale
- Tape measure
- Thermometer
- Sphygmomanometer
- Stethoscope

Subjective Data: Focus Questions

Reason for seeking health care? Major concern about current health? Current age, height, and weight? Recent weight change? Change in pulse or heart rate? Problem with hypertension or hypotension? Difficulty with respirations? Explain. Any pain? See Chapter 5. Pain is considered the fifth vital sign.

Objective Data: Assessment Techniques

When you meet the client, observe the client from head to toe to note any gross abnormalities in appearance or behavior. Assess vital signs (temperature, pulse, respirations, and blood pressure) to detect any severe deviations and to acquire baseline data. Then weigh the client and measure height with shoes and heavy clothing removed.

GENERAL PHYSICAL SURVEY

PROCEDURE	NORMAL FINDINGS	DEVIATIONS FROM NORMAL
Observe the following:		
• Physical development	• Appears to be stated chronological age	• Appears older than age with hard manual labor, chronic illness, or alcoholism/smoking
• Behavior	• Cooperative attitude and behavior	• Uncooperative or bizarre, unpredictable behavior may be seen in angry, mentally ill, or violent client; apathy or crying seen in depression
• Mood	• Mild anxiety or tenseness	• Moderate to severe anxiety and tenseness, restlessness, or fidgeting seen in anxiety states
• Dress	• Dressed for occasion	• Dress bizarre and inappropriate for occasion seen in mentally ill, grieving, depressed, or poor clients
• Gait	• Erect posture, coordinated, smooth and steady gait	• Lordosis, scoliosis, or kyphosis; uncoordinated, shaky, unsteady, or stiff gait seen in Parkinson disease; stiff, rigid gait seen with arthritis
• Body build	• Bilateral, firm, developed muscles	• Lack of subcutaneous fat seen in the undernourished, abdominal ascites seen in starvation, abundant fatty tissue seen in obesity

PROCEDURE

Monitor **temperature.** Electronic thermometers are quicker than glass thermometers. They may be used for oral, rectal, or axillary temperatures depending on the model and type of probe used.

Oral. Place clean thermometer under tongue near vascular bed with lips closed for 5 minutes. Wait 15 minutes before taking temperature if client just drank hot/cold fluids.

Rectal. Lubricate clean thermometer with water-soluble lubricant and insert 1–2 inches into rectum for 3 minutes. Use this method only when other routes are not practical.

NORMAL FINDINGS

Body temperature is usually lowest in early AM and highest in late PM: 96.0–99.9°F (35.6–37.7°C).

Strenuous exercise, stress, and ovulation may elevate temperature to 101.0°F (38.3°C). Hot fluids, smoking, and gum chewing may elevate temperature, while cold fluids may lower it.

0.7–1.0°F (0.4–0.5°C) higher than oral temperature. Strenuous exercise may elevate temperature to 104.0°F (40.0°C).

DEVIATIONS FROM NORMAL

Hypothermia (less than 96.0°F or 35.6°C) may be seen in prolonged exposure to cold, sepsis, hypoglycemia, hypothyroidism, or starvation.

Hyperthermia (more than 100.0°F or 37.8°C) may be seen in viral or bacterial infections, malignancies, trauma, and various blood and immune disorders.

PROCEDURE	NORMAL FINDINGS	DEVIATIONS FROM NORMAL
Axillary. Insert thermometer under axilla with arm down and across chest for 5–10 minutes.	1.0°F (0.5°C) lower than oral temperature. Environmental temperature may alter body temperature, and stress may raise body temperature.	
Tympanic. Use special electronic thermometer for tympanic membrane temperature. Place covered probe very gently at opening of ear canal for 2–3 seconds until temperature appears on digital screen. This is a safe, quick, non-invasive method that may be used with client of any age (Fig. 4-1).	1.4°F (0.8°C) higher than the normal oral temperature.	
Monitor **pulse.**		
Radial. Use middle three fingers to palpate radial pulse for 30 seconds and multiply by two if pulse is regular (Fig. 4-2). If pulse is irregular, take for 1 full minute. Always start counting with zero so that second pulse felt is no. 1.		

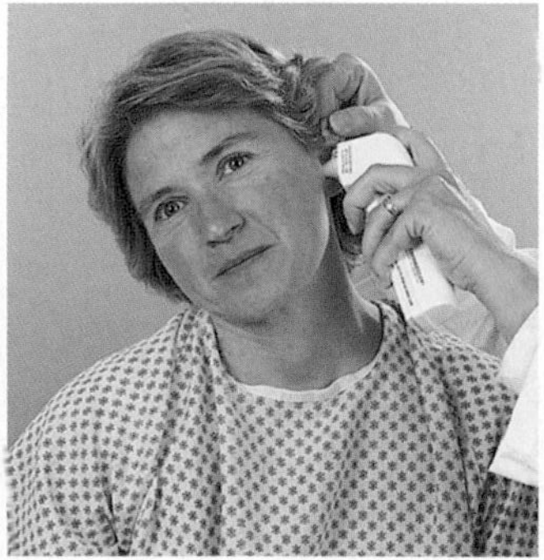

General Physical Survey

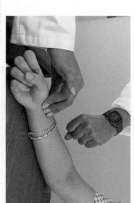

FIGURE 4–1 Taking a tympanic temperature. (© B. Proud.)

FIGURE 4–2 Timing the radial pulse rate. (© B. Proud.)

PROCEDURE	NORMAL FINDINGS	DEVIATIONS FROM NORMAL
Palpate for the following:		
• Rate	• 60–100 bpm (may be as low as 50 bpm in healthy athletes)	• More than 100 bpm equals tachycardia, seen in fever, in stress, and with some medications; less than 60 bpm equals bradycardia, may be seen with prolonged sitting or standing; follow up with cardiac auscultation of apical pulse
• Rhythm (if irregular, feel for full minute)	• Regular	• Irregular (follow up with cardiac auscultation of apical pulse)
• Equality of strength	• Equal bilaterally in strength	• Asymmetrical in strength, bounding, weak, or thready; follow up with palpation of the carotid arteries (one at a time)
Apical. Auscultate heart sounds for 1 minute with stethoscope.		
• Rate	• 60–100 bpm	• More than 100 bpm equals tachycardia; less than 60 bpm equals bradycardia
• Rhythm	• Regular	• Irregular; pulse deficit (difference between apical and radial pulse) may indicate atrial fibrillation, atrial flutter, premature ventricular contractions, and various degrees of heart block

PROCEDURE	NORMAL FINDINGS	DEVIATIONS FROM NORMAL
Monitor **respirations** *1 full minute for the following:* • Rate • Rhythm • Depth See Table 4–1.	• 10–20 breaths/min • Regular and spontaneous • Equal bilateral chest expansion of 1–2 inches	• Less than 12/min, more than 20/min • Irregular • Unequal, shallow, or extremely deep chest expansion
Monitor **blood pressure** after client is seated or supine quietly for 10 minutes. Repeat after 2 minutes. Repeat with client standing. Verify blood pressure in the contralateral arm. Refer to Table 4–2.	Systolic: less than/equal to 139 mm Hg, diastolic: less than/equal to 89 mm Hg; varies with individuals	Higher or lower than normal systolic and diastolic readings (Tables 4–2 and 4–3)
Assess for pain as the fifth vital sign. See Chapter 5.	Absence of pain	Pain of any degree as perceived by the client

TABLE 4-1	TYPES OF RESPIRATIONS	
	Description	**Pattern**
Normal	12–20/min and regular	∿∿∿
Apnea	Absence of respiration	—
Bradypnea	Slow, shallow respiration	⌒⌒
Tachypnea	More than 20/min and regular	∿∿∿∿∿∿
Hyperventilation	Increased rate and increased depth	MMMMM
Hypoventilation	Decreased rate and decreased depth	⌒
Cheyne-Stokes	Periods of apnea and hyperventilation	MM___MM
Kussmaul	Very deep with normal rhythm	MMMMM

TABLE 4–2 CLASSIFICATION AND MANAGEMENT OF BLOOD PRESSURE FOR ADULTS*

BP Classification	SBP* mm Hg	DBP* mm Hg	Lifestyle Modification	Initial Drug Therapy Without Compelling Indication	Initial Drug Therapy With Compelling Indications
Normal	<120	and <80	Encourage		
Prehypertension	120–139	or 80–89	Yes	No antihypertensive drug indicated	Drug(s) for compelling indications[‡]
Stage 1 hypertension	140–159	or 90–99	Yes	Thiazide-type diuretics for most; may consider ACEI, ARB, BB, CCB, or combination	Drug(s) for compelling indications.[‡] Other antihypertensive drugs (diuretics, ACEI, ARB, BB, CCB) as needed
Stage 2 hypertension	≥160	or ≥100	Yes	Two-drug combination for most (usually thiazide-type diuretic and ACEI or ARB or BB or CCB)	

DBP, diastolic blood pressure; SBP, systolic blood pressure.

Drug abbreviations: ACEI, angiotensin converting enzyme inhibitor; ARB, angiotensin receptor blocker; BB, beta-blocker; CCB, calcium channel blocker.

*Treatment determined by highest BP category.

[†]Initial combined therapy should be used cautiously in those at risk for orthostatic hypotension.

[‡]Treat patients with chronic kidney disease or diabetes to BP goal of <130/80 mm Hg.

Source: 7th Report of the Joint National Committee on Prevention, Detection, and Treatment of High Blood Pressure (2003).

TABLE 4–3

CLINICAL TRIAL AND GUIDELINE BASIS FOR COMPELLING INDICATIONS FOR INDIVIDUAL DRUG CLASSES

Compelling Indication*	Recommended Drugs						Clinical Trial Basis[†]
	Diuretic	BB	ACEI	ARB	CCB	Aldo ANT	
Heart failure	•	•	•	•		•	ACC/AHA Heart Failure Guideline, MERIT-HF, COPERNICUS, CIBIS, SOLVD, AIRE, TRACE, ValHEFT, RALES
Postmyocardial infarction		•	•			•	ACC/AHA Post-MI Guideline, BHAT, SAVE, Capricorn, EPHESUS
High coronary disease risk	•	•	•		•		ALLHAT, HOPE, ANBP₂, LIFE, CONVINCE
Diabetes	•	•	•	•	•		NKF-ADA Guideline, UKPDS, ALLHAT
Chronic kidney disease			•	•			NKF Guideline, Captopril Trial, RENAAL, IDNT, REIN, AASK
Recurrent stroke prevention	•		•				PROGRESS

Drug abbreviations: ACEI, angiotensin converting enzyme inhibitor; Aldo ANT, aldosterone antagonist; ARB, angiotensin receptor blocker; BB, beta-blocker; CCB, calcium channel blocker.

*Compelling indications for antihypertensive drugs are based on benefits from outcome studies or existing clinical guidelines. The compelling indication is managed in parallel with the BP.

[†]Conditions for which clinical trials demonstrate benefit of specific classes of antihypertensive drugs.

Source: 7th Report of the Joint National Committee on Prevention, Detection, and Treatment of High Blood Pressure (2003).

PEDIATRIC VARIATIONS

Equipment Needed

- Tape measure
- Growth charts for specific age comparisons (see Appendix 7)

Subjective Data: Focus Questions

Inquire about child's development milestones (see Appendix 3).
Inquire about immunizations (see Appendix 4).
Inquire about parent–child relationships (see Appendix 3).

Objective Data: Assessment Techniques

PROCEDURE	NORMAL VARIATIONS
Observe **physical level of development** and compare with chronological age.	See Appendix 3, Developmental Information—Age 1 Month to 18 Years
Monitor **temperature.**	Temperature fluctuates markedly in infants and young children.
Oral: Caution against biting glass thermometer.	*Infants:* 99.4°F (37.2°C; because of excess heat production) *Children and adolescents:* 98.6°F (37°C)
Note: Take tympanic, axillary, or rectal temperature in children younger than 6 years if they are uncooperative or unconscious.	

General Physical Survey

PEDIATRIC VARIATIONS (continued)

PROCEDURE	NORMAL VARIATIONS

Rectal. Position child prone, supine, or sidelying (may use parent's lap). Insert lubricated thermometer no more than 1 inch into rectum.

Tympanic. Pull pinna down and back.

Monitor **pulse:** Take apical (not radial) pulse in children younger than 2 years (Fig. 4–3). Count pulse for 1 full minute.

Awake and resting pulse rates vary with the age of the child: 1 wk–3 mo, 100–160; 3 mo–2 y, 80–150; 2–10 y, 70–110; 10 y–adult, 55–90.

Athletic adolescents tend to have lower pulse rates.

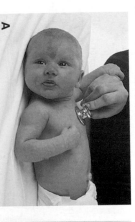 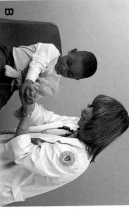

FIGURE 4–3 (A) Auscultating apical pulse rate in child under 2 years. (B) Measuring radial pulse in child over 2 years. (© B. Proud.)

PROCEDURE

Monitor **respirations** by observing abdominal movement in infants and young children

Monitor **blood pressure:** Width of cuff should cover two thirds of upper arm or be 20% greater than diameter of the extremity. Length of bladder should encircle without overlapping.

Measure the following and plot on growth chart:

- Height

  Children under 24 months: Measure length from vertex of head to heel in recumbent position.

  Children over 24 months: Measure standing height in bare feet.

- Weight: For infants and young children, use platform scale.

NORMAL VARIATIONS

Respiratory rates: birth–6 mo, 30–50; 6 mo–2 y, 20–30; 3–10 y, 20–28; 10–18 y, 12–20

Blood pressure rates: *Systolic:* 1–7 years, age in years + 90; 8–18 years, ($2 \times$ age in years) + 90; *Diastolic:* 1–5 years, 56; 6–18 years, age in years + 52

- See Appendix 7 for normal height ranges.

- See Appendix 7. At 1 year of age, the child's weight is usually three times the birth weight.

PROCEDURE

- Head circumference (HC) *Children under 24 months:* Measure slightly above eyebrows, pinna of ears over occipital prominence of skull (see Fig. 4–4).

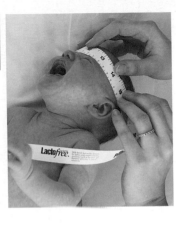

FIGURE 4–4 Measuring the circumference of an infant's head. (© B. Proud.)

NORMAL VARIATIONS

- Plot head circumference on standard growth chart (Appendix 7). Head circumference measurement should fall between the 5th and 95th percentiles, and should be comparable with the child's height and weight percentiles. Those greater than 95% may indicate macrocephaly. Those under the 5th percentile may indicate microcephaly. Increased head circumference in children older than 3 years may indicate separation of cranial sutures due to increased intracranial pressure.

GERIATRIC VARIATIONS

- Dress may be heavier because of a decrease in body metabolism and a loss of subcutaneous fat.
- Posture may indicate kyphosis due to osteoporotic thinning and collapse of vertebrae, decreasing height.
- Steps in gait may shorten with decreased speed and arm swing.
- Normal temperature may range from 95.0°F to 97.5°F (35–36.4°C), and thus temperature may not appear to be elevated with an infection.
- Arteries are more rigid, hard, and bent.
- Systolic blood pressure may be increased.
- Systolic murmurs may be present.

CULTURAL VARIATIONS

- Caucasian men tend to be 0.5 inch taller than African American men.
- African American women consistently weigh more than Caucasian women (Overfield, 1995).
- Blood pressure percentiles of prepubertal children in nonindustrialized countries may fall well below Western percentiles.

Possible Collaborative Problems

- Hypertension
- Hypotension
- Infection
- Dysrhythmia

TEACHING TIPS FOR SELECTED NURSING DIAGNOSES AND COLLABORATIVE PROBLEMS

Adult Client

Nursing Diagnosis: Health-Seeking Behaviors (desire to learn more about health promotion)

Teach client self-assessment procedures (eg, breast self-exam, testicular self-exam) and the importance of regular medical checkups. Refer to community wellness resources and support groups as they relate to client.

Collaborative Problem: Potential complication—hype-tension

Explain the relationships between body weight, diet, exercise, stress, and blood pressure. Explain the possible effects of a low-fat, low-cholesterol diet along with vigorous exercise in reducing the atherosclerotic process. Explain methods of preparing food low in sodium and fat, and high in potassium. Teach clients who drink alcohol to limit their intake. (See Tables 4–2 and 4–3 for follow-up and referral.)

Pediatric Client

Nursing Diagnosis: Risk for Imbalanced Body Temperature related to febrile illness

Instruct parents on proper method to assess temperature and detect fever. Teach proper method of giving tepid sponge baths and using antipyretics to reduce fever. Explain the use of quiet play and increasing fluids during this time.

Instruct parent to notify physician in case of high fever.

Nursing Diagnosis: Ineffective Protection related to loss of passive immunity of placenta (age 6–12 months)

Instruct parents to clothe infant well to decrease exposure to others with illnesses. Encourage use of good hand-washing techniques and complete immunizations throughout childhood.

Geriatric Client

Collaborative Problem: Potential complication—postural hypotension

- Identify postural hypotension in elderly (difference of 20 mm Hg systolic BP and 10 mm Hg diastolic BP from a lying to a standing position). Instruct client to reduce risk of falls by moving from a lying to a sitting position slowly, then standing for 2–3 minutes before proceeding.

Nursing Diagnosis: Risk for Imbalanced Body Temperature—Hypothermia related to decreased cardiac output and decreased subcutaneous tissue secondary to aging processes

- Encourage good heating in homes and added clothing in cold weather. Teach family to observe for signs of hypothermia, including facial edema, pallor, clouding of vision, decreased blood pressure, and decreased heart rate. Refer to community agencies that may provide shelter, clothing, and food when needed.

PAIN ASSESSMENT: THE FIFTH VITAL SIGN

5

EQUIPMENT/TOOLS NEEDED

The main tools used are the Verbal Descriptor Scale (VDS), Wong-Baker Faces scale (FACES), Numeric Rating Scale, and Visual Analog Scale.

Verbal Descriptor Scale (VDS)

The VDS ranges pain on a scale between mild, moderate, and severe (Fig. 5-1).

Wong-Baker Faces Scale (FACES)

The Wong-Baker Faces scale shows various facial expressions. The client is asked to choose the face that best describes the intensity or level of pain being experienced; this works well with pediatric clients (Fig. 5-2).

Numeric Rating Scale (NRS)

The NRS rates pain on a scale from 0 to 10 in which 0 reflects no pain and 10 reflects pain at its worst (Fig. 5-3).

Visual Analog Scale (VAS)

The VAS rates pain on a 10-cm continuum numbered from 0 to 10 in which 0 reflects no pain and 10 reflects pain at its worst (Fig. 5-4).

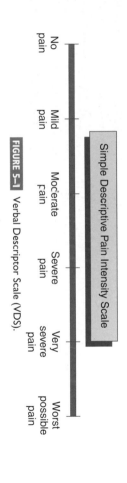

FIGURE 5–1 Verbal Descriptor Scale (VDS).

Simple Descriptive Pain Intensity Scale

No pain   Mild pain   Moderate pain   Severe pain   Very severe pain   Worst possible pain

Wong-Baker FACES Pain Rating Scale

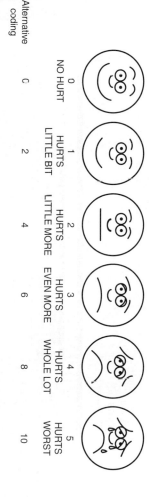

0 NO HURT	1 HURTS LITTLE BIT	2 HURTS LITTLE MORE	3 HURTS EVEN MORE	4 HURTS WHOLE LOT	5 HURTS WORST

Alternative coding	0	2	4	6	8	10

Explain to the person that each face is for a person who feels happy because he has no pain (hurt) or sad because he has some or a lot of pain. Face 0 is very happy because he doesn't hurt at all. Face 1 hurts just a little bit. Face 2 hurts a little more. Face 3 hurts even more. Face 4 hurts a whole lot. Face 5 hurts as much as you can imagine, although you don't have to be crying to feel this bad. Ask the person to choose the face that best describes how he is feeling.

Rating scale is recommended for persons age 3 years and older.

Brief word instructions: Point to each face using the words to describe the pain intensity. Ask the child to choose face that best describes own pain and record the appropriate number.

FIGURE 5–2 FACES pain rating scale (Wong, D. L., Hockenberry-Eaton, M., Wilson, D., Winkelstein, M. L., & Schwartz, P. [2001]. *Wong's essentials of pediatric nursing* [6th ed.]; St. Louis: Mosby, Copyrighted by Mosby, Inc. Reprinted by permission.)

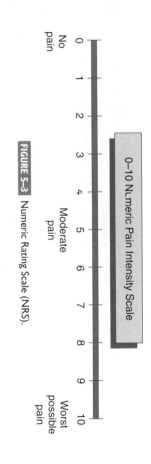

| | | | | | | | | | | |
|0|1|2|3|4|5|6|7|8|9|10|

No
pain

Moderate
pain

Worst
possible
pain

0–10 Numeric Pain Intensity Scale

FIGURE 5-3 Numeric Rating Scale (NRS).

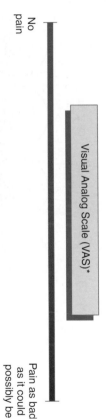

Visual Analog Scale (VAS)*

No
pain

Pain as bad
as it could
possibly be

* A 10-cm baseline is recommended for VAS scales.

FIGURE 5-4 Visual Analog Scale (VAS).

CLASSIFICATION OF PAIN

Pain has many different classifications. Common categories of pain include acute, chronic nonmalignant, and cancer pain.

- Acute pain: usually associated with an injury with a recent onset and duration of less than 6 months and usually lasts less than a month
- Chronic nonmalignant pain: usually associated with a specific cause or injury and is described as a constant pain that persists more than 6 months
- Cancer pain: often due to the compression of peripheral nerves or meninges or from the damage to these structures following surgery, chemotherapy, radiation, or tumor growth and infiltration

Pain is also described as transient pain, tissue injury pain (surgical pain, trauma-related pain, burn pain, or iatrogenic pain as a result of an intervention), and chronic neuropathic pain. Also, pain is viewed in terms of its intensity and location.

PHYSIOLOGIC RESPONSES TO PAIN

Pain elicits a stress response in the human body, triggering the sympathetic nervous system, resulting in physiologic responses such as the following:

- Anxiety, fear, hopelessness, sleeplessness, thoughts of suicide
- Focus on pain, reports of pain, cries and moans, frowns and facial grimaces
- Decrease in cognitive function, mental confusion, altered temperament, high somatization, dilated pupils
- Increased heart rate; peripheral, systemic, and coronary vascular resistance
- Increased respiratory rate and sputum retention resulting in infection and atelectasis
- Decreased gastric and intestinal motility
- Decreased urinary output, fluid overload, depression of all immune responses
- Increased antidiuretic hormone, epinephrine, norepinephrine, aldosterone, and glucagon; decreased insulin and testosterone
- Hyperglycemia, glucose intolerance, insulin resistance, protein catabolism
- Muscle spasm resulting in impaired muscle function and immobility, perspiration

SUBJECTIVE DATA: FOCUS QUESTIONS

There are few objective findings on which the assessment of pain can rely. Pain is a subjective phenomenon, and thus the main assessment lies in the client's reporting. The client's description of pain is quoted. The exact words used to describe the experience of pain are used to help in the diagnosis and management. The pain and its onset, duration, causes, and alleviating and aggravating factors are assessed. Then the quality, intensity, and effects of pain on the physical, psychosocial, and spiritual aspects are questioned. Past experience with pain in addition to past and current therapies are explored. (See Box 5-1 for tips on collecting subjective data.)

BOX 5-1 • Tips for Collecting Subjective Data

- Maintain a quiet and calm environment that is comfortable for the client being interviewed.
- Maintain the client's privacy and ensure confidentiality.
- Ask questions in an open-ended format.
- Listen carefully to the client's verbal descriptions and quote the terms used.
- Watch the client for facial expressions and grimaces during the interview.
- DO NOT put words in the client's mouth.

PRESENT HEALTH CONCERNS

Question

Are you experiencing pain now or have you in the past 24 hours?

Where is the pain located?

Does it radiate or spread?

Are there any other concurrent symptoms accompanying the pain?

When did the pain start?

What were you doing when the pain first started?

Is the pain continuous or intermittent?

If intermittent pain, how often do the episodes occur and for how long do they last?

Rationale

This helps to establish the presence or absence of perceived pain.

The location of pain helps to identify the underlying cause.

Radiating or spreading pain helps to identify the source. For example, chest pain radiating to the left arm is most probably of cardiac origin, while pain that is pricking and spreading in the chest muscle area is probably musculoskeletal in origin.

Accompanying symptoms also help to identify the possible source. For example, right lower quadrant pain associated with nausea, vomiting, and the inability to stand up straight is possibly associated with appendicitis.

The onset of pain is an essential indicator for the severity of the situation and suggests a source.

This helps to identify the precipitating factors and what might have exacerbated the pain.

The pain pattern helps to identify the nature of pain and may assist in identifying the source.

Understanding the course of the pain provides a pattern that may help to determine the source.

Describe the pain in your own words.

Clients are quoted so that terms used to describe their pain may indicate the type and source. The most common terms used are throbbing, shooting, stabbing, sharp, cramping, gnawing, hot/burning, aching, heavy, tender, splitting, tiring/exhausting, sickening, fearful, and punishing.

What factors relieve your pain?
What factors increase your pain?

Relieving factors help to determine the source and the plan of care.
Identifying factors that increase pain helps to determine the source and helps in planning to avoid aggravating factors.

Are you on any therapy to manage your pain?

This question establishes any current treatment modalities and their effect on the pain. This helps in planning the future plan of care.

Is there anything you would like to add?

An open-ended question allows the client to mention anything that has been missed or the issues that were not fully addressed by the above questions

PAST HEALTH HISTORY

Question

Have you had any previous experience with pain?

Rationale

Past experiences of pain may shed light on the previous history of the client in addition to possible positive or negative expectations of pain therapies.

FAMILY HISTORY

Question

Does anyone in your family experience pain?

How does pain affect your family?

Rationale

This helps to assess possible family-related perceptions or any past experiences with persons in pain.
This helps to assess how much the pain is interfering with the client's family relations.

LIFESTYLE AND HEALTH PRACTICES

Question

What are your concerns about pain?

How does your pain interfere with the following?

- General activity
- Mood/emotions
- Concentration
- Physical ability
- Work
- Relations with other people
- Sleep
- Appetite
- Enjoyment of life

Rationale

Identifying the client's fears and worries helps in prioritizing the plan of care and providing adequate psychological support.

These are the main lifestyle factors that pain interferes with. The more that pain interferes with the client's ability to function in his or her daily activities, the more it will reflect on the client's psychological status and thus the quality of life.

COLLECTING OBJECTIVE DATA

Objective data are collected by using one of the pain assessment tools. There are many assessment tools, some of which are specific to special types of pain. The main issues in choosing the tool are its reliability and its validity. Moreover, the tool must be clear and, therefore, easily understood by the client, and it must require little effort from the client and the nurse.

The Joint Commission on Accreditation of Healthcare Organizations (JCAHO) standards for pain management are listed in Box 5-2. Review these JCAHO standards and the points listed in Box 5-3 before performing a physical exam.

BOX 5-2 ● Joint Commission on Accreditation of Healthcare Organizations (JCAHO) Standards for Pain Management

- Recognize clients' rights to appropriate assessment and management of pain.
- Screen for pain and assess the nature and intensity of pain in all clients.
- Record assessment results in a way that allows regular reassessment and follow-up.
- Determine and ensure that staff is competent in assessing and managing pain. Address pain assessment and management when orienting new clinical staff.
- Establish policies and procedures that support appropriate prescribing of pain medications.
- Ensure that pain doesn't interfere with a client's participation in rehabilitation.
- Educate clients and their families about effective pain management.
- Address client needs for symptom management in the discharge planning process.
- Establish a way to collect facility-wide data to monitor the appropriateness and effectiveness of the pain management plan.

Source: JCAHO. Retrieved from: http://www.jcaho.com.

BOX 5-3 ● Key Points to Remember During a Physical Examination

- Choose an assessment tool that is reliable and valid to the client's culture.
- Explain to the client the purpose of rating the intensity of pain.
- Ensure the client's privacy and confidentiality.
- Respect the client's behavior toward pain and the terms used to express it.
- Understand that different cultures express pain differently and maintain different pain thresholds and expectations.

GENERAL OBSERVATION

Inspection

PROCEDURE	NORMAL FINDINGS	DEVIATIONS FROM NORMAL
Observe posture.	Posture is upright when the client appears to be comfortable, attentive, and without excessive changes in position and posture.	Client appears to be slumped with the shoulders not straight (indicates being disturbed/uncomfortable). Client is inattentive and agitated. Client might be guarding affected area and have breathing patterns reflecting distress.
Observe facial expression.	Client smiles with appropriate facial expressions and maintains adequate eye contact.	Client's facial expressions indicate distress and discomfort, including frowning, moans, cries, and grimacing. Eye contact is not maintained, indicating discomfort.
Inspect joints and muscles.	Joints appear normal (no edema); muscles appear relaxed.	Edema of a joint may indicate injury or arthritis. Pain may result in muscle tension.
Observe skin for scars, lesions, rashes, changes, or discoloration.	No inconsistency, wounds, or bruising are noted.	Bruising, wounds, or edema may be the result of injuries or infections, which may cause pain.

VITAL SIGNS

Inspection

PROCEDURE	NORMAL FINDINGS	DEVIATIONS FROM NORMAL
Measure heart rate.	Heart rate ranges from 60 to 100 bpm.	Increased heart rate may indicate discomfort or pain.
Measure respiratory rate.	Respiratory rate ranges from 12 to 20 bpm.	Respiratory rate may be increased, and breathing may be irregular and shallow.
Measure blood pressure.	Blood pressure ranges from 100 to 130 mm Hg (systolic) and 60 to 80 mm Hg (diastolic).	Increased blood pressure often occurs in severe pain.

Note: Refer to Chapter 3, Physical Assessment, appropriate to affected body area. Body system assessments will include techniques for assessing for pain (eg, palpating the abdomen for tenderness or palpating joints for tenderness or pain).

Possible Collaborative Problems

Angina
Decreased cardiac output
Paralytic ileus/small bowel obstruction
Sickling crisis
Peripheral nerve compression
Corneal ulceration

Endocarditis
Peripheral vascular insufficiency
Osteoarthritis
Joint dislocation
Pathologic fractures
Renal calculi

TEACHING TIPS FOR SELECTED NURSING DIAGNOSES

Nursing Diagnosis: Readiness for Enhanced Spiritual Well-Being related to coping with prolonged physical pain

- Encourage client to request interactions with spiritual leaders, and to request forgiveness from family, friends, and others.
- Encourage client to express reverence and awe, and to participate in religious activities.
- Encourage client to spend time outdoors, and to display creative energy (ie, writing, drawing, poetry, etc.).

Nursing Diagnosis: Readiness for Enhanced Comfort Level

- Teach client to identify comfortable positions.
- Teach client to identify uncomfortable postures and to attempt to minimize their occurrences.

Risk Diagnoses

- Risk for Activity Intolerance related to chronic pain and immobility
- Risk for Spiritual Distress related to anxiety, pain, life change, and chronic illness
- Risk for Powerlessness related to chronic pain, health care environment, and pain treatment-related regimen

Actual Diagnoses

- Acute Pain related to injury agents (biological, chemical, physical, or psychological)
- Chronic Pain related to chronic inflammatory process of rheumatoid arthritis
- Disturbed Energy Field related to pain and anxiety
- Fatigue related to stress of handling chronic pain
- Impaired Physical Mobility related to chronic pain
- Self-Care Deficit (bathing/hygiene) related to severe pain (specify)

NUTRITIONAL ASSESSMENT

6

Equipment Needed

- Beam balance scale
- Metric measuring tape
- Skinfold calipers

Subjective Data: Focus Questions

Describe your appetite and nutritional status. Have you had anything to eat or drink during the past 3 days? Do you consider your usual dietary intake to be healthy? What are your food preferences and intolerances? Are you allergic to any foods? Explain. Do you have any food preferences related to your religious or cultural practices? Explain. Who usually shops for food and prepares food for you? Have you ever used particular health foods, vitamins, or diets? Explain. What are your usual activities during a day? Have you had any recent weight loss or gain?

Objective Data: Assessment Techniques

Assessment of the client's nutritional status consists of an overall inspection of muscle mass, distribution of fat, and skeleton. The examiner must determine if abnormalities found during assessment of the skin, thyroid, mouth, lungs, abdomen, and nervous system are related to alterations in nutrition. (Refer to Chapters 7, 8, 11, 12, 14, 16, and 19.)

GENERAL INSPECTION

PROCEDURE	NORMAL FINDINGS	DEVIATIONS FROM NORMAL
Observe the **muscle mass** *over temporal areas, dorsum of hands, and spine for:*		
• Tone	• Firm, developed	• Flaccid, wasted, underdeveloped
• Strength with voluntary movement	• Strength equal bilaterally	• Weak, sluggish, or unequal
Observe **body fat** for distribution over waist, thighs, and triceps.	Equal distribution; some fat under skin	Lack of fat under skin, increased bony prominences, emaciated, cachexic, abundant fatty tissue, abdominal ascites (due to fluid shift in protein)
Observe **posture.**	Erect, no malformations, smooth and coordinated gait	Poor posture, difficulty walking, bow-legged, knock-kneed
Observe **energy level.**	Energetic	Fatigued, irritable
Observe **skin** for color and texture.	Pink, smooth, turgor present	Pale, rough, dry, flaky, petechiae, lacks subcutaneous fat, loss of turgor
Observe **nails** for color and texture.	Nails firm, skin under nails pink	Pale, brittle, opaque, spoon shaped, ridged
Observe **hair** for texture.	Lustrous and shiny	Brittle, dry

PROCEDURE	NORMAL FINDINGS	DEVIATIONS FROM NORMAL
Observe **lips** for color and texture.	Pink, smooth, moist	Swollen, puffy, lesions, fissures at corners of mouth
Observe **tongue** for color and texture.	Deep red with papillae	Beefy red, smooth, swollen, atrophy or hypertrophy; dry tongue seen with dehydration
Observe **teeth** for position and condition.	Straight with no cavities	Missing, malpositioned, cavities
Observe **gums** for condition and color.	Smooth, firm, pink	Inflamed, spongy, swollen, red, bleed easily
Observe **eyes** for moisture, lesions, color.	Clear, moist surfaces, transparent cornea	Pale or red eye; membranes dry, increased vascularity, dull appearance of cornea; sunken eyeballs seen with dehydration
Observe **reflexes.**	Reflexes normal	Loss of or decreased ankle and knee reflexes
Observe **pulse and blood pressure.**	Normal heart rate and blood pressure for age	Tachycardia, hypertension, irregular pulse; blood pressure that drops 20 mm Hg from lying to standing position may indicate fluid volume deficit.

ANTHROPOMETRIC MEASUREMENTS

PROCEDURE	NORMAL FINDINGS	DEVIATIONS FROM NORMAL
Measure **height:** Have client stand erect against wall without shoes. Record height in centimeters and inches.	Compare findings for normal adult height and weight.	Extreme shortness seen with achondroplastic dwarfism and Turner syndrome. Extreme heights are seen with Marfan syndrome, gigantism, and with excessive secretion of growth hormone.
Measure **weight** on a balance beam scale. Ask client to remove shoes and heavy outer clothing and to stand on the scale. Record weight (1 lb = 2.2 kg). If you are weighing a client at home, you may have to use a scale with an automatically adjusting true zero. Determine **ideal body weight** (IBW) and **percentage of IBW.**	Healthy weights for men and women are listed in Table 6–1.	Weight does not fall within range of desirable weights for women and men. Table 6–1 indicates weights in the overweight and obese categories.
Use this formula to calculate the client's IBW: *Female:* 100 lb for 5 ft + 5 lb for each inch over 5 ft ± 10% for small or large frame	Body weight is within 10% of ideal range=.	A current weight that is 80–90% of IBW indicates a lean client and possibly mild malnutrition. Weight that is 70–80% indicates moderate malnutrition; less than 70% may indicate severe

TABLE 6-1 ADULT BODY MASS INDEX (BMI) CHART

Locate the height of interest in the left-most column and read across the row for that height to the weight of interest. Follow the column of the weight up to the top row that lists the BMI. BMI of 19–24 is the healthy weight range, BMI of 25–29 is the overweight range, and BMI of 30 and above is in the obese range. BMI of 40 or above is considered extreme obesity.

BMI	19	20	21	22	23	24	25	26	27	28	29	30	31	32	33	34	35
Height																	
								Weight in Pounds									
4'10"	91	96	100	105	110	115	119	124	129	134	138	143	148	153	158	162	167
4'11"	94	99	104	109	114	119	124	128	133	138	143	148	153	158	163	168	173
5'	97	102	107	112	118	123	128	133	138	143	148	153	158	163	168	174	179
5'1"	100	106	111	116	122	127	132	137	143	148	153	158	164	169	174	180	185
5'2"	104	109	115	120	126	131	136	142	147	153	158	164	169	175	180	186	191
5'3"	107	113	118	124	130	135	141	146	152	158	163	169	175	180	186	191	197
5'4"	110	116	122	128	134	140	145	151	157	163	169	174	180	186	192	197	204

(continued)

TABLE 6–1 ADULT BODY MASS INDEX (BMI) CHART (Continued)

	Healthy Weight						Overweight					Obese				
5'5"	114	120	126	132	138	144	150	156	162	168	174	180	186	192	198	204	210
5'6"	118	124	130	136	142	148	155	161	167	173	179	186	192	198	204	210	216
5'7"	121	127	134	140	146	153	159	166	172	178	185	191	198	204	211	217	223
5'8"	125	131	138	144	151	158	164	171	177	184	190	197	203	210	216	223	230
5'9"	128	135	142	149	155	162	169	176	182	189	196	203	209	216	223	230	236
5'10"	132	139	146	153	160	167	174	181	188	195	202	209	216	222	229	236	243
5'11"	136	143	150	157	165	172	179	186	193	200	208	215	222	229	236	243	250
6'	140	147	154	162	169	177	184	191	199	206	213	221	228	235	242	250	258
6'1"	144	151	159	166	174	182	189	197	204	212	219	227	235	242	250	257	265
6'2"	148	155	163	171	179	186	194	202	210	218	225	233	241	249	256	264	272
6'3"	152	160	168	176	184	192	200	208	216	224	232	240	248	256	264	272	279

Source: Evidence Report of Clinical Guidelines on the Identification, Evaluation, and Treatment of Overweight and Obesity in Adults, 1998. NIH/National Heart, Lung, and Blood Institute (NHLBI).

ANTHROPOMETRIC MEASUREMENTS (continued)

PROCEDURE	NORMAL FINDINGS	DEVIATIONS FROM NORMAL
Male: 106 lb for 5 ft + 6 lb for each inch over 5 ft ± 10% for small or large frame. Calculate the client's percentage of IBW by the following formula: $$actual\ weight \times 100 = \%\ IBW.$$		malnutrition possibly from systemic disease, eating disorders, cancer therapies, and other problems. Weight exceeding 10% of the IBW range is called overweight; weight exceeding 20% of IBW is called obesity.
Measure **body mass index** (BMI). Determine BMI using one of these formulas: $$\frac{Weight\ in\ kilograms}{Height\ in\ meters^2} = BMI$$ or $$\frac{Weight\ in\ pounds}{Height\ in\ inches^2} \times 705 = BMI$$ or Quick Web BMI by accessing the National Institutes of Health's Web Site: http://nhlbisupport.com/bmi/bmicalc.htm	BMI between 18.5 and 24.9 Refer to Table 6–1 for the healthy weight.	BMI < 18.5 is associated with being underweight. BMI between 25 and 29.9 is considered overweight and may lead to health problems. BMI ≥ 30 is considered obese and indicates increased risk of developing health problems such as diabetes and cardiovascular disorders. Refer to Table 6–1.

Nutritional Assessment

ANTHROPOMETRIC MEASUREMENTS (continued)

PROCEDURE	NORMAL FINDINGS	DEVIATIONS FROM NORMAL
Determine **waist circumference.** Have the client stand straight with feet together and arms at the sides. Place the measuring tape snugly around the waist at the umbilicus, yet not compressing the skin. Instruct the client to relax the abdomen and take a normal breath. When the client exhales, record the waist circumference. See Table 6–2 for an interpretation of waist circumference, BMI, and associated risks.	*Females:* Less than or equal to 35 inches (88 cm) *Males:* Less than or equal to 40 inches (102 cm) These findings are associated with reduced disease risk.	*Females:* Greater than 35 inches (88 cm) *Males:* Greater than 40 inches (102 cm) See Table 6–2. Adults with large amounts of visceral fat located mostly around the waist are more likely to develop health-related problems than adults with the fat located in the hips or thighs. Increased risk of type 2 diabetes, abnormal cholesterol and triglyceride levels, hypertension, and cardiovascular disease such as heart attack or stroke may occur.
Measure **mid-arm circumference** (MAC; Fig. 6–1). The MAC measurement evaluates skeletal muscle mass and fat stores. Have the client dangle the non-dominant arm freely next to the body. Locate the arm's midpoint (halfway between the top of the acromion process and the ole-cranion process and the ole-		Compare the client's current MAC to prior measurements and compare to standard reference MAC measurements for the client's age and sex listed in Table 6–3. The standard reference is 29.3 cm for men and 28.5 cm for women.
		Measurements less than 90% of the standard reference are in the category of moderately malnourished. Measurements less than 60% of the standard reference indicates severe malnourish-ment. See Table 6–3.

TABLE 6-2 CLASSIFICATION OF OVERWEIGHT AND OBESITY BY BMI, WAIST CIRCUMFERENCE, AND ASSOCIATED DISEASE RISK*

	BMI (kg/m²)	Obesity Class	Disease Risk* (Relative to Normal Weight and Waist Circumference)	
			Men <40 in (≤ 102 cm) Women ≤ 35 in (≤ 88 cm)	>40 in (> 102 cm) > 35 in (> 88 cm)
Underweight	< 18.5			
Normal†	18.5–24.9			
Overweight	25.0–29.9		Increased	High
Obesity	30.0–34.9	I	High	Very High
	35.0–39.9	II	Very High	Very High
Extreme Obesity	≥ 40	III	Extremely High	Extremely High

*Disease risk for type 2 diabetes, hypertension, and cardiovascular disease.
†Increased waist circumference can also be a marker for increased risk even in persons of normal weight.

Adapted from Preventing and Managing the Global Epidemic of Obesity: Report of the World Health Organization Consultation of Obesity. WHO. Geneva, June 1997.
Reprinted from *The practical guide. Identification, evaluation, and treatment of overweight and obesity in adults.* NIH Publication Number 00-4084, October 2000.

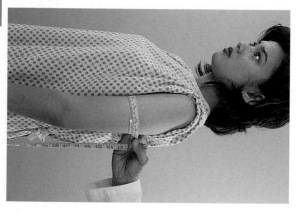

FIGURE 6–1 Measuring mid-arm circumference. (© B. Proud.)

TABLE 6-3 MID-ARM CIRCUMFERENCE (MAC) STANDARD REFERENCE

Adult MAC (cm)	Standard Reference	60% of Standard Reference—Moderately Malnourished	Severely Malnourished
Men	29.3	26.3	17.6
Women	28.5	25.7	17.1

PROCEDURE	NORMAL FINDINGS	DEVIATIONS FROM NORMAL

cranon process). Mark the midpoint and measure the MAC, holding the tape measure firmly around, but not pinching, the arm.

Measure **triceps skinfold thickness** (TSF; Fig. 6–2). Take the TSF measurement to evaluate the degree of fat stores. Instruct the client to stand and hang the nondominant arm freely. Grasp the skinfold and subcutaneous fat between the thumb and forefinger midway between the acromion process and the tip of the elbow. Pull the skin away from the muscle (ask client to flex arm—if you feel a contraction with this maneuver, you still have the muscle) and apply the calipers. Repeat three times.

Compare the client's current measurement to past measurements and to standard TSF measurements for the client's age and sex listed in Table 6–4. Standard reference is 12.5 mm for men and 16.5 mm for women.

Fat stores decrease in malnutrition and increase in obesity. See Table 6–4 for criteria indicating moderate to severe malnourishment. Measurements greater than 120% of the standard indicate obesity.

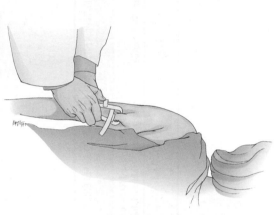

FIGURE 6-2 Measuring triceps skinfold thickness.

Nutritional Assessment

TABLE 6-4 TRICEPS SKINFOLD THICKNESS (TSF) STANDARD REFERENCE

Adult TSF (mm)	Standard Reference	90% of Standard Reference— Moderately Malnourished	60% of Standard Reference— Severely Malnourished
Men	12.5	11.3	7.5
Women	16.5	14.9	9.9

ANTHROPOMETRIC MEASUREMENTS (continued)

PROCEDURE	NORMAL FINDINGS	DEVIATIONS FROM NORMAL
and average the three measurements. *Note:* A more accurate measurement can be obtained from the suprailiac region of the abdomen or the subscapular area. Calculate **mid-arm muscle circumference** (MAMC). The MAMC calculation determines skeletal muscle reserves from MAC and TSF measurements by this formula: MAMC (cm) = MAC (cm) − (0.314 × TSF)	Compare the client's current MAMC to past measurements and to data percentiles with the client's age and sex listed in Table 6–5. Standard reference is 25.3 cm for men and 23.2 cm for women.	The MAMC decreases to the lower percentiles with malnutrition and in obesity if TSF is high. If the MAMC is in a lower percentile and the TSF is in a higher percentile, the client may benefit from muscle-building exercises that increase muscle mass and decrease fat. Malnutrition Mild—MAMC of 90–99% Moderate—MAMC 60–90% Severe—MAMC < 60% as seen in protein-calorie malnutrition. See Table 6–5.

TABLE 6-5 MID-ARM MUSCLE CIRCUMFERENCE (MAMC) STANDARD REFERENCE

Adult MAMC (cm)	Standard Reference	90% of Standard Reference—Moderately Malnourished	60% of Standard Reference—Severely Malnourished
Men	25.3	22.8	15.2
Women	23.2	20.9	13.9

DIETARY ASSESSMENT

Assess client's dietary requirements and intake by asking client to keep 3-day diary of food and fluid intake. You may also use Box 6–1, Speedy Checklist for Nutritional Health.

PROCEDURE	NORMAL FINDINGS	DEVIATIONS FROM NORMAL
Estimate client's daily caloric requirements. See Table 6–6 for estimated daily calorie needs.	Meets caloric requirements	Consumes more or less than caloric requirements for age, height, body build and weight
Compare client's intake with USDA-recommended food guidelines (Fig. 6–3) MyPyramid (2005).	See Table 6–6 for daily amount of food from each group. Compare with Figure 6–4 Asian and Latin American pyramids.	Consumes more or less than recommended Compare with Figure 6–3 and Figure 6–4 Asian and Latin American pyramids

BOX 6-1 • Speedy Checklist for Nutritional Health

Some warning signs of poor nutritional health are noted in this checklist. Use it to find out if your client is at nutritional risk. Read the statements below. Circle the number in the yes column for those that apply to the client. For each yes answer, score the number in the box. Total the nutrition score.

	YES
Illness or condition that made client change the kind and/or amount of food eaten	2
Eats fewer than two meals per day	3
Eats few fruits or vegetables, or milk products	2
Has three or more drinks of beer, liquor, or wine almost every day	2
Has tooth or mouth problems that make it hard to eat	2
Does not always have enough money to buy the food needed	4
Eats alone most of the time	1
Takes three or more different prescribed or over-the-counter drugs a day	1
Without wanting to, has lost or gained 10 lb in the last 6 months	2
Is not physically able to shop, cook, and/or feed self	2

TOTAL _____

Total the nutritional score.

0–2   Good. Recheck the score in 6 months.

3–5   Moderate nutritional risk. See what can be done to improve eating habits and lifestyle. Recheck score in 3 months.

6 or more   High nutritional risk. Consult with physician, dietitian, or other qualified health or social service professional.

Note: Remember that warning signs suggest risk but do not represent diagnosis of any condition.

TABLE 6–6 ESTIMATED DAILY CALORIE NEEDS

To determine which food intake pattern to use for an individual, the following chart gives an estimate of individual calorie needs. The calorie range for each age/sex group is based on physical activity level, from sedentary to active.

Calorie Range	Sedentary	→	Active
Children			
2–3 yr	1,000	→	1,400
Females			
4–8 yr	1,200	→	1,800
9–13	1,600	→	2,200
14–18	1,800	→	2,400
19–30	2,000	→	2,400
31–50	1,800	→	2,200
51+	1,600	→	2,200

Calorie Range	Sedentary	→	Active
Males			
4–8 yr	1,400	→	2,000
9–13	1,800	→	2,600
14–18	2,200	→	3,200
19–30	2,400	→	3,000
31–50	2,200	→	3,000
51+	2,000	→	2,800

Sedentary means a lifestyle that includes only the light physical activity associated with typical day-to-day life.
Active means a lifestyle that includes physical activity equivalent to walking more than 3 miles per day at 3 to 4 miles per hour, in addition to the light physical activity associated with typical day-to-day life.

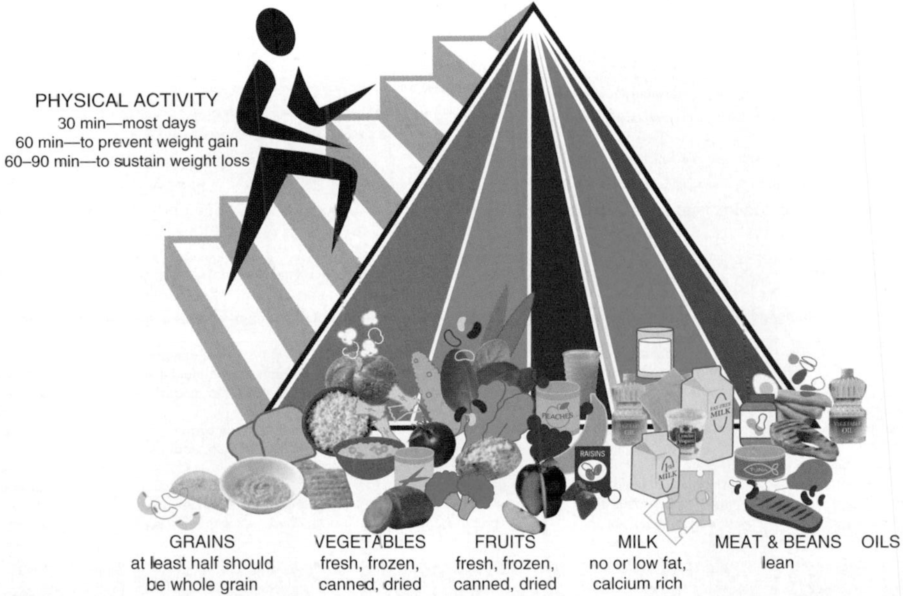

FIGURE 6-3 USDA food pyramid. (U.S. Department of Agriculture, Center for Nutrition Policy and Promotion, April 2005, CNPP-15.)

PHYSICAL ACTIVITY
30 min—most days
60 min—to prevent weight gain
60–90 min—to sustain weight loss

GRAINS
at least half should
be whole grain

VEGETABLES
fresh, frozen,
canned, dried

FRUITS
fresh, frozen,
canned, dried

MILK
no or low fat,
calcium rich

MEAT & BEANS
lean

OILS

GRAINS Make half your grains whole	VEGETABLES Vary your veggies	FRUITS Focus on fruits	MILK Get your calcium-rich foods	MEAT & BEANS Go lean with protein
Eat at least 3 oz. of whole-grain cereals, breads, crackers, rice, or pasta every day	Eat more dark-green veggies like broccoli, spinach, and other dark leafy greens	Eat a variety of fruit	Go low fat or fat free when you choose milk, yogurt, and other milk products	Choose low-fat or lean meats and poultry
	Eat more orange vegetables like carrots and sweet potatoes	Choose fresh, frozen, canned, or dried fruit	If you don't or can't consume milk, choose lactose-free products or other calcium sources such as fortified foods and beverages	Bake it, broil it, or grill it
1 oz. is about 1 slice of bread, about 1 cup of breakfast cereal, or ½ cup of cooked rice, cereal, or pasta	Eat more dry beans and peas like pinto beans, kidney beans, and lentils	Go easy on fruit juices		Vary your protein routine – choose more fish, beans, peas, nuts, and seeds

For a 2,000-calorie diet, you need the amounts below from each food group. To find the amounts that are right for you, go to MyPyramid.gov.

Eat 6 oz. every day	Eat 2½ cups every day	Eat 2 cups every day	Get 3 cups every day; for kids aged 2 to 8, it's 2	Eat 5½ oz. every day

Find your balance between food and physical activity

- Be sure to stay within your daily calorie needs.
- Be physically active for at least 30 minutes most days of the week.
- About 60 minutes a day of physical activity may be needed to prevent weight gain.
- For sustaining weight loss, at least 60 to 90 minutes a day of physical activity may be required.
- Children and teenagers should be physically active for 60 minutes every day, or most days.

Know the limits on fats, sugars, and salt (sodium)

- Make most of your fat sources from fish, nuts, and vegetable oils.
- Limit solid fats like butter, stick margarine, shortening, and lard, as well as foods that contain these.
- Check the Nutrition Facts label to keep saturated fats, trans fats, and sodium low.
- Choose food and beverages low in added sugars. Added sugars contribute calories with few, if any, nutrients.

FIGURE 6-3 (Continued)

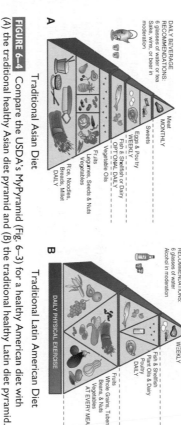

FIGURE 6-4 Compare the USDA's MyPyramid (Fig. 6-3) for a healthy American diet with (A) the traditional healthy Asian diet pyramid and (B) the traditional healthy Latin diet pyramid.

A

Traditional Asian Diet

DAILY BEVERAGE RECOMMENDATIONS:
6 glasses of water or tea
Sake, wine, or beer in moderation

Meat MONTHLY

Sweets

Eggs & Poultry WEEKLY

Fish & Shellfish or Dairy OPTIONAL DAILY

Vegetable Oils

Fruits

Legumes, Seeds & Nuts

Vegetables

Rice, Noodles, Breads, Millet DAILY

B

Traditional Latin American Diet

DAILY BEVERAGE RECOMMENDATIONS:
6 glasses of water
Alcohol in moderation

Meat, Sweets, & Eggs WEEKLY

Fish & Shellfish
Plant Oils & Dairy
Poultry DAILY

DAILY PHYSICAL EXERCISE

Fruits

Whole Grains, Tubers, Beans, & Nuts

Vegetables

AT EVERY MEAL

PEDIATRIC VARIATIONS

Physiologic Growth Patterns

- See Appendix 7 for height/weight parameters.
- Growth is most rapid during the first year of life.
- Birth weight doubles at age 4 to 6 months and triples by 1 year.
- Length increases 50% the first year of life.
- Teeth erupt first year of life.
- Growth decreases from ages 1 to 6 years, but biting, chewing, and swallowing abilities increase.
- Muscle mass and bone density increase from ages 1 to 6 years.
- There is a latent uneven period of growth from ages 1 to 12 years.
- Permanent teeth erupt at ages 6 to 12 years.
- School-age children tolerate larger, less frequent meals.
- Nutritional needs increase during growth spurts (ages 10–15 years for girls and ages 12–19 years for boys).

Dietary Requirements

- Allow 1000 calories plus 100 more per each year of age (eg, a 5-year-old needs 1500 calories per day).
- Children need three milks, two meats, four fruits or vegetables, and four grains per day.
- Adolescents need four milks, two meats, four fruits or vegetables, and four grains per day.
- The American Academy of Pediatrics (2005) recommends infants be breast-fed for at least the first year of life. Exclusive breast-feeding is sufficient for optimal growth and development for approximately the first 6 months. Solid foods should not be introduced before age 6 months, and they should be iron enriched.

Assessment Techniques

- *Infants*: Use pediatric pain scale. Obtain weight, length, and head circumference. Identify type of feeding and iron source.
- *Children and adolescents*: Weigh child and obtain height. Identify adequacy of meals and snacks and sources of iron, calories, and protein.

GERIATRIC VARIATIONS

- Elderly clients may have atrophy on dorsum of hands even with good nutrition.
- Assess for poor-fitting dentures and decreased ability to taste.
- Body weight may decrease with aging because of a loss of muscle or lean body tissue.
- Elderly tend to consume less food and eat more irregularly as they get older. This tends to increase with social isolation.
- Elderly have decreased peristalsis and nerve sensation, which may lead to constipation. Encourage fluids and dietary bulk to avoid laxative abuse.
- Caloric requirements decrease in response to a decreased basal metabolic rate, decreased activity, and change in body composition. A 10% decrease in calories is recommended for people ages 51 to 75 years and a 20 to 25% decrease in calories for people older than 75 years.
- A decrease in mobility and vision may impair the ability to purchase and prepare food. Sensory taste losses may lead to anorexia.
- Fifty percent of elderly are thought to be economically deprived, which may affect nutrition when meats and milks are omitted from diet to save money.
- Dietary recall may be difficult for the elderly.
- Skinfold measurements are often inaccurate owing to changes in subcutaneous fat.

CULTURAL VARIATIONS

- Great variations may be seen in nutritional preferences, eating habits, and patterns of various groups (Andrews & Boyle, 2002; Giger & Davidhizar, 2003).
- Foods, beverages, and medications are classified as hot/cold by many Asians and Hispanics (eg, yin/yang by Chinese); it is very important to these clients to seek a balanced consumption based on these theories.
- Many people, especially of non-northern European descent, have some degree of lactose intolerance.*
- Classifications of "food" and "nonfood" items vary in cultures.
- Cultural or religious dietary rules or laws are of great importance to some groups (eg, Orthodox Jews).
- Some groups may have diseases precipitated by certain foods or medications (eg, glucose-6-phosphate dehydrogenase [G-6-PD] deficiency, lactose deficiency).
- Some cultural food preferences are contraindicated in specific disease states (eg, Japanese client with hypertension who consumes high-sodium soy sauce).

Possible Collaborative Problems

Hypoglycemia
Hyperglycemia
Electrolyte imbalance
Anemia

---

*Clients with lactose intolerance may be able to consume yogurt, buttermilk, fermented cheese, and acidophilus milk, or they may use products such as chewable tablets or liquid drops to act in place of the lactose enzyme.

TEACHING TIPS FOR SELECTED NURSING DIAGNOSES

Adult Client

Nursing Diagnosis: Readiness for enhanced nutritional-metabolic pattern

 Encourage proper oral hygiene. Teach nutritional guidelines:

- Eat a variety of foods.
- Balance the food you eat with physical activity—maintain or improve your weight. All adults should be more active and get at least 30 minutes of moderate physical activity most or all days of the week. Regular physical activity is important for a healthy body, enhancing psychological well-being, and preventing premature death (Healthy People 2010).
- Choose a diet with more dark green and orange vegetables, legumes, fruits, whole grains, low-fat milk, and milk products.
- Choose a diet with less total fats.
- Choose a diet with less added sugar and calories
- Choose a diet with less salt and sodium.
- If you drink alcoholic beverages, do so in moderation. According to Healthy People 2010, alcohol as well as illegal drug use is linked to violence, injury, and HIV infection. Indicators set forth by Healthy People 2010 include: increasing the proportion of adolescents not using alcohol or any illicit drugs and reducing the proportion of adults using any illicit drug during the past 30 days.

Teach client how to get the most for his or her food dollar, how to read food labels, and ways to maintain nutrients in foods:

- Buy frozen vegetables and ripe produce.
- Encourage proper food storage and preparation to retain nutritional value.
- Prepare low-fat foods—suggest substituting applesauce or yogurt for butter when baking. Use bouillon or tomato juice instead of oil for sautéing. Use herbs and spices to replace the fat with flavor.

(Recommended by U.S. Department of Agriculture, U.S. Department of Health and Human Services [2005]. Nutrition and your health: Dietary guidelines for Americans.)

Nursing Diagnosis: Imbalanced Nutrition: more than body requirements

Provide client with information on social support groups. Teach client self-assessment and rewarding techniques when proper nutrition is followed. Teach client how to calculate caloric intake and caloric expenditure and how to explore forms of exercise that meet client's needs. Assist client to replace frequent unhealthy snacking with nutritious snacks. Teach dietary guidelines and food choices for Americans recommended by the U.S. Department of Agriculture, Center for Nutrition Policy and Promotion (April, 2005).

Pediatric Client

Nursing Diagnosis: Imbalanced Nutrition: risk for more than body requirements

Teach parents to avoid overfeeding infants. Encourage proper formula dilution. Teach avoidance of empty caloric foods. Discourage use of food for rewarding behavior.

Nursing Diagnosis: Imbalanced Nutrition: risk for less than body requirements

Teach parents to avoid restricting normal intake of fat. Teach that low-fat diets are dangerous to growing infants because fat is essential to metabolism of some vitamins and other substances and to hormone production associated with growth and development. The Dietary Guidelines for Americans (2005) recommends that children get at least 60 minutes of physical activity each day. Furthermore, inactive forms of play such as television viewing and computer gaming should be limited.

SKIN, HAIR, AND NAIL ASSESSMENT

ANATOMY OVERVIEW

The skin is composed of three layers, the epidermis, dermis, and subcutaneous tissue (Fig. 7–1). The skin is a physical barrier that protects the underlying tissues and structures.

Hair consists of layers of keratinized cells found over much of the body except for the lips, nipples, soles of the feet, palms of the hands, labia minora, and penis.

The nails, located on the distal phalanges of fingers and toes, are hard, transparent plates of keratinized epidermal cells that grow from a root underneath the skin fold called the cuticle (Fig. 7–2).

Equipment Needed

- Adequate lighting (natural daylight is best)
- Comfortable room temperature
- Gloves
- Penlight
- Magnifying glass
- Centimeter rule

7

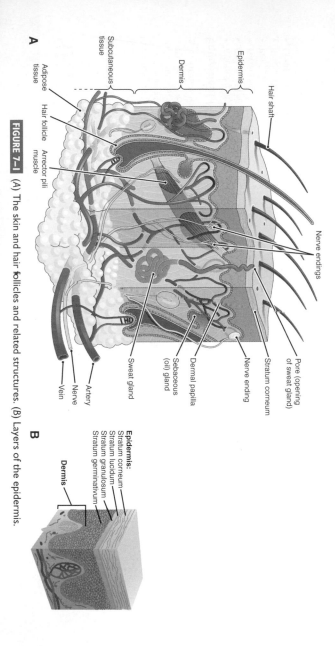

FIGURE 7-1 (A) The skin and hair follicles and related structures. (B) Layers of the epidermis.

A

Subcutaneous tissue

Dermis

Epidermis

Hair shaft

Adipose tissue

Hair follicle

Arrector pili muscle

Nerve endings

Pore (opening of sweat gland)

Stratum corneum

Sweat gland

Sebaceous (oil) gland

Dermal papilla

Nerve ending

Vein

Nerve

Artery

B

Dermis

Epidermis:
Stratum corneum
Stratum lucidum
Stratum granulosum
Stratum germinativum

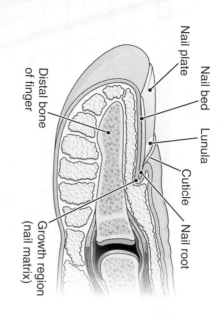

Nail plate

Nail bed

Distal bone
of finger

Lunula

Cuticle

Nail root

Growth region
(nail matrix)

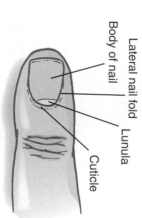

Body of nail

Lateral nail fold

Lunula

Cuticle

FIGURE 7-2 The nail and related structures.

Subjective Data: Focus Questions

Skin rashes, lesions, itching, dryness, oiliness, bruising (location; onset; precipitating factors: stress, weather, drugs, exposure to allergens)? Methods of relief (eg, medications, lotions, soaks)? Changes in skin color, lesions, bruising (onset, type of change)? Scalp lesions, itching, infections? History of skin disorders? Surgical excision of skin lesions? Describe. Changes in texture, condition, and amount of hair? Changes in condition of nails and cuticles? Nail breaking, splitting? Cuticle inflammation? Changes in body odor? Skin, hair, and nail care habits; bathing patterns; soaps and lotions used? Shampoo, hair spray, coloring, nail enamels used? Amount of sun/tanning exposure (type of oils and lotions used)? Exposure to chemicals?

Risk Factors. Risk for skin cancer related to repeated, intermittent sun exposure with sunburn beginning at early age; use of tanning booths; medical therapies (PUVA and radiation); genetic susceptibility; fair skinned; immunosuppression

Objective Data: Assessment Techniques

Review Figure 7–1 for a diagram of the skin and related structures.

SKIN INSPECTION AND PALPATION

Expose the body part to be inspected (cleanse skin if necessary).

PROCEDURE	NORMAL FINDINGS	DEVIATIONS FROM NORMAL
Inspect skin for the following:		
• Generalized color	• *In white skin:* Light to dark pink	• *In white skin:* Extreme pallor, flushed, bluish (cyanosis).
	• *In dark skin:* Light to dark brown, olive	• *In dark skin:* Loss of red tones in pallor; ashen gray in cyanosis. Bluish color

SKIN INSPECTION AND PALPATION (continued)

PROCEDURE	NORMAL FINDINGS	DEVIATIONS FROM NORMAL
• Color variations in patches on body	• *In white skin:* Sun-tanned areas, white patches (vitiligo) • *In dark skin:* Lighter colored palms, soles, nail beds, and lips; black/blue area over lower lumbar area (mongolian spot); frecklelike pigmentation of nail beds and sclerae	ored palms, soles, lips, nails, earlobes are seen with cyanosis. Cyanosis is seen in vasoconstriction, myocardial infarction, or pulmonary insufficiency. Pallor is seen in arterial insufficiency and anemia. • *In white skin:* Generalized pale yellow to pumpkin color (jaundice). • *In dark skin:* Yellow color may appear in sclerae, oral mucous membranes, hard and soft palates, palms, and soles. Increased pigmented areas; decreased pigmented areas; reddened, warm areas (erythema); black and blue marks (ecchymosis); tiny red spots (petechiae). Jaundice is often seen in liver or gall-bladder disease, hemolysis, or anemia.
Palpate skin for the following: • Texture	• Smooth, soft	• Rough, thick. Dry skin is seen in hypothyroidism.

SKIN INSPECTION AND PALPATION (continued)

PROCEDURE	NORMAL FINDINGS	DEVIATIONS FROM NORMAL
• Temperature and moisture: feel with back of hand.	• Warm, dry	• Extremely cool or warm, wet, oily. Cold skin is seen in shock, hypotension, arterial insufficiency. Very warm skin is seen in fever and hyperthyroidism.
• Turgor: Pinch up skin on sternum or under clavicle.	• Pinched-up skin returns immediately to original position.	• Pinched-up skin takes 30 seconds or longer to return to original position. Turgor is decreased in dehydration.
• Edema: Press firmly for 5–10 seconds over tibia and ankle.	• No swelling, pitting, or edema	• Swollen, shallow to deep pitting, ascites. Generalized edema is seen in congestive heart failure or kidney disease. Unilateral, localized edema is seen in peripheral vascular problems such as venous stasis, obstruction, or lymphedema.
If a skin lesion is detected, inspect and palpate for size, location, mobility, consistency, and pattern (circular, clustered, or straight-lined).	Silver-pink stretch marks (striae), moles (nevi), freckles, birthmarks	Primary lesions (Fig. 7–3) arise from normal skin owing to disease or irritation. Secondary lesions (Fig. 7–4) arise from changes in primary lesions. Vascular lesions (Fig. 7–5) may be seen with increased venous pressure, aging, liver disease, or pregnancy. Skin cancer can manifest as either primary or secondary lesions.

Nonpalpable Lesion

Macule: Flat and colored (Example: Freckle, petechia)

Palpable Lesions

Papule: Elevated and superficial (Example: Mole)

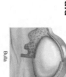
Macule

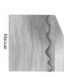
Papule

Palpable Lesions With Fluid

Bulla, vesicle: Elevated and filled with fluid (Example: Blister)

Cyst: Encapsulated, filled with fluid or semisolid mass (Example: Epidermoid cyst)

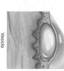
Bulla

Vesicle

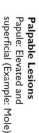
Cyst

Nodule, tumor: Elevated and firm, has dimension of depth (Example: Lipoma)

Wheal: Localized edema (Example: Insect bite)

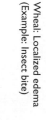
Tumor

Wheal

Pustule: Elevated and filled with pus (Example: Acne)

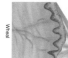
Pustule

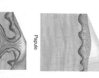

FIGURE 7-3 Primary skin lesions.

Ulcer: Skin surface loss, often bleeds

Ulcer

Atrophy: Thin, shiny, taut skin

Atrophy

Crust: Dried pus or blood

Crust

Lichenification: Thickened, roughened skin

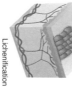

Lichenification

Scale: Thin, flaky skin

Scales

Keloid: Hypertrophied scar

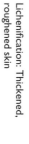

Keloid

FIGURE 7–4 Secondary skin lesions (changes in primary lesions).

Cherry angioma: Ruby red; flat or raised

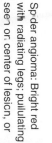

Spider angioma: Bright red with radiating legs; pulsating seen or center of lesion, or legs, or arms, and upper trunk; blanches when pressure is applied to center

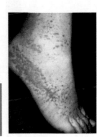

Petechiae: Round red or purple macules.

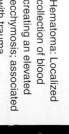

Spider vein: Bluish; may have radiating legs; seen mostly on legs

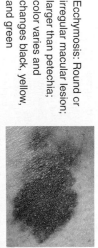

Ecchymosis: Round or irregular macular lesion; larger than petechia; color varies and changes black, yellow, and green

Hematoma: Localized collection of blood creating an elevated ecchymosis; associated with trauma

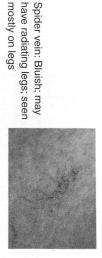

FIGURE 7-5 Vascular lesions.

HAIR INSPECTION AND PALPATION

PROCEDURE	NORMAL FINDINGS	DEVIATIONS FROM NORMAL
Inspect and palpate hair for the following:		
• Color	• Varies	• Patchy gray areas are seen in nutritional deficiencies. Copper-red hair in an African American child may indicate severe malnutrition.
• Amount and distribution	• Vary	• Sudden loss of hair (alopecia) or increase in facial hair in females (hirsutism). Hirsutism is seen in Cushing syndrome; general hair loss seen in infections, nutritional deficiencies, hormonal disorders, some types of chemotherapy, or radiation therapy; patchy loss seen with scale infection and lupus erythematosus.
• Texture	• Fine to coarse, pliant	• Change in texture, brittle. Dull, dry hair is seen in hypothyroidism and malnutrition.
• Presence of parasites	• None	• Lice (body or head), eggs attached to hair shaft, usually accompanied by severe itching.

SCALP INSPECTION AND PALPATION

PROCEDURE	NORMAL FINDINGS	DEVIATIONS FROM NORMAL
Inspect and palpate scalp for the following:		
• Symmetry	• Symmetrical	• Asymmetrical
• Texture	• Smooth, firm	• Bumpy, scaly, excoriated. Scaly, dry flakes are seen in dermatitis; gray scaly patches seen in fungal infections; dandruff seen with psoriasis.
• Lesions	• None	• Open or closed lesions

NAIL INSPECTION AND PALPATION

PROCEDURE	NORMAL FINDINGS	DEVIATIONS FROM NORMAL
Inspect and palpate nails for the following:		
• Color	• Pink nail bed *In dark skin:* may have small or large pigmented deposits, streaks, freckles	• Pale or cyanotic nails are seen in hypoxia or anemia; yellow discoloration seen in fungal infections or psoriasis; splinter hemorrhages (vertical lines) seen in trauma; Beau's lines (horizontal)

PROCEDURE	NORMAL FINDINGS	DEVIATIONS FROM NORMAL
		seen in acute trauma; nail pitting seen in psoriasis.

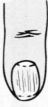

Splinter hemorrhages

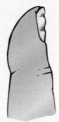

Beau's lines
(acute illness)

NAIL INSPECTION AND PALPATION (continued)

PROCEDURE	NORMAL FINDINGS	DEVIATIONS FROM NORMAL
• Shape	• Round nail with 160° nail base	• Clubbing: 180° or more nail base is seen with hypoxia. Spoon nails occur with iron deficiency anemia.

160°

Normal angle

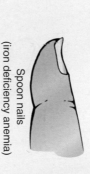

Spoon nails
(iron deficiency anemia)

180

Early clubbing
(oxygen deficiency)

>180

Late clubbing
(oxygen deficiency)

Skin, Hair, and Nail Assessment

NAIL INSPECTION AND PALPATION (continued)

PROCEDURE	NORMAL FINDINGS	DEVIATIONS FROM NORMAL
• Texture	• Nail is round, hard, immobile *In dark skin:* may be thick	• Thickened nails are seen with decreased circulation.
• Condition of nail bed	• Smooth, firm, and pink	• Paronychia (inflamed nail head) indicates infection. Onycholysis (detached nail plate from nail bed) indicates infection or trauma.

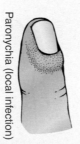

Paronychia (local infection)

PEDIATRIC VARIATIONS

Subjective Data: Focus Questions

Skin eruptions or rashes and relationship to any allergies (eg, food, formula, type of diapers used, diaper creams, soaps, dust)? Bathing routines and soap used? Play injuries (cuts, abrasions, bruises)? Indicators of physical abuse (bruises)? Exposure to communicable diseases? Exposure to pets, stuffed animals? Eczema (onset, precipitating factors, treatment)? Acne (during adolescence; location: face, back, chest; onset; precipitating factors; treatment)? Excessive nail biting? Twirling of hair? History of communicable diseases? Immunization history (see Appendix 4)?

Objective Data: Assessment Techniques

PROCEDURE	NORMAL FINDINGS	DEVIATIONS FROM NORMAL
Inspect the following:		
• Skin color	• Infant's skin is lighter shade than parents'; Mongolian spot is common hyperpigmentation variation in African Americans, Native Americans, Latin Americans, and Asians. Body piercing may be cultural or a fad. Excessive piercing or tattooing that is "homemade" may increase risk for hepatitis B or HIV from infected needles.	• Yellow skin is seen in jaundice or with ingestion of too many yellow/orange vegetables.
• Oiliness and acne	• Adolescents have increased sebaceous gland activity.	• Cystic acne
• Skin lesions	• None	• Crusted or ruptured vesicles are seen in impetigo. Fruitic macular–papular skin eruptions that become vesicular are seen in chicken pox. Pink to red macular–papular rash is seen in measles.

PROCEDURE

- Hand creases: Assess dermatoglyphics by inspecting flexion creases in palm.

- Hair

NORMAL FINDINGS

- Three flexion creases present in palm

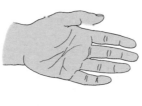

Normal creases

- Lustrous, strong, elastic

DEVIATIONS FROM NORMAL

- More or fewer than three flexion creases with varied pattern in palm (eg, one horizontal crease in palm [Simian crease])

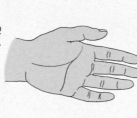

Simian creases

GERIATRIC VARIATIONS

Skin

- Thinning epithelium
- Wrinkles, decreased turgor and elasticity
- Dry, itchy skin due to decrease in activity of eccrine and sebaceous glands
- Seborrheic or senile keratosis (tan to black macular–papular lesions on neck, chest, or back)
- Senile lentigines ("liver spots" or "age spots"—flat brown maculae on hands, arms, neck, face)
- Cherry angiomas (small, round, red elevated spots)
- Senile purpura (vivid purple patches)
- Acrochordons (soft, light-pink to brown skin tags)
- Prominent veins due to thinning epithelium

Hair

- Loss of pigment; fine, brittle texture
- Alopecia, especially in men; sparse body hair
- Coarse facial hair, especially in women
- Decreased axillary, pubic, and extremity hair

Nails

- Thickened, yellow, brittle nails
- Ingrown toenails

CULTURAL VARIATIONS

- Infants and newborns of African American, Native American, or Asian descent often have mongolian spots, a blue-black or purple macular area on buttocks and sacrum; sometimes this pattern appears on the abdomen, thighs, or upper extremities.

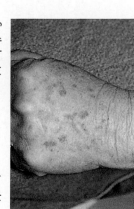

Senile lentigines are common on aging skin.

- Dark-skinned clients tend to have lighter colored palms, soles, nail beds, and lips. They may also have frecklelike pigmentation of nail beds and sclera. Nails may also be thick.
- Females of certain cultural groups shave or pluck pubic hair.
- Pallor is assessed in the dark-skinned client by observing the absence of underlying red tones. (Brown skin appears yellow-brown; black skin appears ashen-gray.)
- Erythema is detected by palpation of increased warmth of skin in dark-skinned clients.
- Cyanosis is detected in dark-skinned clients by observing the lips and tongue, which become ashen-gray.
- Inspect for petechiae in the oral mucosa or conjunctiva of the dark-skinned client, because they are difficult to see in dark-pigmented areas; also observe the sclerae, hard palate, palms, and soles for jaundice.
- Presence of body piercing may be a fad or a cultural norm.

Possible Collaborative Problems

Skin infections	Burns	Allergic reactions (skin)
Skin rashes	Graft rejection	Insect-animal bite
Skin lesions	Hemorrhage	

TEACHING TIPS FOR SELECTED NURSING DIAGNOSES

Adult Client

Nursing Diagnosis: Readiness for Enhanced Skin Integrity

- Teach client that regular exercise improves circulation and oxygenation of skin.
  Encourage protective clothing and boots when walking in wooded areas.
- Reduce sun exposure.
- Always use sunscreen (SPF 15 or higher) when sun exposure is anticipated.

- Wear long-sleeved shirts and wide-brimmed hats.
- Avoid sunburns.
- Avoid intermittent tanning.
- Understand the link between sun exposure and skin cancer and the accumulating effects of sun exposure on developing cancers.
- Teach skin self-assessment (Appendix 8). If there is anything unusual, seek professional advice as soon as possible.

Nursing Diagnosis: Ineffective Health Maintenance related to lack of hygienic care of skin, hair, and nails, and/or excessive piercing/tattooing performed with "homemade" materials

📖 Assess hair, nail, and skin care, and instruct client on appropriate hygiene measures as necessary (eg, use mild soap, lotion for dry skin; wash oily areas with warm soap and water three times a day).

Teach dangers of hepatitis B and HIV when using contaminated needles.

Nursing Diagnosis: Risk for Impaired Skin Integrity related to prolonged sun exposure

📖 Caution client against prolonged sun exposure or tanning lamp, and instruct that proper use of sunscreen agents can decrease the risk of skin pathologies. Teach client to report a change in the size or appearance of a mole, nodule, pigmented area, new growth on the skin; to limit or avoid sun exposure between 10 AM and 4 PM, when the sun's ultraviolet rays are strongest; to use a sunscreen with a solar protection factor (SPF) of at least 15; to wear protective clothing and hats (American Cancer Society, 2003).

Nursing Diagnosis: Risk for Impaired Nail Integrity related to prolonged use of nail polish

📖 Caution client of potential nail damage caused by prolonged use of nail polish.

Pediatric Client

Nursing Diagnosis: Risk for Impaired Skin Integrity: "diaper rash" related to parental knowledge deficit of skin care for diapered infant or child

- Inform parents of products available for treatment of rash and importance of frequent diaper changes and cleansing of skin with mild soap (eg, Ivory or Dove).

Nursing Diagnosis: Impaired Skin Integrity: related to improper care of acne lesions

- Teach adolescents proper skin cleansing, to avoid squeezing lesions, and the significance of adequate rest, moderate exercise, and balanced diet.

Geriatric Client

Nursing Diagnosis: Risk for Impaired Skin Integrity related to immobility, decreased production of natural oils, and thinning skin

- Teach client and family the benefits of turning of client, range-of-motion (ROM) exercises, massage, and cleaning of skin for reducing risk of skin breakdown. Teach family and client how to observe for reddened pressure areas. Encourage the use of lotions to replace skin oils. Massage skin with lotions. Instruct client to decrease the frequency of baths and use a humidifier during the cold seasons. Explain the effects of proper nutrition and adequate fluids on skin integrity.

Nursing Diagnosis: Risk for Impaired Tissue Integrity related to thickened, dried toenails

- Instruct client to soak nails 15 minutes in warm water prior to cutting. Use good scissors and lighting. Refer to podiatrist as necessary. Ascertain whether shoes fit correctly.

HEAD AND NECK ASSESSMENT

ANATOMY OVERVIEW

The framework of the head is the skull, which can be divided into two subsections, the cranium and the face (Fig. 8–1).

The structure of the neck is composed of muscles, ligaments, and the cervical vertebrae. Contained within the neck are the hyoid bone, several major blood vessels, the larynx, the trachea, and the thyroid gland (Fig. 8–2).

The sternomastoid (sternocleidomastoid) and trapezius muscles are two of the paired muscles that allow movement and provide support to the head and neck (Fig. 8–3).

The thyroid gland is the largest endocrine gland in the body. The first upper tracheal ring, called the cricoid cartilage, has a small notch in it. The thyroid cartilage (Adam's apple) is larger and located just above the cricoid cartilage. The hyoid bone, which is attached to the tongue, lies above the thyroid cartilage and under the mandible (see Fig. 8–2). Several lymph nodes are located in the head and neck (Fig. 8–4).

Equipment Needed

- Clean gloves
- Small cup of water for client during thyroid exam

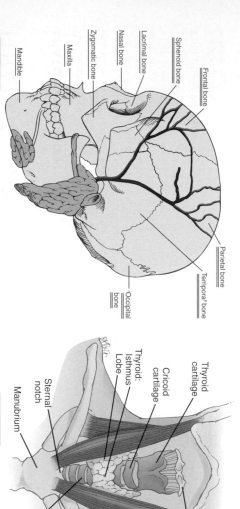

FIGURE 8–1 Bones and sutures of the skull (<u>face</u> and <u>cranium</u>).

Mandible

Maxilla

Zygomatic bone

Lacrimal bone

Nasal bone

Sphenoid bone

Frontal bone

Parietal bone

Temporal bone

Occipital bone

FIGURE 8–2 Structures of the neck.

Thyroid cartilage

Thyroid:
Isthmus
Lobe

Cricoid cartilage

Sternal notch

Manubrium

Trachea

Clavicle

Sternomastoid muscle

Hyoid bone

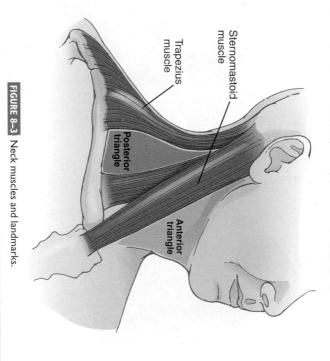

FIGURE 8–3 Neck muscles and landmarks.

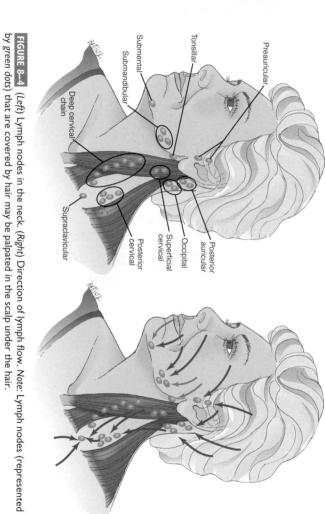

FIGURE 8–4 (*Left*) Lymph nodes in the neck. (*Right*) Direction of lymph flow. *Note:* Lymph nodes (represented by *green dots*) that are covered by hair may be palpated in the scalp under the hair.

Preauricular

Tonsillar

Submental
Submandibular

Deep cervical chain

Supraclavicular

Posterior cervical

Superficial cervical

Occipital

Posterior auricular

Subjective Data: Focus Questions

Lumps (onset, location, size, texture)? Limited movement of neck? Describe. Facial pain/neck pain/headaches (location, onset, duration, precipitating factors, relief)? See Table 8–1 for kinds and characteristics of headaches. Prior neck injuries (date, related to work, recreation, treatment)? Prior radiation therapy to head or neck? Prior thyroid surgery? Family history of head/neck cancer, migraines? Head and neck self-care: posture; use of helmet, seat belts, tobacco products?

Risk Factors. For head injury: high-risk sports, lack of protective devices (eg, seatbelts, helmet), violence, falls (especially after age 65). For thyroid disease: radiation to upper body; family history. For lymphatic enlargement: immunosuppression, chronic disease, malnutrition.

Objective Data: Assessment Techniques

See Figures 8–1 to 8–4 for diagrams of the anatomy of the head, neck, and lymph nodes.

SCALP, FACE, AND NECK INSPECTION AND PALPATION

PROCEDURE	NORMAL FINDINGS	DEVIATIONS FROM NORMAL
Inspect and palpate **scalp** *for the following:*		
• Size	• Varies somewhat	• Extremely large or small. Scalp is thick in acromegaly (increase in growth hormones); large, acorn-shaped in Paget disease.
• Shape	• Symmetrical and round	• Asymmetrical

TABLE 8–1	KINDS AND CHARACTERISTICS OF HEADACHES		
Migraine	**Cluster**	**Tension**	**Tumor Related**
Character			
Accompanied by nausea, vomiting, and sensitivity to noise or light	May be accompanied by tearing, eyelid drooping, reddened eyes, or runny nose	Symptoms of anxiety, tension, and depression may be present	Neurologic and mental symptoms and nausea and vomiting may develop
Onset and Precipitating Factors			
• May have prodromal stage (visual disturbances, vertigo, tinnitus, numbness or tingling of fingers or toes) • Precipitated by emotional disturbances, anxiety, or ingestion of alcohol, cheese, chocolate, or other foods and substances to which client is sensitive	• Sudden onset • May be precipitated by ingesting alcohol	• No prodromal stage • May occur with stress, anxiety, or depression	• No prodromal stage • May be aggravated by coughing, sneezing, or sudden movements of the head
Location			
Located around eyes, temples, cheeks, or forehead	Localized in the eye and orbit and radiating to the facial and temporal	Usually located in the frontal, temporal, or occipital region	Varies with location of tumor

Duration			
Lasts up to 3 days	Typically occurs in the late evening or night	Lasts days, months, or years	Commonly occurs in the morning and lasts for several hours
Severity			
Throbbing, severe, recurring	Intense and stabbing	Dull, aching, tight, diffuse	Aching, steady, variable in intensity
Pattern			
Rest may bring relief	Movement or walking back and forth may relieve the discomfort	Symptomatic relief may be obtained by local heat, massage, analgesics, antidepressants, and muscle relaxants	Headache usually subsides later in the day
Associated Factors			
Migraines occur more often in women	Cluster headaches occur more in young males	Tension headaches affect women more often than men	

SCALP, FACE, AND NECK INSPECTION AND PALPATION (continued)

PROCEDURE	NORMAL FINDINGS	DEVIATIONS FROM NORMAL
• Consistency	• Hard and smooth	• Bumpy or soft. Lumps or lesions are seen in cancer and trauma.
*Observe **face** for the following:*		
• Symmetry	• Symmetrical	• Asymmetrical. Face is asymmetrical with parotid gland enlargement or Bell palsy, mask face in Parkinson disease.
• Facial features	• Features vary	• Distorted features: mask face in Parkinson disease; tightened, hard face in scleroderma; sunken, hollow face in cachexia; swollen face in nephrotic syndrome; moon shape with red cheeks, facial hair in Cushing's syndrome.
	• Symmetrical, centered head position	

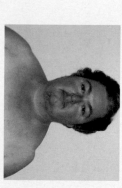

A moon-shaped face with reddened cheeks and increased facial hair may

SCALP, FACE, AND NECK INSPECTION AND PALPATION (continued)

PROCEDURE	NORMAL FINDINGS	DEVIATIONS FROM NORMAL
*Observe **neck** for the following:* • Appearance	• Smooth, controlled movements; range of motion (ROM) from upright position: Flexion = 45° Extension = 55° Lateral abduction = 40° Rotation = 70°	• Asymmetrical head position, masses or scars present. Swelling is seen in cancer, enlarged thyroid, or inflamed lymph nodes.
• Movement		• Rigid, jerky movements; ROM less than normal values; pain on movement. Limited ROM, stiffness, and rigidity are seen with muscle spasms, inflammation, meningitis, cervical arthritis.

TRACHEA, THYROID, AND LYMPH NODE PALPATION

Palpate first the trachea, then the thyroid using the guidelines described in Figure 8–5. After the thyroid, palpate the cervical lymph nodes.

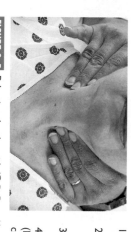

1. Stand behind client and position your hands with thumbs on nape of client's neck.
2. Ask client to flex neck forward and to the right, and use fingers of your left hand to displace thyroid to the right.
3. Palpate the right lobe using your right fingers while client swallows—offer small sips of water.
4. Repeat procedure to examine the left lobe. (Note: Ability to see or palpate the thyroid varies considerably with client thyroid size and body fluid.)

FIGURE 8–5   Palpating the thyroid. (© B. Proud.)

TRACHEA, THYROID, AND LYMPH NODE PALPATION (continued)

PROCEDURE	NORMAL FINDINGS	DEVIATIONS FROM NORMAL
Palpate **trachea** for position and landmarks (tracheal rings, cricoid and thyroid cartilage) (see Fig. 8-2 for location).	Midline position; symmetrical; landmarks identifiable	Asymmetrical. Position deviates from the midline with tumor, enlarged thyroid, aortic aneurysm, pneumothorax, atelectasis, or fibrosis.
Palpate **thyroid** *(see Fig. 8-5) for the following:*		
• Position	• Midline	• Deviates from the midline if obscured by masses or growths
• Characteristics, landmarks	• Smooth, firm, nontender	• Enlarged lobes, irregular consistency, tender on palpation. Diffuse enlargement is seen in hyperthyroidism, Graves disease, or endemic goiter; rapid enlargement of a single nodule suggests malignancy.
Note: Ability to see or palpate the thyroid size varies considerably with client's thyroid size and body build.		
Palpate **cervical lymph nodes** *(see Figure 8-4 for location) for the following:*		
• Size and shape	• Cervical lymph nodes are usually not palpable. If palpable, they should be 1 cm or less and round.	• Enlarged nodes with irregular borders. Enlarged nodes greater than 1 cm are

TRACHEA, THYROID, AND LYMPH NODE PALPATION (continued)

PROCEDURE	NORMAL FINDINGS	DEVIATIONS FROM NORMAL
• Delineation • Mobility • Consistency • Tenderness	• Discrete • Mobile • Soft • Nontender	seen in acute or chronic infection, autoimmune disorders, or metastatic disease; hard, fixed, enlarged, unilateral nodes seen in metastasis; tender, enlarged nodes seen in acute infections; enlarged occipital nodes seen in HIV infection. • Confluent • Fixed to tissue • Hard, firm • Client verbalizes pain on palpation.

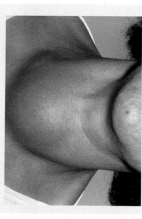

Diffuse enlargement of the thyroid gland.

PEDIATRIC VARIATIONS

PROCEDURE	NORMAL FINDINGS	DEVIATIONS FROM NORMAL
Observe **head shape, size** (see Appendix 7 for head circumference norms), **and symmetry.**	Normocephalic and symmetrical, features appropriate for size. Head may have odd shape due to molding during birth.	Uneven molding, asymmetrical masses, enlarged head. Hydrocephalus is seen with increased cerebrospinal fluid. Microcephaly is a head circumference less than norms.
Observe **head control.**	Holds head erect in midline by 4 months; moves head up and down, side to side	Resistance to movement (head lag after 6 months seen with cerebral injury)
Palpate **skull and fontanelles** very gently when infant is quiet in sitting position.	Smooth, fused except for fontanelles	Ecchymotic areas on scalp; loss of hair in spots; posterior fontanelle (triangular) open after 2 months of age; anterior fontanelle open after 12–18 months of age. Bulging fontanelle is seen in increased intracranial pressure; depressed fontanelles seen in dehydration or malnutrition; delayed fusion of fontanelles seen with hydrocephalus, Down syndrome, hypothyroidism, or rickets; third fontanel seen in Down syndrome; limited ROM seen in torticollis (wryneck).

PEDIATRIC VARIATIONS (continued)

PROCEDURE	NORMAL FINDINGS	DEVIATIONS FROM NORMAL
Palpate **neck** for lymph nodes.	Moderate number of small (> 3 mm), shotty, firm lymph nodes in child (age 3–12 years)	Diffuse large lymph nodes, asymmetrical placement. Enlarging supraclavicular lymph nodes are seen with Hodgkin disease.

GERIATRIC VARIATIONS

- Bones of face and nose are more angular in appearance.
- Muscle atrophy and loss of fat cause shortening of neck.

Possible Collaborative Problems

Lymphedema
Hypercalcemia
Hypocalcemia

TEACHING TIPS FOR SELECTED NURSING DIAGNOSES

Adult Client

Nursing Diagnosis: Risk for Injury to Head and Neck related to poor posture

 Teach correct posture and body mechanics for sitting, lifting, and pushing.

Nursing Diagnosis: Risk for Injury to **Head and Neck** related to not wearing protective devices (eg, head gear during contact sports, seat belts, eye goggles).

👉 Teach risk reduction tips:

- Use safe driving techniques.
- Wear protective gear such as helmets and seat belts, especially when riding a bicycle or motorcycle.
- Avoid violent or potentially violent environments when possible.
- Modify one's residence to prevent falls.
- Avoid dangerous contact sports likely to cause brain injury; wear protective equipment when engaging in such activity.

Pediatric and Adolescent Clients

Nursing Diagnosis: Risk for Injury related to open fontanelles

👉 Teach parents normal development of fontanelles and how to protect infants from pressure and injury.

Nursing Diagnosis: Ineffective Health Maintenance related to a knowledge deficit on the effects of smokeless tobacco

👉 Teach that "dipping snuff" is highly addictive and increases the risk of cheek and gum cancer nearly 50-fold among long-term snuff users. Explain that this is *not* a healthy substitute for smoking cigarettes (American Cancer Society, 2000).

Nursing Diagnosis: Risk for Injury to **Teeth and Oral Mucous Membrane** related to tongue piercing and wearing metal balls

👉 Teach risks of teeth chipping and hepatitis B and HIV virus when done with contaminated needles.

EYE ASSESSMENT

ANATOMY OVERVIEW

External Structures of the Eye

The *eyelids* (upper and lower) are two movable structures composed of skin and two types of muscle—striated and smooth (Fig. 9–1). The palpebral conjunctiva lines the inside of the eyelids, and the bulbar conjunctiva covers most of the anterior eye, merging with the cornea at the limbus.

The *lacrimal apparatus* consists of glands and ducts that serve to lubricate the eye (Fig. 9–2). The *lacrimal gland*, located in the upper outer corner of the orbital cavity just above the eye, is responsible for tear production. Tears are channeled into the *nasolacrimal sac*, through the *nasolacrimal duct*, into the nasal meatus.

The *extraocular muscles* are the six muscles attached to the outer surface of each eyeball (Fig. 9–3).

Internal Structures of the Eye

The eyeball is composed of three separate coats or layers (Fig. 9–4). The outermost layer consists of the *sclera* and *cornea*. The *iris* is a circular disc of muscle that contains pigments that determine eye color. The central aperture of the iris is called the pupil.

The *lens* is a biconvex, transparent, avascular, encapsulated structure located immediately posterior to the iris. The innermost layer, the *retina*, extends only to the ciliary body anteriorly and consists of numerous layers of nerve cells, including the cells commonly called rods and cones.

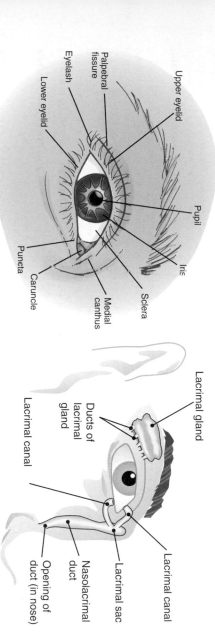

FIGURE 9–1 External structures of the eye.

Upper eyelid

Palpebral fissure

Eyelash

Lower eyelid

Puncta

Caruncle

Medial canthus

Sclera

Iris

Pupil

FIGURE 9–2 The lacrimal apparatus consists of tear (lacrimal) glands and ducts.

Lacrimal gland

Ducts of lacrimal gland

Lacrimal canal

Lacrimal sac

Nasolacrimal duct

Lacrimal canal

Opening of duct (in nose)

Eye Assessment

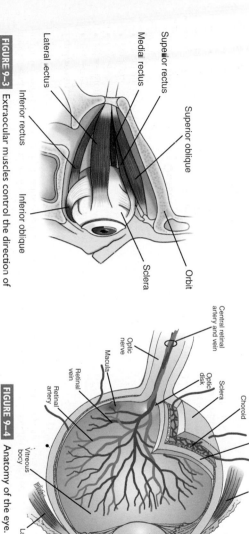

FIGURE 9-3 Extraocular muscles control the direction of eye movement.

- Lateral rectus
- Media rectus
- Superior rectus
- Inferior rectus
- Superior oblique
- Inferior oblique
- Orbit
- Sclera

FIGURE 9-4 Anatomy of the eye.

- Central retinal artery and vein
- Optic nerve
- Macula
- Retinal vein
- Retinal artery
- Vitreous body
- Optic disk
- Sclera
- Choroid
- Retina
- Medial rectus muscle
- Conjunctiva
- Lens
- Pupil
- Anterior chamber
- Iris muscle
- Cornea
- Ciliary muscle
- Lateral rectus muscle

The *optic disc* is a cream-colored, circular area located on the retina toward the medial or nasal side of the eye (Fig. 9–5). A small circular area that appears slightly depressed is referred to as the *physiologic cup*.

The *retinal vessels* can be readily viewed with the aid of an ophthalmoscope. Four sets of *arterioles* and *venules* travel through the optic disc, bifurcate, and extend to the periphery of the fundus. Vessels are dark red and grow progressively narrower as they extend out to the peripheral areas. A retinal depression known as the fovea centralis is located adjacent to the optic disc in the temporal section of the fundus (see Fig. 9–5). This area is surrounded by the macula, which appears darker than the rest of the fundus.

Equipment Needed

- Eye chart (Snellen or handheld Rosenbaum)
- Near-vision chart or newsprint
- Cover card or occluder
- Penlight
- Ophthalmoscope
- Ruler

Subjective Data: Focus Questions

Recent changes in vision? (Spots? Floaters? Blind spots? Halos? Rings? Difficulty with night vision? Double vision? Blurred vision? Strabismus?) Eye pain? Redness or swelling? Eye discharge? Excessive watering or tearing? History of prior eye surgery? Trauma? Use of corrective glasses or contact lenses? Date of last eye exam? Eye care habits? (Use of sunglasses? Safety glasses? Work around chemicals, sparks, smokes, fumes, or dust?) Have visual changes affected work or ability to care for self?

Risk Factors. Risk for glaucoma related to diabetes mellitus, myopia, age older than 75 years, or family history of glaucoma. Risk for cataracts related to increasing age, ultraviolet light exposure, diabetes mellitus, smoking, alcohol use, diet low in antioxidant vitamins.

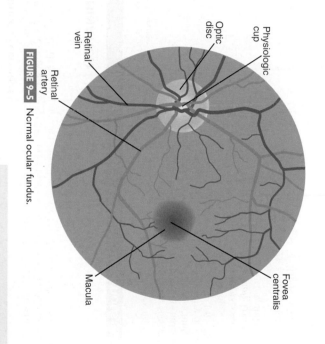

FIGURE 9-5 Normal ocular fundus.

Physiologic cup

Optic disc

Retinal vein

Retinal artery

Macula

Fovea centralis

Objective Data: Assessment Techniques

Review Figures 9–1 through 9–5 for diagrams of the anatomy of the internal and external eye structures.

Client should be seated comfortably in a well-lighted room that can be darkened for ophthalmic examination. First, the external eye structures are examined. Then eye function is tested, followed by the ophthalmic examination, using the following guidelines:

EXTERNAL EYE EXAMINATION

PROCEDURE	NORMAL FINDINGS	DEVIATIONS FROM NORMAL
Inspect eyelids and lashes (see Figure 9-1) for the following:		
• Position and appearance	• Lid margins moist and pink; lashes short, evenly spaced, and curled outward; lower margins at bottom edge of iris; upper margins of lid cover approximately 2 mm of iris	• Crusting; scales; lashes absent or curled inward; edema or xanthelasma present; itching; ulcerative lesions; asymmetry of lids; weak muscles
		See Box 9–1 for illustrations of the following:
		Ectropion: Lower lids turn outward.
		Entropion: Lower lids turn inward.
		Chalazion: Inflammation of meibomian glands
		Hordeolum: Stye or inflammation of glands in lid

BOX 9–1 • External Eye Examination: Deviations from Normal

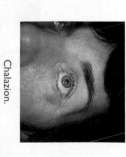

Ectropion.

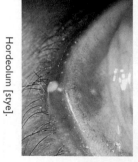

Entropion.

Chalazion.

Hordeolum [stye].

BOX 9-1 • (continued)

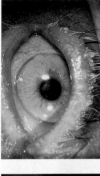

Blepharitis.

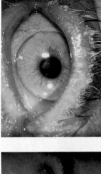

Ptosis.

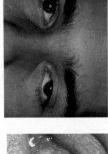

Conjunctivitis. (© 1995
Dr. P. Marazzi/Science Photo
Library/CMSP.)

BOX 9-1 • (continued)

Miosis.

Anisocoria.

Mydriasis.

PROCEDURE	NORMAL FINDINGS	DEVIATIONS FROM NORMAL
• Blinking	• Blinking symmetrical, involuntary, at approximately 15 blinks/min	*Blepharitis:* Waxy white scales (seborrheic) or inflammation of hair follicles (*Staphylococcus*)
		Ptosis: Drooping of lids; seen with oculomotor nerve damage, myasthenia gravis. Protrusion of eyeballs with retracted lids seen with hyperthyroidism
		• Asymmetrical blink, incomplete closure, rapid blinking
Inspect **conjunctiva** (bulbar and palpebral) and **sclera** for clarity and appearance by separating lids with thumb and index finger and asking the client to look up, down, and to either side.	Bulbar conjunctiva is clear with tiny vessels visible; palpebral conjunctiva is pink with no discharge; sclera is blue-white	Lesions, nodules, discharge, crusting, foreign body present. Marked redness of the conjunctiva is seen with conjunctivitis (see Box 9–1). Sclera with petechiae; marked jaundice
Inspect **cornea** (using oblique lighting) for appearance.	Transparent, smooth, moist	Lesions, opacities, irregular light reflections, or foreign body present. Rough or dry cornea is seen with trauma or allergic responses.

PROCEDURE	NORMAL FINDINGS	DEVIATIONS FROM NORMAL
Inspect **iris and pupil** for the following:		
• Shape	• Round	• Irregular. Miosis is constricted, fixed pupils; mydriasis (see Box 9–1).
• Equality	• Equal	• Unequal; anisocoria is abnormal when difference in pupil size becomes greater during pupillary reaction tests (see Box 9–1).
Inspect **lens** for clarity.		
• Color (iris)	• Uniform color	• Inconsistent color
	• Clear	Cloudy; opacities are seen with cataracts (see page 158).
Inspect and palpate **lacrimal apparatus** (see Fig. 9–2) for the following:		
• Appearance	• Puncta (small elevations on the nasal side of the upper and lower lids), mucosa pink	• Puncta markedly reddened and edematous with infection, blockage, or inflammation
• Response to pressure applied at nasal side of lower orbital rim	• No tenderness or discharge noted when pressure is applied	• Fluid or purulent discharge expressed with pain on palpation with duct blockage

EYE FUNCTION TESTING

PROCEDURE	NORMAL FINDINGS	DEVIATIONS FROM NORMAL
Check **visual acuity:**		
• Check distance vision with Snellen chart 20 feet from client. 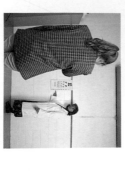	• 20/20 OD and OS with no hesitation, frowning, or squinting	• Any letters missed on 20/20 line or above; client reads chart by leaning forward, with head tilted, or squinting. *Myopia*, impaired far vision, occurs when second number is larger than first number (eg, 20/40).
• Check near vision with newspaper approximately 14 inches from client's head	• Client reads print at 14 inches without difficulty.	• Client reads print by holding it closer or farther away than 14 inches. *Presbyopia*, impaired near vision, is seen when client moves reading material farther away to read owing to decreased accommodation of lenses.

PROCEDURE	NORMAL FINDINGS	DEVIATIONS FROM NORMAL
Check **peripheral vision:** Face client at a distance of 2–3 feet; client and examiner look directly ahead and cover eye directly opposite each other.	Client and examiner report seeing object at the same time as it approaches from the periphery.	With reduced peripheral vision, client does not report seeing object at the same time as the examiner.
Check **accommodation.** (Fig. 9–6): Ask client to stare at an object 3–4 feet away, and move object in toward client's nose.	Pupils converge and constrict as object moves in toward the nose; pupil responses are uniform.	Pupils do not converge or constrict. Pupil responses are unequal.

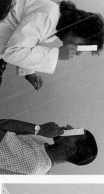

Checking peripheral vision. (© B. Proud.)

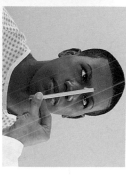

FIGURE 9–6 Testing accommodation of pupils. (© B. Proud.)

EYE FUNCTION TESTING (continued)

PROCEDURE

Check **extraocular movements** (Fig. 9–7): Ask client to follow object as it is moved in six cardinal fields.

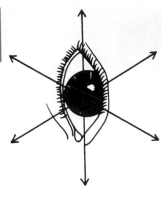

FIGURE 9–7 Six cardinal fields for checking extraocular movements.

NORMAL FINDINGS

Both eyes move in a smooth, coordinated manner in all directions.

DEVIATIONS FROM NORMAL

Jerky eye movements (nystagmus) are seen with inner ear disorders, multiple sclerosis, brain lesions, or narcotics use; failure to follow object with one or both eyes indicates muscle weakness or cranial nerve dysfunction.

EYE FUNCTION TESTING (continued)

PROCEDURE	NORMAL FINDINGS	DEVIATIONS FROM NORMAL
Check response to light:		
• Check corneal light reflex by asking client to look straight ahead and then shining light toward facial midline.	• Reflections of light noted at same location on both eyes.	• Light reflections noted at different areas on both eyes occur with deviation in alignment of eyes due to muscle weakness or paralysis.
• Check direct pupil response by asking client to look straight ahead and approaching each eye from the client's side with a penlight.	• Illuminated pupils constrict.	• Illuminated pupils fail to constrict.
• Check consensual pupil response by asking client to look straight ahead and approaching each eye from the client's side with a penlight.	• Pupil opposite the one illuminated constricts simultaneously.	• Pupil opposite the one illuminated fails to constrict; monocular blindness is seen when light directed to blind eye results in no response in either pupil.
Check for **abnormal eye movement** using cover-uncover test (Fig. 9–8):		
Ask client to look straight ahead, covering one eye with a cover card, and observe uncovered eye for movement.	Uncovered eye does not move as opposite eye is covered. Covered eye does not move as cover is removed.	Uncovered eye moves to focus when opposite eye is covered. Covered eye moves to focus when cover is removed. These findings are seen with eye muscle weakness and deviation in alignment of eyes. *Esotropia* is turning in of eyes, *exotropia* is turning outward of eyes, and *strabismus* is constant malalignment of eyes.

PROCEDURE	NORMAL FINDINGS	DEVIATIONS FROM NORMAL

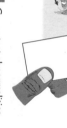

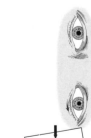

Strabismus (or tropia).

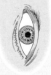

FIGURE 9–8 Cover test abnormalities.

Ophthalmic Examination

Use ophthalmoscope according to the following guidelines:

Guidelines for Using the Ophthalmoscope

The examiner can rotate the lenses that are labeled with a negative or positive number. Red numbers indicate a negative diopter and are used for myopic (nearsighted) clients. Black numbers indicate a positive diopter and are used for hyperopic (farsighted) clients. The zero lens is used if neither the examiner nor the client has a refractive error.

1. Turn ophthalmoscope on and select the aperture with the large, round beam of white light.

2. Ask the client to remove glasses. Remove your glasses. Contact lenses can be left in the eyes of the client or examiner.

3. Ask the client to fix gaze on an object that is straight ahead and slightly upward.

4. Darken the room to allow pupils to dilate.

5. Hold the ophthalmoscope in your right hand with your index finger on the lens wheel and place the instrument to your right eye (braced between the eyebrow and nose). Examine the client's right eye. Use your left hand and left eye to examine the client's left eye.

6. Begin about 10–15 inches from the client at a 15° angle to the client's side.

7. Keep focused on the red reflex as you move in closer, and then rotate the diopter setting to see the optic disc.

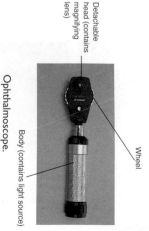

Ophthalmoscope.

Detachable head (contains magnifying lens)

Wheel

Body (contains light source)

Ophthalmic Examination (continued)

PROCEDURE	NORMAL FINDINGS	DEVIATIONS FROM NORMAL
Inspect **red reflex** for shape and color.	Red reflex is round, bright, with red-orange glow	Red reflex has decreased color or abnormal shape; dark spots are seen with cataracts.

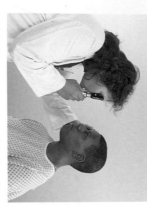

Inspecting the red reflex. (© B. Proud.)

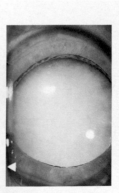

Nuclear cataracts appear gray when seen with a flashlight; they appear as a black spot against the red reflex when seen through an ophthalmoscope.

Ophthalmic Examination (continued)

*Inspect **optic disc** (see Fig. 9–5)
for the following:*
- Shape

PROCEDURE	NORMAL FINDINGS	DEVIATIONS FROM NORMAL
	Round or slightly oval disc with sharply defined margins	Irregularly shaped disc, blurred margins. A swollen disc with blurred margins is papilledema and is seen with hypertension or increased intracranial pressure. Optic atrophy is a white-colored disc without vessels and is seen with the death of optic nerves.

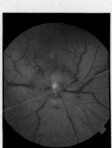

Papilledema.

Ophthalmic Examination *(continued)*

PROCEDURE	NORMAL FINDINGS	DEVIATIONS FROM NORMAL
• Color	• Creamy pink (lighter than retina)	• Pallor of entire disc or one section
• Size	• Approximately 1.5 mm size, symmetrical in both eyes	• Size of disc not equal in both eyes
• Physiologic cup	• Small area is noted as paler than disc located just temporal of center of disc; occupies $\frac{4}{10}$ to $\frac{5}{10}$ of the diameter of the disc.	• Cup location and size are not symmetrical in both eyes; cup occupies more than $\frac{5}{10}$ diameter of the disc.
Inspect **retinal vessels** *for the following:*		
• Appearance	*Arteries:* Light red and smaller than veins	• Arteries less than $\frac{2}{3}$ size of veins; arteries pale
	Veins: Darker in color and larger than arteries	• Arterioles widen and have copper color in hypertension; with long-standing hypertension arterioles have silver color.
• Distribution	• Vessels regular in shape and decreasing in size as they branch and move toward the periphery; crossing of arteries and veins show no changes in the diameter of the underlying vessel.	• Vessels irregular in shape and uneven in distribution; narrowing of underlying vessels at crossings of arteries and veins; abnormal arteriole venous crossings are seen with hypertension and arteriosclerosis.
Inspect **retinal background** *for appearance*	Fine texture with pink, uniform color	Pallor of the fundus; soft or hard exudates (cotton-wool patches) seen in

Ophthalmic Examination (continued)

PROCEDURE	NORMAL FINDINGS	DEVIATIONS FROM NORMAL
Inspect **macula** for appearance.	Darker than remainder of retina; fovea seen as a tiny bright light in the center of macula	hypertension and diabetes; red spots or streaks may be microaneurysms or hemorrhages. Abnormalities in color or vessels; lesions present. Clumped pigment is seen with detached retinas or injuries.

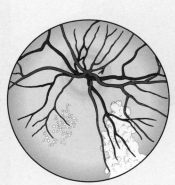

Exudates.

Eye Assessment

DEVIATIONS FROM NORMAL

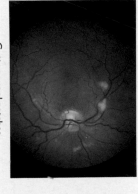

Cotton-wool patches.

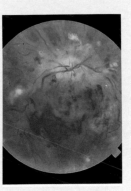

Retinal hemorrhages.

PEDIATRIC VARIATIONS

Objective Data: Assessment Techniques

Explain procedure to decrease child's fear when room is darkened.

PROCEDURE	NORMAL FINDINGS	DEVIATIONS FROM NORMAL
Inspect **placement of light** on cornea.	Light falls symmetrically within each pupil.	Asymmetrical location of light reflection on pupil signals strabismus.
Observe **placement and alignment of eyes** *by doing the following:* • Measure inner canthal distance.	• Average distance 3 cm (1.2 inches)	• Wide-set eyes, upward slant, and thick epicanthal folds may suggest Down syndrome.
• Assess palpebral slant.	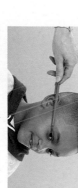 • Outer canthus aligns with tips of pinna (except in Asian children). Outer canthus is in alignment with the tip of the pinna. (© B. Proud.)	• Presence of upward slant in non-Asians • Upper lid that lies above iris ("setting-sun" sign) suggests hydrocephalus. Black and white speckling of iris (Brush-field spots) seen in Down syndrome

Eye Assessment

PROCEDURE	NORMAL FINDINGS	DEVIATIONS FROM NORMAL
• Observe placement of lids.	• With eye open, lids lie between upper iris and pupil.	
Inspect **iris.**	Color varies from brown to green to blue.	
Inspect **lacrimal apparatus.**	Lacrimal meatus not present until 3 months of age	
Perform **visual acuity tests.** Use E chart for preschoolers.	Children can differentiate colors by age 5 years.	A one-line difference indicates visual impairment and should be referred; may be due to congenital defects, chronic disease, or refractive errors.

GERIATRIC VARIATIONS

External eye examination reveals the following:

• Conjunctiva thins and becomes yellowish.
• White ring around iris (arcus senilis)—does not affect vision
• Dry eyes due to decreased tear production
• Drooping eyelids (senile ptosis)
• Entropion and ectropion common in the older adult
• Clouding of lens (cataracts)
• Yellowish nodules on bulbar conjunctiva (pinguecula) common

Visual examination reveals the following:

• Presbyopia (decreased near vision due to decreased elasticity of lens) common in clients older than 45 years
• Slowed pupillary response and slowed accommodation
• Poorer night vision and decreased tolerance to glare

Visual field examination reveals the following:

• Decreased peripheral vision
• Difficulty differentiating blues from greens

Funduscopic examination reveals the following:

• Pale, narrowed arterioles

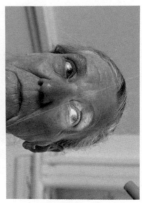

Observe the pupils. With a penlight or similar device, test pupillary reaction to light.
(© B. Proud.)

CULTURAL VARIATIONS

- Asians and members of some other groups may have common variation of epicanthal folds or narrowed palpebral fissures.
- Dark-skinned clients may have sclera with yellow or pigmented freckles.

Possible Collaborative Problems

Visual changes   Glaucoma
Eye infections   Impaired functioning of lacrimal apparatus
Cataracts   Corneal abrasions

TEACHING TIPS FOR SELECTED NURSING DIAGNOSES

Adult Client

 Nursing Diagnosis: Ineffective Health Maintenance related to lack of knowledge of necessity for eye examinations
Recommend the following guidelines for frequency of eye evaluations for adults without risk factors:

Age (years)	Frequency of Evaluation
65 or older	Every 1–2 years
55–64	Every 1–3 years
40–54	Every 2–4 years
Under 40	5–10 years

Interim eye evaluations, consisting of vision examinations (refractions, spectacles, contact lens evaluations, etc.), may be performed during these periods as well. Patients with risk factors for disease or symptoms and signs of eye disease, and patients who desire an examination, may have additional evaluations during these periods. (Reprinted with permission from the American Academy of Ophthalmology. [2005]. *Comprehensive adult eye evaluation, preferred practice patterns*. San Francisco.)

? Table 9–1 for guidelines for patients with risk factors.

Condition/Risk Factor	Frequency of Evaluation*	
Diabetes Mellitus	Recommended Time of First Examination	Recommended Follow-up*
Type 1	5 years after onset	Yearly
Type 2	At time of diagnosis	Yearly
Prior to pregnancy (Type 1 or 2)	Prior to conception or early in the first trimester	No retinopathy to mild or moderate NPDR: every 3–12 months. Severe NPDR or worse: every 1–3 months.

Condition/Risk Factor	Frequency of Evaluation*
Risk factors for glaucoma (eg, elevated IOP, family history of glaucoma, African or Hispanic/Latino descent)	
Age 65 or older	Every 6–12 months
Age 55–64	Every 1–2 years
Age 40–54	Every 1–3 years
Under 40	Every 2–4 years

*Abnormal findings may dictate more frequent follow-up examinations.
IOP, intraocular pressure; NPDP, nonproliferative diabetic retinopathy.
(Reprinted with permission from the American Academy of Ophthalmology. [2005]. *Comprehensive adult medical eye evaluation, preferred practice patterns.* San Francisco.)

Nursing Diagnosis: Ineffective Health Maintenance related to inadequate knowledge of eye infection care

Instruct client on proper administration of eye drops and ointments. Discuss proper cleansing from inner to outer canthus and changing of cleansing cloth to prevent cross-contamination (from eye to eye).

Pediatric Client

Nursing Diagnosis: Readiness for Enhanced Knowledge of Eye Care During the Growing Years

Teach parents the following schedule for eye exams:

In the newborn nursery: Pediatricians or family physicians should examine all high-risk infants.

By age 6 months: Pediatricians, family physicians, or ophthalmologists should screen all infants.

At age 3 years: Pediatricians, family physicians, or ophthalmologists should examine all children. Focus should be on visual acuity.

At age 5 years: Pediatricians, family physicians, or ophthalmologists should evaluate vision and alignment. Further screening should be done at routine school checks or after the appearance of symptoms.

(Reprinted from American Academy of Ophthalmology. [2002]. *Pediatric eye evaluations [preferred practice pattern].* San Francisco.)

Geriatric Client

Nursing Diagnosis: Ineffective Protection related to decreased tear production secondary to the aging process

Instruct client on the use of artificial tears as necessary.

Nursing Diagnosis: Ineffective Protection related to impaired vision secondary to the aging process

Explore with client aids for independent living (eg, magnifying glasses, cane). Encourage further evaluation if necessary. Instruct family to keep furniture in same place and to provide better lighting. Provide community resources (eg, "talking" books and magazines available in libraries).

Adults age 65 years or older with no risk factors should have an ophthalmologic eye examination every 1–2 years. To promote this goal, the National Eye Care Project is a nationwide outreach program sponsored by the American

Academy of Ophthalmology as a public service. It is designed to help the disadvantaged elderly obtain medical eye care. The toll-free phone number is 1-800-222-EYES. To be eligible, a person must be a U.S. citizen or legal resident, age 65 years or older, who does not have access to an ophthalmologist he or she may have seen in the past.

Clients should wear sunglasses and hats in the sun. This is important because even on bright cloudy days, ultraviolet light can penetrate clouds. Squinting does not eliminate ultraviolet light entering the eye.

Adults with diabetes mellitus should have an ophthalmologic eye examination at the time of diagnosis and yearly thereafter. Abnormal findings may require more frequent examinations.

Following are eye disorders commonly seen in older clients. Discuss symptoms of each with the client.

- Presbyopia (difficulty reading printed material)
- Floaters (moving specks or clouded vision)
- Cataracts (painless blurring of vision, glare or light sensitivity, poor night vision, double vision in one eye, needing brighter light to read, fading or yellowing of colors)
- Glaucoma (Symptoms of glaucoma are not noticeable until damage has already occurred. Early diagnosis and treatment are keys to preventing blindness.)
- Macular degeneration (words on a page look blurred in the center; straight lines look distorted, especially toward the center; a dark or empty area appears in the center of vision; colors look dim)

(Source: American Academy of Ophthalmology. [2003]. *Seeing well as you grow older: a closer look.* San Francisco.)

EAR ASSESSMENT

ANATOMY OVERVIEW

The external ear is composed of the auricle or pinna and the external auditory canal (Fig. 10–1). A translucent, pearly gray, concave membrane, the tympanic membrane, or eardrum, serves as a partition stretched across the inner end of the auditory canal, separating it from the middle ear. The distinct landmarks (Fig. 10–2) of the tympanic membrane include:

- Handle and short process of the malleus
- Umbo
- Cone of light
- Pars flaccida
- Pars tensa

The middle ear, or tympanic cavity, is a small, air-filled chamber in the temporal bone. It is separated from the external ear by the eardrum and from the inner ear by a bony partition containing two openings, the round and oval windows. The middle ear contains three auditory ossicles: the malleus, the incus, and the stapes (see Fig. 10–1).

The inner ear, or labyrinth, is fluid filled and is made up of the bony labyrinth and an inner membranous labyrinth. The bony labyrinth has three parts: the cochlea, the vestibule, and the semicircular canals.

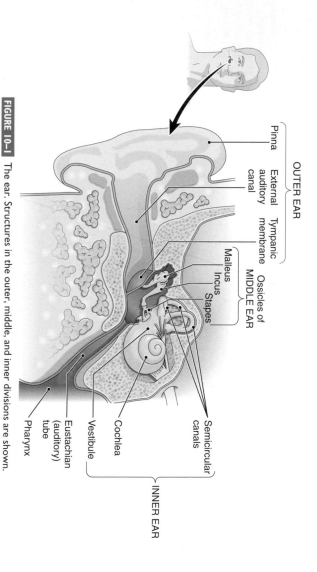

10

FIGURE 10–1 The ear. Structures in the outer, middle, and inner divisions are shown.

OUTER EAR

Pinna

External auditory canal

Tympanic membrane

Ossicles of MIDDLE EAR

Malleus

Incus

Stapes

Semicircular canals

Cochlea

Vestibule

Eustachian (auditory) tube

Pharynx

INNER EAR

Ear Assessment

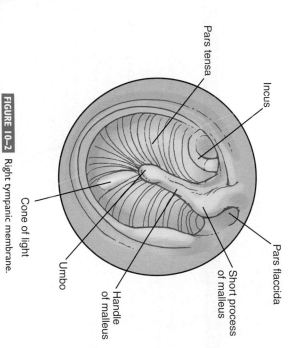

FIGURE 10–2 Right tympanic membrane.

Pars tensa

Incus

Pars flaccida

Short process
of malleus

Handle
of malleus

Umbo

Cone of light

Equipment Needed

- Otoscope with good batteries (pneumatic bulb device for young children)
- Tuning fork (512 and 1024 Hz)

Subjective Data: Focus Questions

Recent changes in hearing? All or some sounds affected? Ear drainage? Type? Ear pain? Occurrence? Relief? Associated factors such as sore throat, sinus infection, or gum/teeth problems? Ringing or cracking in ears (tinnitus)? Dizziness, unbalanced or spinning (vertigo)? History of prior ear surgery? Trauma? Use of ototoxic medications? Last hearing examination?

Risk Factors. Risk for hearing loss related to genetic predisposition, congenital anomalies, otitis media, fluid in inner ear, loud noises, ototoxic medications, aging (presbycusis), trauma to eardrum, otosclerosis, viral inner ear infections, impacted cerumen.

Objective Data: Assessment Techniques

Review Figures 10–1 to 10–2 for the anatomy of the external, middle, and inner ear.

Client should be comfortably seated in such a way that you can easily visualize both ears. First examine the external ear, then examine the ear canal and tympanic membrane with the otoscope, and finally assess hearing function.

PROCEDURE	NORMAL FINDINGS	DEVIATIONS FROM NORMAL
Inspect **external ear** (Fig. 10–3) *for the following:*		
• Size and shape	• Ears of equal size and similar appearance	• Ears of unequal size or configuration (smaller than 4 cm or larger than 10 cm)

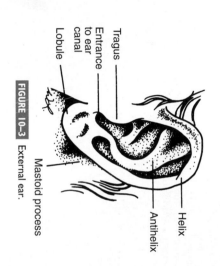

FIGURE 10-3 External ear.

Tragus

Entrance
to ear
canal

Lobule

Mastoid process

Antihelix

Helix

ANATOMY OVERVIEW (continued)

PROCEDURE	NORMAL FINDINGS	DEVIATIONS FROM NORMAL
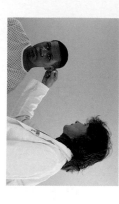 Inspecting the external ear. (© B. Proud.)		
• Position	• Alignment of pinna with corner of eye and within 10° angle of vertical position	• Pinna positioned below a line from corner of eye, or unequal alignment. Malaligned or low-set ears are seen with chromosomal defects or genitourinary disorders.
• Lesions and discolorations	• Skin smooth and without nodules; color pink	• Erythema, edema, nodules, or areas of discoloration. Postauricular cysts are seen with blocked sebaceous glands;

PROCEDURE	NORMAL FINDINGS	DEVIATIONS FROM NORMAL
Palpate **external ear** (see Fig. 10–3).	Nontender auricle, tragus	ulcerated crusted nodules may be malignant; pale-blue color seen in frostbite. Painful auricle or tragus associated with otitis externa or postauricular cyst. Tenderness behind ear is associated with otitis media.
*Palpate **mastoid process** for the following:* • Tenderness • Temperature • Edema	• No tenderness or pain when palpated • Warm • Mastoid process easily palpated	• Pain on palpation of mastoid process with mastoiditis • Erythema • Actual process difficult to palpate; ear displaced outward owing to edema
*Inspect **auditory canal** using otoscope (Fig. 10–4) for the following:* • Cerumen	• *Color:* Black, dark red, gray, or brown *Consistency:* Waxy, flaky, soft or hard *Odor:* None	• Impacted cerumen (obstructs visualization of membrane); bloody purulent discharge is seen in otitis media with perforated eardrum; foul-smelling discharge associated with otitis externa or impacted foreign body

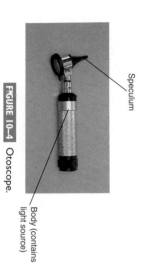

FIGURE 10—4 Otoscope.

Speculum

Body (contains light source)

PROCEDURE	NORMAL FINDINGS	DEVIATIONS FROM NORMAL
• Appearance	• Canal walls pink and uniform with tympanic membrane (TM) visible	• Lesions, foreign body, erythema, or edema present in canal. Red, swollen canals are seen with otitis media; polyps (Box 10–2) or nonmalignant nodular swellings can block the view of the eardrum.

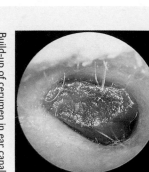

Build-up of cerumen in ear canal.

ANATOMY OVERVIEW (continued)

PROCEDURE

- Tenderness

*Inspect **tympanic membrane**, using otoscope (Box 10–1), for the following:*

- Color

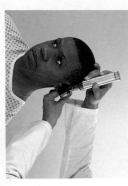

Inspecting the external canal and tympanic membrane. (© B. Proud.)

NORMAL FINDINGS

- Little or no discomfort on manipulation of pinna; inner two thirds of canal very tender if touched with speculum

- Pearly gray, shiny, and translucent

DEVIATIONS FROM NORMAL

- Moderate to severe pain when pinna is moved or otoscope speculum is inserted

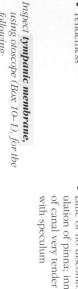

- Dull appearance: blue (blood) or pink/red (inflammation). Red, bulging TM is seen with acute otitis media (see Box 10–2); yellow bulging TM seen with serous otitis media; blue or dark color seen in trauma when there is blood behind the TM.

BOX 10-1 • Using Otoscope to Inspect Tympanic Membrane

1. Ask clients to sit comfortably with the back straight and the head tilted slightly away from you toward their opposite shoulder.

2. Choose the largest speculum that fits comfortably into the ear canal (usually 5 mm in the adult) and attach it to the otoscope. Hold otoscope in your dominant hand and turn the otoscope light to "on."

3. Use thumb and fingers of your opposite hand to grasp client's auricle firmly but gently. Pull out, up, and back to straighten the external auditory canal. Do not alter this position during the exam.

4. Grasp the otoscope handle between your thumb and fingers. Hold otoscope up or down, whichever is comfortable for you.

5. Steady your hand holding the otoscope against the client's head or face.

6. Insert the speculum gently down and forward into the ear canal (approximately 0.5 inch). Be careful not to touch the inner portion of the sensitive canal wall.

7. Position your eye against the lens.

Ear Assessment

BOX 10-2 • Ear Assessment: Deviations from Normal

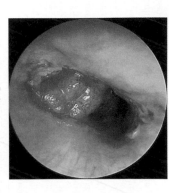

Polyp.

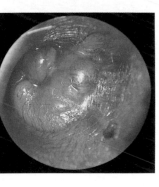

Acute otitis media.

BOX 10-2 • (continued)

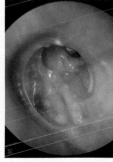

Perforated tympanic membrane.
(© 1992 Science Photo
Library/CMSP.)

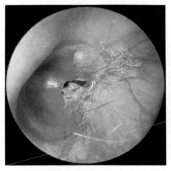

Scarred tympanic membrane.

PROCEDURE	NORMAL FINDINGS	DEVIATIONS FROM NORMAL
• Consistency	• Intact; may show movement when swallowing	• *Perforations, scarring* (see Box 10–2), or immobility. White spots are seen with scarring of the TM.
• Landmarks (see Fig. 10–2)	• Cone of light, umbo, handle of malleus, and short process of malleus easily visualized	• Retracted TM accentuates landmarks; bulging TM partially occludes land-marks. Prominent landmarks indicate TM retraction due to negative pressure from obstructed eustachian tube, whereas obscured landmarks indicate thickened TM due to chronic otitis media.
*Assess **auditory function** for the following:*		
• Gross hearing ability: Whisper words 1–2 feet behind client; hold watch 1–2 inches from client's ear.	• Client is able to hear whispered words from 1–2 feet; able to hear watch tick from 1–2 inches.	• Client is unable to hear whispered words or watch tick; unequal response.
• Lateralization of sound—Weber test: Place activated tuning fork on center top of client's head (Fig. 10–5A).	• Vibration heard equally in both ears	• Vibratory sound lateralized to poor ear in conductive loss and to good ear in sensorineural loss.

ANATOMY OVERVIEW (continued)

PROCEDURE	NORMAL FINDINGS	DEVIATIONS FROM NORMAL
• Comparison of air conduction (AC) to bone conduction (BC)—Rinne test: Place tuning fork on mastoid process until no longer heard, and then move it to front of ear (Fig. 10–5B, C).	• AC > BC (AC is twice as long as BC)	• BC ≥ AC: BC heard longer than or equal to AC in conductive loss; AC longer than, but not twice as long as, BC in sensorineural loss

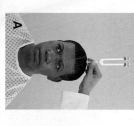
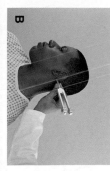
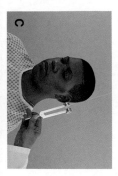

FIGURE 10–5 Using a tuning fork to assess auditory function. (A) Weber test. (B) Rinne test: bone conduction. (C) Rinne test: air conduction. (© B. Proud.)

PROCEDURE	NORMAL FINDINGS	DEVIATIONS FROM NORMAL
Perform **Romberg test for equilibrium** by having client stand with feet together first with eyes open, then with eyes closed (put your arms around client to prevent fall).	Client stands straight with minimal swaying.	Client sways and moves feet apart to prevent fall—may indicate vestibular disorder.

PEDIATRIC VARIATIONS

Objective Data: Assessment Techniques

PROCEDURE	NORMAL FINDINGS	DEVIATIONS FROM NORMAL
Observe for **placement and alignment of pinna.**	Pinna slightly crosses the horizontal line (Fig. 10–6A), extends slightly forward from skull symmetrically.	Pinna falls below horizontal line (Fig. 10–6B); low ears with vertical alignment greater than 10° angle suggest mental retardation or congenital syndrome; abnormal shape indicates renal pathology.

PEDIATRIC VARIATIONS (continued)

PROCEDURE	NORMAL FINDINGS	DEVIATIONS FROM NORMAL
Note on otoscopic exam: For examination of infants and young children, restraint may be necessary to accomplish a safe, effective assessment (Fig. 10–7). In infants and young children, examination with the otoscope should be last in the assessment because this part of the examination is often distressing to clients of this age group.		
Observe **inner canal.**		
Child younger than 3 years: Restrain; pull pinna downward and backward.		
Children older than 3 years: Pull pinna upward and backward.		
Inspect **TM** using otoscope with pneumatic device.	TM moves with introduction of air.	TM does not move with introduction of air.

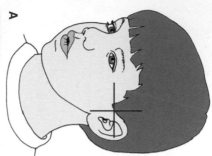

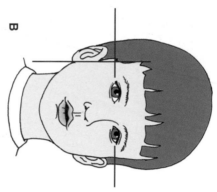

FIGURE 10–6 Placement and alignment of pinna in children. (A) Normal. (B) Low-set ears with alignment greater than 10° angle.

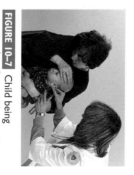

FIGURE 10–7 Child being restrained in the upright position. (© B. Proud.)

GERIATRIC VARIATIONS

- Elongated lobule with linear wrinkles
- Tuft of wirelike hair may be present at entrance of ear canal.
- More cerumen buildup; drier, harder cerumen due to rigid cilia in ear canal
- Perception of consonants (Z, T, F, G) and high-frequency sounds (S, Sh, Ph, K) decreases.
- Dull, retracted TM—may be cloudy with more prominent landmarks owing to normal aging process
- Diminished hearing acuity (presbycusis)

CULTURAL VARIATIONS

- Ear wax varies. Dry, gray, flaky wax is usual in Asians and Native Americans. Wetter, light-honey to orange to dark-brown wax is most common in African Americans and Caucasians.

Possible Collaborative Problems

Otitis media: acute, chronic, serous otitis externa
Perforated tympanic membrane
Hearing impairment

TEACHING TIPS FOR SELECTED NURSING DIAGNOSES

Adult Client

Nursing Diagnosis: Risk for Disturbed Sensory Perception (hearing) related to working in loud, noisy environment
- Teach client to wear protective hearing device when in environment with loud noises such as music, loud engines, aircraft, explosives, or firearms.

Nursing Diagnosis: Risk for Injury related to decreased auditory perception

🖐 Teach safety measures (eg, burglar alarms, lights on telephone and alarms, phone designed for hearing impaired). Explore availability of resources for hearing aids, and refer client to reading materials or sign language learning if appropriate. Encourage client to ask others to repeat what is not heard.

Nursing Diagnosis: Readiness for Enhanced Auditory Perception

🖐 Teach client to cleanse ears with damp cloth and to avoid use of cotton-tipped applicators for cleaning internal auditory canal. Encourage use of sunscreen on external ear. Teach client to shake head to remove water in ear and to dry ear after swimming to prevent swimmer's ear.

Pediatric Client

Nursing Diagnosis: Risk for Injury related to attempts to insert foreign objects in ear

🖐 Teach parents and child (as appropriate for age) dangers of insertion of foreign objects in ear. Teach parents to avoid toys with small, removable parts. Also, teach parents to avoid putting infant to bed with bottle filled with formula, juices, or sugar water, because this can settle in the oral pharynx and provide medium for bacterial growth and cause middle ear infections. Encourage yearly ear screening with physical examination during growing years.

Geriatric Client

Nursing Diagnosis: Disturbed Sensory Perception (auditory) related to aging process

🖐 Speak clearly, and allow client to see your lips. Speak within distance of 3–6 feet.

MOUTH, THROAT, NOSE, AND SINUS ASSESSMENT

11

ANATOMY OVERVIEW

The mouth or oral cavity is formed by the lips, cheeks, hard and soft palates, uvula, and the tongue and its muscles (Fig. 11–1).

Contained within the mouth are the tongue, teeth, gums, and openings of the salivary glands (parotid, submandibular, and sublingual). The gums (gingiva) are covered by mucous membrane and normally hold 32 permanent teeth in the adult (Fig. 11–2).

Three pairs of salivary glands secrete saliva (watery, serous fluid containing salts, mucus, and salivary amylase) into the mouth (Fig. 11–3): The submandibular glands and the sublingual glands.

The throat (pharynx), located behind the mouth and nose, serves as a muscular passage for food and air. The upper part of the throat is the nasopharynx. Below the nasopharynx lies the oropharynx, and below the oropharynx lies the laryngopharynx (Fig. 11–4).

The superior, middle, and inferior turbinates are bony lobes, sometimes called conchae, that project from the lateral walls of the nasal cavity. These three turbinates serve to increase the surface area that is exposed to incoming air (see Fig. 11–4).

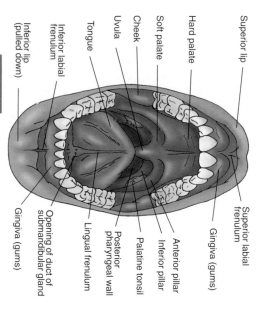

FIGURE 11-1 Structures of the mouth.

Superior lip

Hard palate

Soft palate

Cheek

Uvula

Tongue

Inferior labial frenulum

Inferior lip (pulled down)

Superior labial frenulum

Gingiva (gums)

Anterior pillar

Inferior pillar

Palatine tonsil

Posterior pharyngeal wall

Lingual frenulum

Opening of duct of submandibular gland

Gingiva (gums)

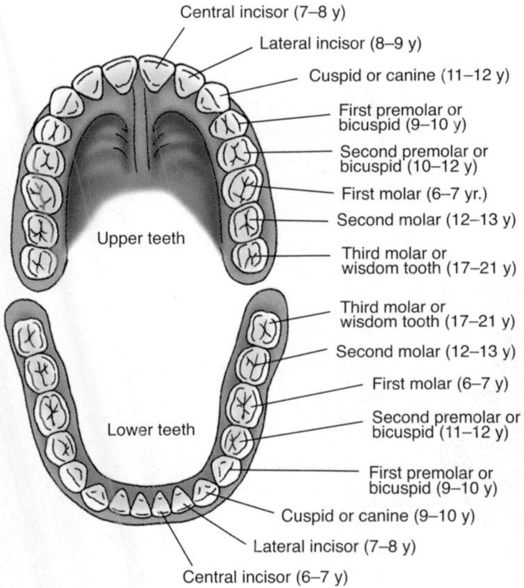

FIGURE 11-2 Teeth.

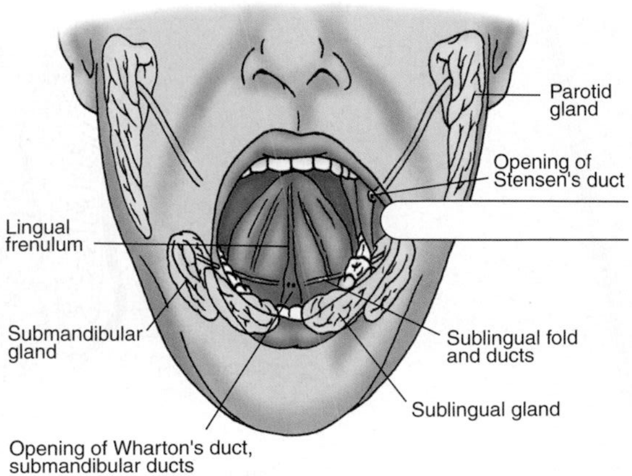

Upper teeth

Central incisor (7–8 y)
Lateral incisor (8–9 y)
Cuspid or canine (11–12 y)
First premolar or bicuspid (9–10 y)
Second premolar or bicuspid (10–12 y)
First molar (6–7 y)
Second molar (12–13 y)
Third molar or wisdom tooth (17–21 y)

Lower teeth

Third molar or wisdom tooth (17–21 y)
Second molar (12–13 y)
First molar (6–7 y)
Second premolar or bicuspid (11–12 y)
First premolar or bicuspid (9–10 y)
Cuspid or canine (9–10 y)
Lateral incisor (7–8 y)
Central incisor (6–7 y)

FIGURE 11-3 Salivary glands.

Lingual frenulum
Submandibular gland
Opening of Wharton's duct, submandibular ducts
Sublingual fold and ducts
Sublingual gland
Opening of Stensen's duct
Parotid gland

Mouth, Throat, Nose, and Sinus Assessment

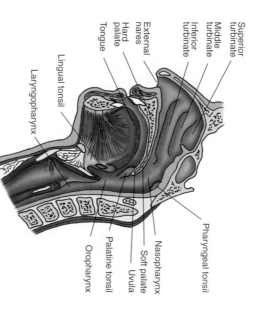

FIGURE 11–4 Nasal cavity and throat structures.

Superior turbinate
Middle turbinate
Inferior turbinate
External nares
Hard palate
Tongue
Lingual tonsil
Laryngopharynx
Oropharynx
Palatine tonsil
Soft palate
Uvula
Nasopharynx
Pharyngeal tonsil

MOUTH AND OROPHARYNX ASSESSMENT

Equipment Needed

- Penlight
- Tongue blade
- Small gauze (2 × 2-inch)
- Clean gloves

Subjective Data: Focus Questions

Prior dental problems? Dentures? Lip or oral lesions? Redness or swelling (location, occurrence, relief)? Sore throat? Dysphagia? Hoarseness? History of mouth, nose, or throat cancer in family? Smoking or use of smokeless tobacco? Dental care practices? Brushing, flossing, dental checkups?

Risk Factors. Risk for oral cancer related to smoking or use of smokeless tobacco; family history; alcoholism; working with wood, nickel refining, or textile fibers.

Objective Data: Assessment Techniques

Review Figures 11–1 through 11–4 for diagrams of the mouth, oropharynx, and nose.

INSPECTION AND PALPATION

PROCEDURE	NORMAL FINDINGS	DEVIATIONS FROM NORMAL
Inspect **open and closed mouth** for symmetry and alignment.	Lips and surrounding tissue relatively symmetrical in net position and with smiling. No lesions, tumors, infections, or dental abnormalities or poorly fitting dentures. Upper teeth resting on top of lower teeth with upper incisors slightly overriding lower ones	Asymmetrical mouth may indicate neurologic condition (eg, Bell palsy, stroke), tumors, infections, or dental abnormalities or poorly fitting dentures. Malocclusion of teeth, separation of individual teeth, or protrusion of upper or lower incisors
Wearing gloves, inspect and palpate **lips** for the following: • Color	• In white skin: Pink In dark skin: May have bluish hue or frecklelke pigmentation	• Cyanotic, pale lips in shock or anemia; reddish in ketoacidosis or carbon menoxide poisoning
• Consistency	• Moist, smooth with no lesions	• Dry, cracked; nodules, fissures, or lesions present; cheilosis (cracking in the corners) seen in riboflavin deficiencies; broken vesicles with crusting in herpes simplex type 1; scaly nodular lesions or ulcers occur with lip carcinoma

Note: Ask client to remove any dentures or dental appliances prior to continuing examination.

INSPECTION AND PALPATION (continued)

PROCEDURE	NORMAL FINDINGS	DEVIATIONS FROM NORMAL
Wearing gloves, inspect and palpate **buccal mucosa** for the following: • Color	• Pink (increased pigmentation often noted in dark-skinned clients) • Smooth, moist, without lesions	• Pale, cyanotic, or reddened mucosa • Ulcers, dry mucosa, bleeding, or white patches are present. Thick, elevated white patches (leukoplakia) that do not scrape off are precancerous; white, curdy patches that scrape off and bleed indicate thrush; red spots over red mucosa (Koplik spots) indicate measles. Canker sores (painful vesicles that erupt) are seen with allergies and stress.

Inspecting the buccal mucosa.
(© B. Proud.)

INSPECTION AND PALPATION (continued)

PROCEDURE	NORMAL FINDINGS	DEVIATIONS FROM NORMAL
• Landmarks	• Parotid duct (Stensen duct) openings are seen as small papillae located near upper second molar	• Elevated, markedly reddened area near upper second molar
Wearing gloves, retract client's lips to inspect and palpate **gums** *for the following:*		
• Color	• Pink	• Pale, markedly reddened. Swollen gums that bleed are seen with gingivitis; recessed red gums with tooth loss seen with periodontitis; bluish black gum line present in lead poisoning.

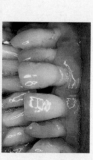

Receding gums (periodontitis).
(Courtesy of Dr. Michael Bennett.)

PROCEDURE	NORMAL FINDINGS	DEVIATIONS FROM NORMAL
• Consistency	• Moist, clearly defined margins	• Dry, edema, ulcers, bleeding, white patches, tenderness
Wearing gloves, inspect and palpate **teeth** *for the following:*		
• Number (see Fig. 11–2)	• 32 teeth	• Missing teeth
• Position and condition	• Stable fixation, smooth surfaces and edges	• Loose or broken teeth, jagged edges, dental caries
• Color	• Pearly white and shiny	• Darkened, brown, or chalky white discoloration. Teeth may be yellow-brown in clients who use excessive coffee, tea, tobacco, or fluoride. Chalky white area is seen with beginning cavity.

INSPECTION AND PALPATION *(continued)*

PROCEDURE	NORMAL FINDINGS	DEVIATIONS FROM NORMAL

Inspect protruded **tongue** *for:*

- Symmetry and texture

- Moist; papillae present; symmetrical appearance; midline fissures present. *Common variations:* Fissured; geographic tongue

- Dry; nodules, ulcers present; papillae or fissures absent, asymmetrical. Deep fissures are seen in dehydration; black hairy tongue with use of some antibiotics; smooth, red, shiny tongue seen in niacin or vitamin B_{12} deficiency.

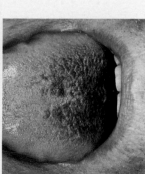

Black hairy tongue. (Courtesy of Dr. Michael Bennett.)

INSPECTION AND PALPATION (continued)

PROCEDURE	NORMAL FINDINGS	DEVIATIONS FROM NORMAL
• Movement	• Smooth	• Jerky or unilateral movement
• Color	• Pink	• Markedly reddened; white patches; pale
Inspect **ventral surface of the tongue and mouth floor** *for the following:*		
• Color	• Pink, slightly pale	• Markedly reddened, cyanotic, or extreme pallor
• Landmarks	• Submandibular duct openings (Wharton ducts) are located on both sides of the frenulum. Tongue is free of lesions or increased redness; frenulum is centered (see Fig. 11–3).	• Lesions, ulcers, nodules, or hypertrophied duct openings are present on either side of the frenulum.

Mouth, Throat, Nose, and Sinus Assessment

INSPECTION AND PALPATION (continued)

PROCEDURE	NORMAL FINDINGS	DEVIATIONS FROM NORMAL
Inspect and palpate **sides of tongue** for color and lesions.	Pink, smooth, moist; no lesions	White or reddened areas, ulcerations, or indurations present. Leukoplakia indicates precancerous lesions; may see canker sores.
		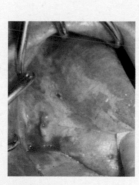

Leukoplakia (ventral surface). |
| Inspect **hard and soft palate** (see Fig. 11–3) for the following: | | |
| • Color | *Hard palate:* Pale *Soft palate:* Pink | • Extreme pallor, white patches, or markedly reddened areas |

INSPECTION AND PALPATION (continued)

PROCEDURE	NORMAL FINDINGS	DEVIATIONS FROM NORMAL
• Consistency		• *Hard palate:* Firm with irregular transverse rugae; *common variation:* palatine torus (bony protuberance) on hard palate. *Soft palate:* Spongy texture with symmetrical elevation or phonation
		• Softened tissue over hard palate; lesions present; absence of elevation; soft palate asymmetrical elevation with phonation. Thick, white plaques are seen in *Candida* infection; deep, purple lesions may indicate Kaposi sarcoma.

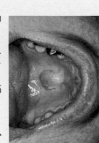

Torus palatinus. (Courtesy of Dr. Michael Bennett.)

INSPECTION AND PALPATION (continued)

PROCEDURE	NORMAL FINDINGS	DEVIATIONS FROM NORMAL
Inspect **oropharynx** (see Fig. 11–1) for the following:		
• Color	• Pink	• Markedly reddened with exudate seen in pharyngitis; yellow mucus seen with postnasal sinus drainage
• Landmarks	• Tonsillar pillars symmetrical; tonsils present (unless surgically removed) and without exudate; uvula at midline and rises on phonation	• Enlarged tonsils (tonsils are red, enlarged, and covered with exudate in tonsillitis); see tonsillitis grading scale (Fig. 11–5); asymmetrical; uvula deviates from midline; edema, ulcers, lesions.

In a client who has both tonsils and a sore throat, tonsillitis can be identified and ranked with a grading scale from 1 to 4 as follows:

1+ Tonsils are visible.
2+ Tonsils are midway between tonsillar pillars and uvula.
3+ Tonsils touch the uvula.
4+ Tonsils touch each other.

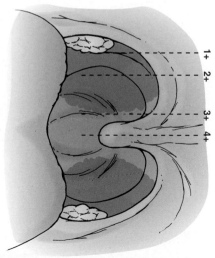

FIGURE 11–5 Detecting and grading tonsillitis.

PEDIATRIC VARIATIONS

Subjective Data: Focus Questions

Number of teeth, time of eruptions? Thumb sucking, use of pacifier (type)? Sore throats? Use of bottle? Fluoridated water?

Objective Data: Assessment Techniques

Observe for eruption of deciduous teeth (Fig. 11–6).

Observe for eruption of permanent teeth (see Fig. 11–2).

Inspect dental caries; may be due to bottle caries syndrome.

Note: A sucking pad inside upper lip of infant may be apparent due to sucking friction.

Tonsils reach adult size by age 6 years and continue to grow. By age 10 to 12 years, they are twice the adult size. By the end of adolescence they begin to atrophy back to normal adult size.

GERIATRIC VARIATIONS

- Worn teeth, abraded enamel, and yellowing teeth
- Gums recede and undergo fibrotic changes.
- Poor-fitting dentures may cause facial asymmetry and poor eating habits.
- Oral mucosa is drier owing to decreased production of saliva.
- Tongue may be fissured and have varicose veins on ventral surface.
- Decreased taste sensations due to a decrease in number of taste buds

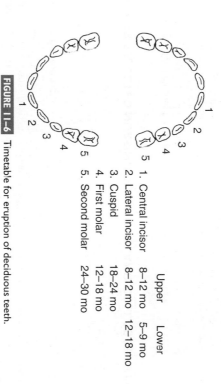

FIGURE 11–6 Timetable for eruption of deciduous teeth.

		Upper	Lower
1.	Central incisor	8–12 mo	5–9 mo
2.	Lateral incisor	8–12 mo	12–18 mo
3.	Cuspid	18–24 mo	
4.	First molar	12–18 mo	
5.	Second molar	24–30 mo	

CULTURAL VARIATIONS

- Dark-skinned clients may have lips with bluish hue or freckle-like pigmentation.
- Some groups have reduced teeth number; Australian aborigines have four extra molars.
- Dark-skinned clients may have dark pigment or freckling on side or ventral surface of tongue and floor of mouth; hard and soft palate may also be darkly pigmented.
- Some groups (especially Asians) may have mandibular torus (lump) on inner mandible near second premolar.
- Native Americans and Asians may have a split uvula.

Possible Collaborative Problems

Stomatitis
Gingivitis
Oral lesions
Periodontal (gum) disease (periodontitis)

TEACHING TIPS FOR SELECTED NURSING DIAGNOSES AND COLLABORATIVE PROBLEMS

Adult Client

Nursing Diagnosis: Impaired Oral Mucous Membrane related to inadequate mouth care

Instruct client on proper brushing and flossing. (Client should brush teeth at least twice a day and floss once a day to remove plaque from under gum line and sides of teeth.)

Recommend a toothbrush with soft rounded end or polished bristles, to be replaced every 3–4 months or sooner when frayed, in addition to an "American Dental Association–accepted" fluoride toothpaste and mouth rinse. Explain the role of fluoride in decreasing tooth decay. Refer to dentist for fluoride protection advice if client's water supply is not fluoridated. Explain the significance of a well-balanced diet in decreasing tooth decay and periodontal (gum) disease. Dry mouth can cause problems with oral health. Refer to dentist or physician for possible recommendation of artificial saliva or fluoride mouth rinse.

Collaborative Problem: Potential complication: Periodontal (gum) disease

📋 *Teach client warning signs:*

- Gums that bleed with brushing
- Red, swollen, tender gums or gums that pull away from teeth
- Pus between teeth and gums
- Loose or separating teeth
- Change in position of teeth or denture fit
- Persistent bad breath

Teach prevention:

- Brush twice daily and floss every day
- Schedule regular dental visits (American Dental Association, 2006).

Collaborative Problem: Potential complication: Oral cancer

📋 *Teach client warning signs:*

- Sore in mouth that does not heal
- White scaly patches in mouth
- Swelling or lumps in mouth/in throat/on lips
- Numbness or pain in mouth/in throat/on lips
- Repeated bleeding in mouth
- Difficulty chewing, swallowing, speaking, or moving tongue or jaw
- Change in bite

Teach client to:

- Stop smoking
- Limit alcohol consumption
- Eat a healthy, balanced diet

Teach client that there is no safe tobacco use:

- Spit tobacco (chewing tobacco) leads to gum inflammation, tooth loss, and oral cancer.
- Cigar smoking leads to mouth, throat, and lung cancer (Healthy People 2010).

Pediatric Client

Nursing Diagnosis. Impaired Dentition related to lack of proper mouth care

Instruct parents not to put child to bed with a bottle filled with formula, milk, juices, or sugar water, because these liquids pool around teeth and promote decay. Use only water in bottles when putting child to bed, to prevent so-called baby bottle tooth decay. Teach the importance of fluoride in drinking water and proper nutrition to prevent decay. Fluoride drops are recommended for infants and fluoride tablets for children up through age 14 years if adequate fluoride is not in water. Refer child who sucks thumb past age 4 years. Explain the benefits of using a small, cool spoon rubbed over gums or using teething rings during teething period. Instruct parents to start brushing child's teeth with eruption of first tooth. Begin flossing when primary teeth have erupted (2–2½ years). Parents should be taught to brush and floss child's teeth until child can be taught to do this alone (approximately age 7 years for brushing and age 10 years for flossing). Encourage a dental exam by a dentist when child is between 6 and 12 months of age.

Nursing Diagnosis: Risk for Injury to teeth related to developmental age and play activities

In case of broken or knocked-out tooth, instruct parent to rinse the tooth in cool water (do not scrub it); when possible, insert back in socket and hold in place. If this cannot be done, put tooth in cup of milk or water, or wrap it in wet cloth and take child to dentist at once for possible replacement. Recommend use of mouth guards to prevent injuries in contact sports.

Geriatric Client

Nursing Diagnosis: Imbalanced Nutrition: Less Than Body Requirements related to decreased appetite secondary to decreased senses of taste and smell

Explore food preferences with client and use visual appeal of food to enhance appetite.

NOSE AND SINUS ASSESSMENT

Equipment Needed

- Penlight
- Nasal speculum or otoscope with short, broad-tipped speculum

Subjective Data: Focus Questions

Change in ability to smell? Nosebleeds? Difficulty breathing through nostrils? Past sinus infections? Past oral, nasal, or sinus surgery? Trauma? Obstructed nares? Use of nasal sprays? Frequent infections? Allergies? Headaches located in sinus areas? Postnasal drip?

Objective Data: Assessment Techniques

See Figure 11–1 for a diagram of the nasal cavity.

INSPECTION

The external nose is inspected; then the internal nose is inspected, using the following guidelines.

Guidelines for Using Nasal Speculum

- Tilt client's head back to facilitate speculum insertion and visualization.
- Hold speculum in hand and brace your index finger against client's nose.
- Insert the speculum tip approximately 1 cm and dilate the naris as much as possible.
- Use the other hand to position client's head and hold penlight.

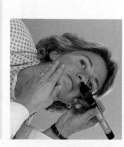

INSPECTION

PROCEDURE	NORMAL FINDINGS	DEVIATIONS FROM NORMAL
Observe **external nose** *for the following:* • Skin appearance • Shape • Nares	• *Color:* Same as face • *Consistency:* Smooth • Symmetrical appearance • Symmetrical appearance; no changes in nares with respiration; dry with no crusting; septum midline	• Nodules, lesions, erythema, visible vasculature • Asymmetry • Asymmetry; flaring nares; discharge, crusting; displaced septum
Inspect **internal nose** *for the following:* • Appearance	• Mucosa pink and moist with uniform color and no lesions	• Mucosa markedly red, dry, or cracked; areas of discoloration; polyps, masses. Mucosa is swollen, pale pink or bluish gray with allergies; nasal mucosa red and swollen with upper respiratory infection; ulcers seen with trauma, infection, nose-picking, or cocaine use; polyps seen with chronic allergies.

INSPECTION (continued)

PROCEDURE	NORMAL FINDINGS	DEVIATIONS FROM NORMAL
• Landmarks: Turbinates, septum (Fig. 11-7)	• Turbinates and middle meatus visible and same color as mucosa, moist and free of lesions; septum symmetrical and uniform without lesion	• Turbinates are not visible owing to edema or occlusion; turbinates pale or markedly reddened; polyps, lesions, copious discharge, bleeding, perforation, deviation present.

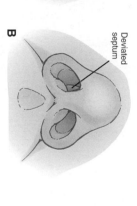

Middle turbinate

Inferior turbinate

A

B

Deviated septum

FIGURE 11-7 Structures of the internal nose. (A) Normal internal nose. (B) Deviated septum.

Assess function of nose for patency (with client's mouth closed and one naris occluded, feel for air).	Air is felt being exhaled through opposite naris; noiseless	Noisy or obstructed exhalation when mouth is closed and one naris is occluded

Mouth, Throat, Nose, and Sinus Assessment

PALPATION

PROCEDURE	NORMAL FINDINGS	DEVIATIONS FROM NORMAL
Palpate **external nose** for firmness.	Solid placement; no nodules, masses, or pain reported on palpation	Unstable placement; nodules or masses present; client verbalizes pain on palpation. Nasal tenderness is seen with local infection.
Palpate **sinuses,** both frontal and maxillary (Fig. 11–8), for tenderness.	Nontender on palpation	Client verbalizes pain or discomfort on palpation with allergies or sinus infection.

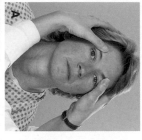

FIGURE 11–8 Palpation of frontal and maxillary sinuses. (A) The frontal sinuses. (B) The maxillary sinuses. (© B. Proud.)

PERCUSSION

PROCEDURE	NORMAL FINDINGS	DEVIATIONS FROM NORMAL
Percuss sinuses for resonance.	Hollow tone elicited	Flat, dull tone elicited; client expresses pain on percussion.

GERIATRIC VARIATIONS

• Decreased senses of taste and smell due to progressive atrophy of olfactory bulbs

Possible Collaborative Problem

Nosebleed

TEACHING TIPS FOR SELECTED NURSING DIAGNOSES AND COLLABORATIVE PROBLEMS

Adult Client

Nursing Diagnosis: Ineffective Health Maintenance related to a lack of information regarding over-the-counter nasal medications

⊙ Instruct client on use, proper dosage, and effects of overuse of nasal sprays.

Collaborative Problem: Potential complication: Nosebleed

⊙ Instruct client to apply pressure for 5 minutes while breathing through mouth and leaning forward. Caution against blowing nose for several hours afterward. Refer as necessary.

Pediatric Client

Nursing Diagnosis: Risk for Injury related to insertion of foreign bodies into nasal cavity

⊙ Caution and give instructions to parents about child's interest in inserting objects into body openings such as the nose. Instruct on common objects to remove from child's reach.

THORACIC AND LUNG ASSESSMENT

12

ANATOMY OVERVIEW

Thorax

The term *thorax* identifies the portion of the body extending from the base of the neck superiorly to the level of the diaphragm inferiorly. This thoracic cage is constructed of the sternum, 12 pairs of ribs, 12 thoracic vertebrae, muscles, and cartilage. The thorax consists of the anterior thoracic cage (Fig. 12–1) and the posterior thoracic cage (Fig. 12–2).

The sternum, or breastbone, lies in the center of the chest anteriorly and is divided into three parts: the manubrium, the body, and the xiphoid process. The clavicles (collar bones) extend from the manubrium to the acromion of the scapula. The manubrium connects laterally with the clavicles and the first two pairs of ribs. A U-shaped indentation located on the superior border of the manubrium is an important landmark known as the *suprasternal notch*. A few centimeters below the suprasternal notch, a bony ridge can be palpated at the point where the manubrium articulates with the body of the sternum. This landmark is referred to as the *sternal angle* (or angle of Louis).

Ribs (seven through 10) connect to the cartilages of the pair lying superior to them rather than to the sternum (see Fig. 12–1). This configuration forms an angle between the right and left costal margins meeting at the level of the xiphoid process, referred to as the *costal angle*.

Each pair of ribs articulates with its respective thoracic vertebra. The spinous process of the seventh cervical vertebra (C7), also called the *vertebra prominens*, can be easily felt with the client's neck flexed. The lower tip of each scapula is at the level of the seventh or eighth rib when the client's arms are at his or her side (see Fig. 12–2).

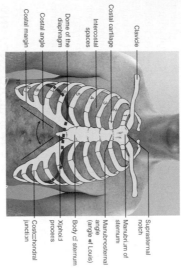

Clavicle

Suprasternal
notch

Manubrium of
sternum

Costal cartilage

Manubriosternal
angle
(angle of Louis)

Intercostal
spaces

Body of sternum

Dome of the
diaphragm

Xiphoid
process

Costal angle

Costochondral
junction

Costal margin

FIGURE 12–1 Anterior thoracic cage.

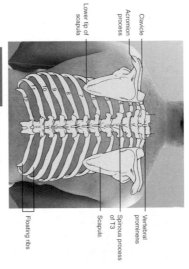

Clavicle

Vertebral
prominens

Acromion
process

Spinous process
of T3

Lower tip of
scapula

Scapula

Floating ribs

FIGURE 12–2 Posterior thoracic cage.

To describe a location around the circumference of the chest wall, imaginary lines running vertically on the chest wall are used.

On the anterior chest, these lines are known as the *midsternal line* and the *right and left midclavicular lines* (Fig. 12–3A).

The posterior thorax includes the vertebral (or spinal) line and the right and left scapular lines, which extend through the inferior angle of the scapulae when the arms are at the client's side (Fig. 12–3B).

The lateral aspect of the thorax is divided into three parallel lines. The *midaxillary line* runs from the apex of the axilla to the level of the 12th rib. The *anterior axillary line* extends from the anterior axillary fold along the anterolateral aspect of the thorax, whereas the *posterior axillary line* runs from the posterior axillary fold down the posterolateral aspect of the chest wall (Fig. 12–3C).

Thoracic Cavity

The thoracic cavity consists of the mediastinum and the lungs.

The lungs are two cone-shaped, elastic structures suspended within the thoracic cavity. The *apex* of each lung extends slightly above the clavicle, whereas the *base* is at the level of the diaphragm. At the point of the midclavicular line on the anterior surface of the thorax, the lung extends to approximately the sixth rib. Laterally, lung tissue reaches the level of the eighth rib, and, posteriorly, the lung base is at about the 10th rib (Fig. 12–4).

The thoracic cavity is lined by a thin, double-layered serous membrane collectively referred to as the pleura (Fig. 12–5). The *parietal pleura* lines the chest cavity, whereas the *visceral pleura* covers the external surfaces of the lungs. The *pleural space* lies between the two pleural layers.

The trachea lies anterior to the esophagus and is approximately 10 to 12 cm long in an adult (see Fig. 12–5). At the level of the sternal angle, the trachea bifurcates into the right and left main bronchi.

Inspired air travels through the trachea into the main bronchi and continues through the system as the bronchi repeatedly bifurcate into smaller passageways known as *bronchioles*. Eventually, the bronchioles terminate at the alveolar ducts, and air is channeled into the alveolar sacs, which contain the alveoli (see Fig. 12–5).

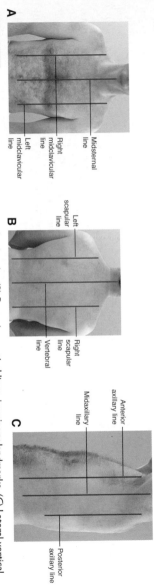

FIGURE 12-3 (A) Anterior vertical lines, imaginary landmarks. (B) Posterior vertical lines, imaginary landmarks. (C) Lateral vertical lines, imaginary landmarks.

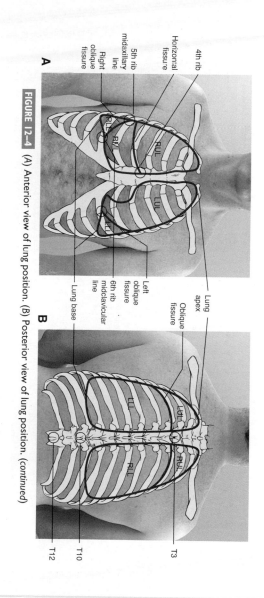

FIGURE 12-4 (A) Anterior view of lung position. (B) Posterior view of lung position. (continued)

The following labels appear in the figure:

Figure A (Anterior view):
- 4th rib
- Horizontal fissure
- 5th rib midaxillary line
- Right oblique fissure
- RUL
- RML
- RLL
- LUL
- LLL
- Left oblique fissure
- 6th rib midclavicular line
- Lung apex
- Oblique fissure

Figure B (Posterior view):
- Lung base
- LUL
- LLL
- RUL
- RLL
- T3
- T10
- T12

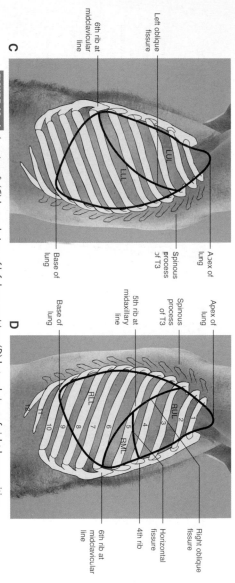

FIGURE 12–4 (continued) (C) Lateral view of left lung position. (D) Lateral view of right lung position.

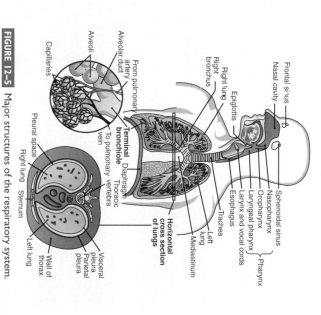

FIGURE 12-5 Major structures of the respiratory system.

Frontal sinus
Nasal cavity
Sphenoidal sinus
Nasopharynx
Oropharynx
Laryngeal pharynx
Larynx and vocal cords
Esophagus
Epiglottis
Right lung
Right bronchus
Trachea
Left lung
Mediastinum

Alveoli
Capillaries
Alveolar duct
From pulmonary artery
Terminal bronchiole
Diaphragm
Thoracic vertebra
To pulmonary vein

Pleural space
Right lung
Sternum
Wall of thorax
Left lung
Visceral pleura
Parietal pleura

Horizontal cross section of lungs

Equipment Needed

- Stethoscope
- Tape measure with centimeters
- Marking pen

Subjective Data: Focus Questions

Difficulty breathing? Timing? Associated factors? Precipitating factors? Relieving factors? Difficulty breathing when sleeping? Use of more than one pillow to sleep? Coughing (productive, nonproductive)? Sputum (type and amount)? Allergies? Dyspnea or shortness of breath (at rest or on exertion)? Chest pain? Location, timing? Associated factors? Precipitating factors? Relieving factors? History of asthma, bronchitis, emphysema, tuberculosis? Exposure to environmental inhalants (chemicals, fumes)? History of smoking (amount and length of time)? Efforts to quit?

Risk Factors. Risk for respiratory disease related to smoking, immobilization or sedentary lifestyle, aging, environmental exposures, and morbid obesity; risk for lung cancer related to cigarette smoking and genetic predisposition, asbestos, or radon exposure.

Objective Data: Assessment Techniques

Review Figures 12–1 through 12–5 for anatomy of the thorax and lungs. Expose anterior, posterior, and lateral chest with patient in sitting position. Locate landmarks (see Fig. 12–3).

INSPECTION

PROCEDURE	NORMAL FINDINGS	DEVIATIONS FROM NORMAL
Inspect anterior, posterior, and lateral thorax for the following:		
• Color	• Pink	• Pallor, cyanosis
• Intercostal spaces	• Even and relaxed	• Bulging, retracting
• Chest symmetry	• Equal	• Unequal
• Rib slope	• Less than 90° downward	• Horizontal or ≥90°
• Respiration patterns (rate, rhythm, depth) (Table 12-1)	• Even, 14–20/min, unlabored	• Uneven, labored, <12/min or >20/min, shallow, deep
• Anterior-posterior to lateral diameter	• 1:2 ratio	• >1:2 ratio (barrel chest seen in emphysema) or <1:2 ratio
• Shape and position of sternum	• Level with ribs	• Depressed or projecting
• Position of trachea	• Midline	• Deviated to one side
• Chest expansion	• 3 inches with deep inspiration	• Less than 3 inches with deep inspiration. Decreased chest excursion is seen with chronic obstructive pulmonary disease.

PALPATION

Drape anterior chest and use finger pads or palms to palpate posterior chest. Have client fold arms across anterior chest and lean forward to increase area of lungs. First palpate, percuss, and auscultate the posterior lungs and thorax while the client is sitting. Then palpate, percuss, and auscultate lateral lungs and thorax while the client is in the supine position.

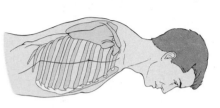

Normal cross section of thorax

Cross section of thorax.

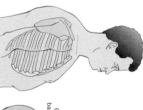

Cross section of barrel-shaped thorax

Cross section of barrel-shaped thorax.

TABLE 12–1 RESPIRATION PATTERNS

Type	Description	Pattern	Clinical Indication
Normal	14–20/min and regular		Normal breathing pattern
Tachypnea	>24/min and shallow		May be a normal response to fever, anxiety, or exercise. Can occur with respiratory insufficiency, alkalosis, pneumonia, or pleurisy
Bradypnea	<10/min and regular		May be normal in well-conditioned athletes. Can occur with medication-induced depression of the respiratory center, diabetic coma, neurologic damage
Hyperventilation	Increased rate and increased depth		Usually occurs with extreme exercise, fear, or anxiety. Kussmaul's respirations are a type of hyperventilation associated with diabetic keto-acidosis. Other causes of hyperventilation include disorders of the central nervous system, an overdose of the drug salicylate, or severe anxiety.

(continued)

TABLE 12-1   RESPIRATION PATTERNS (continued)

Type	Description	Pattern	Clinical Indication
Hypoventilation	Decreased rate, decreased depth, irregular pattern		Usually associated with overdose of narcotics or anesthetics
Cheyne-Stokes respiration	Regular pattern characterized by alternating periods of deep, rapid breathing followed by periods of apnea		May result from severe congestive heart failure, drug overdose, increased intracranial pressure, or renal failure. May be noted in elderly persons during sleep, not related to any disease process
Biot's respiration	Irregular pattern characterized by varying depth and rate of respirations followed by periods of apnea		May be seen with meningitis or severe brain damage

PALPATION (continued)

PROCEDURE	NORMAL FINDINGS	DEVIATIONS FROM NORMAL
Palpate thorax at three levels for the following:		
• Sensation	• No pain or tenderness	• Pain, tenderness. Pain over thorax is seen with inflamed fibrous connective tissue; pain over intercostal area seen with inflamed pleura.
• Vocal fremitus as client says "99"	• Vibration decreased over periphery of lungs and increased over major airways	• Vibration increased over lung with consolidation; vibration decreased over airway with obstruction, pleural effusion, or pneumothorax
Palpate thorax for thoracic expansion by the following methods:	• 2- to 3-inch symmetrical thoracic expansion	Less than 2- to 3-inch thoracic expansion; asymmetrical expansion seen with atelectasis or pneumonia
• Place hands on posterior thorax at level of 10th vertebra. Gently press skin between thumbs and have client take deep breath. Observe thumb movement (Fig. 12–6A).	• Symmetrical expansion (thumbs move apart equal distance in both directions)	• Asymmetrical expansion (thumb movement apart is unequal)
• Anteriorly, press skin together at lower sternum and have patient take deep breath. Observe thumb movement (Fig. 12–6B).	• Symmetrical expansion (thumbs move apart equal distance in both directions)	• Asymmetrical expansion (thumb movement apart is unequal)

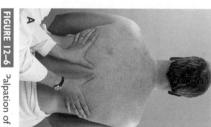

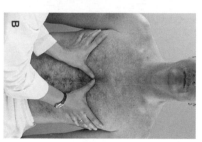

FIGURE 12–6 Palpation of thoracic expansion. (A) Posterior. (B) Anterior. (© B. Proud.)

PERCUSSION

Use mediate percussion over shoulder apices and intercostal spaces. Compare both for symmetry of percussion notes, while moving from apex to base of lungs as illustrated (see Fig. 12–7).

PROCEDURE	NORMAL FINDINGS	DEVIATIONS FROM NORMAL
Percuss over shoulder apices and at posterior, anterior, and lateral intercostal spaces as illustrated (see Fig. 12–7). See Figure 12–4 to determine which lung areas are being percussed.	Resonance	Hyperresonance is heard over emphysematous lungs; dullness heard over solid masses or fluid, eg, in lobar pneumonia, pleural effusion, or tumor.
Percuss for posterior, diaphragmatic excursions bilaterally, as illustrated (Fig. 12–8).	Diaphragm descends 3–6 cm from T10 (with full expiration held) to T12 (with full inspiration held).	Diaphragm descends less than 3 cm owing to atelectasis of lower lobes, emphysema, ascites, or tumors.

AUSCULTATION

Using diaphragm of stethoscope, exert firm pressure over intercostal space. Instruct client to take slow, deep breaths through the mouth. Listen for two full breaths and compare symmetrical sides of thorax while moving stethoscope from apex to base of lungs.

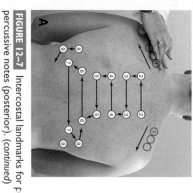

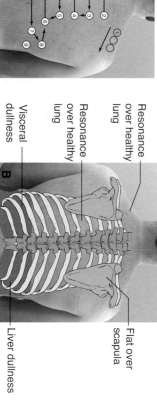

Resonance
over healthy
lung

Resonance
over healthy
lung

Visceral
dullness

Flat over
scapula

Liver dullness

FIGURE 12–7 Intercostal landmarks for percussion and auscultation of thorax. (A) Posterior. (B) Normal percussive notes (posterior). (continued)

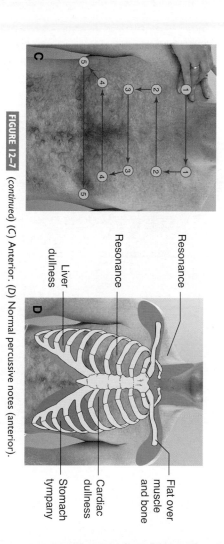

FIGURE 12-7 (continued) (C) Anterior. (D) Normal percussive notes (anterior).

Resonance

Resonance

Liver
dullness

Resonance

Flat over
muscle
and bone

Cardiac
dullness

Stomach
tympany

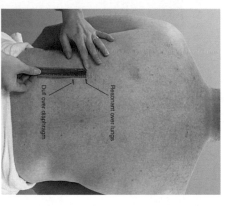

FIGURE 12–8 Percussing bilaterally for diaphragmatic excursions.

Resonant over lungs

Dull over diaphragm

AUSCULTATION (continued)

PROCEDURE	NORMAL FINDINGS	DEVIATIONS FROM NORMAL

*Auscultate **breath sounds** over the following:*

- Trachea

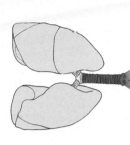

- Large-stem bronchi

- Bronchial (loud, tubular) breath sounds heard over trachea; expiration longer than inspiration; short silence between inspiration and expiration

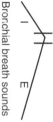

Bronchial breath sounds

- Bronchovesicular breath sounds heard over mainstem bronchi: below clavicles and between scapulae (inspiratory phase equal to expiratory phase)

- Bronchial sounds heard over lung periphery

- Bronchovesicular breath sounds heard over lung periphery

PROCEDURE	NORMAL FINDINGS	DEVIATIONS FROM NORMAL

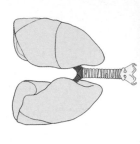

Bronchovesicular breath sounds

- Lung periphery

- Vesicular (low, soft, breezy) breath sounds heard over lung periphery (inspiration longer than expiration)

Lungs clear to auscultation on inspiration and expiration

- Decreased breath sounds with obstruction, pleural thickening, pleural effusion, or pneumothorax

Crackles usually are auscultated during inspiration. They occur late in inspiration with pneumonia and congestive heart failure; occur early in inspiration with bronchitis, asthma, and emphysema. Fine crackles are popping, high-pitched, and very brief (5–10 msec).

Auscultate breath sounds for **adventitious sounds** (crackles, wheezes). If an abnormal sound is heard, ask client to cough. Note if adventitious sound is still present or if it cleared with cough.

AUSCULTATION (continued)

PROCEDURE

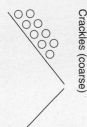

NORMAL FINDINGS

I   E

Vesicular breath sounds

DEVIATIONS FROM NORMAL

Crackles (fine)

Crackles (coarse)

AUSCULTATION (continued)

DEVIATIONS FROM NORMAL

Coarse crackles are bubbling sounds, lower in pitch, and not quite so brief (20-30 msec). Heard with pneumonia, pulmonary edema, and fibrosis. Sibilant wheezes (high-pitched musical sounds) are heard on inspiration or expiration in acute asthma and chronic emphysema. Sonorous wheezes are low-pitched moaning sounds heard mostly on expiration in bronchitis, single obstruction, and snoring before sleep apnea.

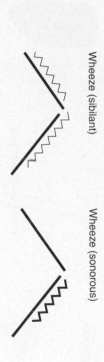

Wheeze (sibilant)

Wheeze (sonorous)

AUSCULTATION (continued)

PROCEDURE	NORMAL FINDINGS	DEVIATIONS FROM NORMAL
Auscultate for **altered voice sounds** over lung periphery where any previous lung abnormality is noted.		
• Bronchophony (client says "99" while examiner auscultates).	• Sounds muffled	• Sounds loud and clear over consolidation from pneumonia, atelectasis, or tumor
• Whispered pectoriloquy (client whispers "one, two, three" while examiner auscultates).	• Sounds muffled	• Sounds loud and clear over areas of consolidation
• Egophony (client says "ee" while examiner auscultates).	• Sounds like muffled "ee"	• Sounds like "ay" over areas of consolidation or compression

Adapted from Bickley, L. S., & Szilagyi, P. G. (2003). *Bates' guide to physical examination and history taking*. 8th ed. Philadelphia: Lippincott Williams & Wilkins.

PEDIATRIC VARIATIONS

Subjective Data: Focus Questions

History of wheezing, asthma, or other breathing problems? Exposure to passive smoke? Occurrence of sudden infant death syndrome (SIDS) in family? Frequent colds or congestion?

Objective Data: Assessment Techniques

Inspection

In infants, anteroposterior (AP) diameter is equal to transverse diameter (1:1)—shape is nearly circular. By age 5 to 6 years, the AP diameter reaches that of the adult 1:2 or 5:7 ratio. Chest wall is thin with bony and cartilaginous rib cage soft and pliant. *Respirations* should be unlabored and quiet; rate varies according to age (Table 12–2).

TABLE 12-2	RESPIRATORY RATES IN CHILDREN
Age	Respiratory Rate (breaths/min)
Newborn	30–60
Early childhood	20–40
Late childhood	15–25
Age 15 years and older	14–20

Adapted from Bickley, L. S., & Szilagyi, P. G. (2003). *Bates' guide to physical examination and history taking,* 8th ed. Philadelphia: Lippincott Williams & Wilkins.

Percussion

In infants and young children, normally hyperresonant throughout because of thinness of chest wall. Any decrease in resonance is equal to dullness in the adult.

Auscultation

Bell or small diaphragm should be used to localize findings, especially in infants and young children. Breath sounds will be louder and harsher owing to close proximity to origin of sounds from thin chest wall. Wheezes and rhonchi occur more frequently in infants and young children.

GERIATRIC VARIATIONS

- Increase in normal respiratory rate (16–25)
- Loss of elasticity, fewer functional capillaries, and loss of lung resiliency
- Decreased ability to cough effectively due to weaker muscles and rigid thoracic wall
- Accentuated dorsal curve (kyphosis) of thoracic spine
- Sternum and ribs may be more prominent owing to loss of subcutaneous fat
- Decreased thoracic expansion due to calcification of costal cartilages and loss of the accessory musculature
- Increased diaphragmatic breathing due to anatomic changes
- Hyperresonance of thorax due to age-related emphysemic changes
- Decreased breath sounds and increased retention of mucus due to decreased pulmonary function
- Increased AP diameter (up to 5:7 AP-to-transverse diameter ratio) due to loss of resiliency and loss of skeletal muscle strength
- Resonance of percussive may increase

CULTURAL VARIATIONS

- Thoracic cavity size varies among cultural groups. The tendency is for Caucasians to have larger thoraxes than blacks, Asians, and Native Americans.

Possible Collaborative Problems

Respiratory insufficiency/failure

Pneumonia

Pulmonary edema

Airway obstruction/atelectasis

Laryngeal edema

Pleural effusion

Atelectasis

Asthma

Chronic obstructive pulmonary disease

Oxygen toxicity

Carbon dioxide toxicity

Pneumothorax

Respiratory acidosis

Respiratory alkalosis

Tracheal necrosis

Tracheobronchial constriction

TEACHING TIPS FOR SELECTED NURSING DIAGNOSES

Adult Client

Nursing Diagnosis: Readiness for Enhanced Respiratory Function

Encourage client to participate in a daily exercise program and to eat a healthy, low-cholesterol diet with adequate vitamin E and lutein. Provide client with information on the risks of secondhand smoke and how to decrease one's exposure. The Indoor Air Quality Information Hotline provides free information (phone 1-800-438-4318). Encourage client not to start smoking and to limit exposure to air pollution and dangerous substances.

Nursing Diagnosis: Ineffective Airway Clearance related to shallow coughing and thickened mucus

🖐 Instruct client on effective deep breathing and coughing. Encourage liquid intake of 2–3 quarts/day. Caution client to use protective measures to prevent spread of infections.

Nursing Diagnosis: Impaired Gas Exchange related to chronic lung tissue damage

🖐 Teach client diaphragmatic and pursed-lip breathing.

Nursing Diagnosis: Ineffective Airway Clearance related to chronic allergy

🖐 Provide literature on environmental control. Assess whether client has kit to deal with emergencies (eg, bee stings). If allergy is produced by unknown food, assist client with keeping a diary of allergy attacks to determine cause.

Nursing Diagnosis: Ineffective Breathing Pattern: hyperventilation related to hypoxia and lack of knowledge of controlled breathing techniques

🖐 Teach client how to become aware of breathing patterns and how to assess what aggravates hyperventilation (eg, fatigue, stress). Teach controlled breathing techniques.

Nursing Diagnosis: Impaired Gas Exchange related to smoking and/or frequent exposure to air pollution or dangerous substances

🖐 Explain effects of smoking and how it is a primary risk factor for lung cancer. Assess client's desire to quit and refer to community agencies for self-help on smoking cessation programs. Discuss alternate methods of coping. Wear mask if job requires exposure to dangerous inhalants

Thoracic and Lung Assessment

Pediatric Client

Nursing Diagnosis: Ineffective Airway Clearance related to bronchospasm and increased pulmonary secretions

Postural drainage and percussion may be used with children of various ages. Teach parents safety measures when using vaporizers. Teach alternate ways of humidifying air. For example, have parent run hot water in shower and close bathroom door. Sit with child in this room for approximately 10 minutes to liquefy secretions by steam (child must not be left alone in room). Teach parents the importance of throat cultures for upper respiratory infections to identify streptococcal infections. *If child has asthma:* Asthma attacks decrease with increasing age of child. Assist parents with letting child have more independence and avoiding overprotection. Teach family how to decrease allergens (eg, dust) in home by using smooth surfaces that are easy to clean.

Geriatric Client

Nursing Diagnosis: Impaired Gas Exchange related to poor muscle tone and decreased ability to remove secretions

Teach client the importance of mobility and exercise to maintain adequate respiratory hygiene. Encourage client to discuss consideration of the flu shot with the physician.

BREAST ASSESSMENT

13

ANATOMY OVERVIEW

The breasts are paired mammary glands that lie over the muscles of the anterior chest wall, anterior to the pectoralis major and serratus anterior muscles (Fig. 13–1). The male and female breasts are similar until puberty, when female breast tissue enlarges in response to hormones.

For assessment purposes, the breasts are divided into four quadrants by drawing horizontal and vertical imaginary lines that intersect at the nipple (Fig. 13–2).

The skin of the breasts is smooth and varies in color. The nipple contains the tiny openings of the lactiferous ducts. The areola surrounds the nipple and contains elevated sebaceous glands (Montgomery glands).

Female breasts consist of three types of tissue: glandular, fibrous, and fatty (adipose; Fig. 13–3). The amount of glandular, fibrous, and fatty tissue varies according to various factors including the client's age, body build, nutritional status, hormonal cycle, and whether she is pregnant or lactating.

The major axillary lymph nodes consist of the anterior (pectoral), posterior (subscapular), lateral (brachial), and central (mid-axillary) nodes, supraclavicular, and infraclavicular (Fig. 13–4).

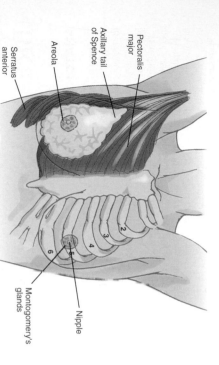

FIGURE 13–1 Anatomic breast landmarks and their position in the thorax.

Pectoralis
major

Axillary tail
of Spence

Areola

Serratus
anterior

Montogomery's
glands

Nipple

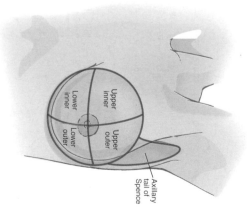

FIGURE 13–2 Breast quadrants. The upper outer quadrant is the area most targeted by breast cancer.

Upper
inner

Lower
inner

Lower
outer

Upper
outer

Axillary
tail of
Spence

Breast Assessment

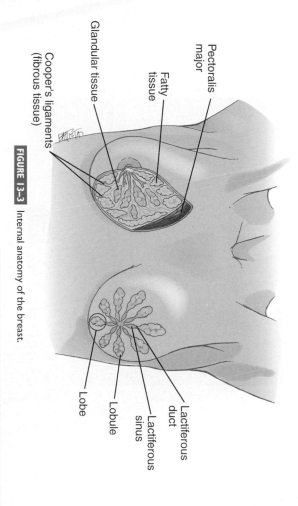

FIGURE 13–3 Internal anatomy of the breast.

Pectoralis major

Fatty tissue

Glandular tissue

Cooper's ligaments (fibrous tissue)

Lactiferous duct

Lactiferous sinus

Lobule

Lobe

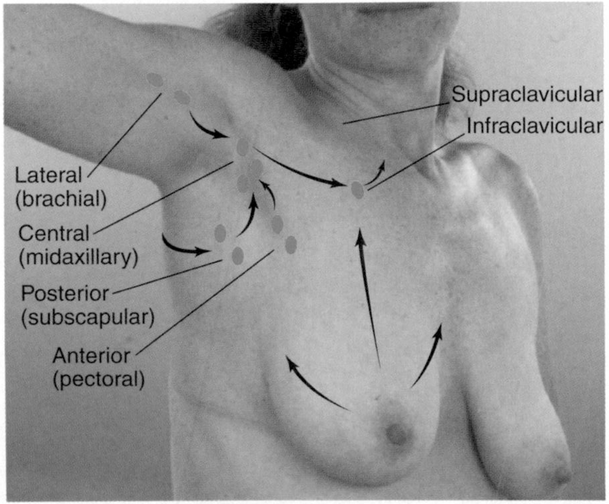

FIGURE 13–4 The lymph nodes drain impurities from the breasts (arrows show direction).

Lateral (brachial)

Central (midaxillary)

Posterior (subscapular)

Anterior (pectoral)

Supraclavicular

Infraclavicular

Equipment Needed

• Centimeter ruler
• Small pillow
• Breast self-examination brochure
• Gloves and slide for specimen if nipple discharge is present

Subjective Data: Focus Questions

Any lumps or lesions (location, size) or swelling in breasts? Change in size or firmness? Redness, warmth, or dimpling of breasts? Tenderness? Pain? Timing in menstrual cycle? Change in position of nipple or nipple discharge? Age of menstruation? Birth to children and age? Previous breast surgeries? History of breast cancer in family? Self-care: Breast self-examination (frequency and time performed)? Use of hormones, birth control, or antidepressants? Exposure to radiation, benzene, or asbestos? Use of alcohol, caffeine? Diet and daily exercise routine? Last breast exam? Last mammogram?

Risk Factors. Risk for breast cancer related to increasing age, personal history of breast cancer, family history of breast cancer, early menarche and late menopause, no natural children, first child after age 30 years, higher education and socioeconomic status, regular alcohol intake (2–5 drinks daily), previous breast irradiation, hormone replacement with progesterone, no or poor breast self-examination, poor screening.

Objective Data: Assessment Techniques

See Figures 13–1 through 13–8 for illustrations of the breasts and regional lymphatics.

INSPECTION

The breasts should be inspected with client in sitting position with arms at sides, arms overhead, hands pressed on hips, palms pressed together, and arms extended straight ahead as client leans forward (Fig. 13–5). The areolae and nipples should also be inspected.

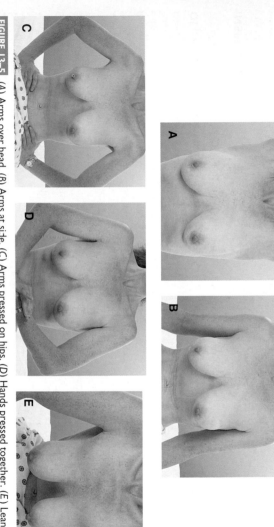

FIGURE 13-5 (A) Arms over head. (B) Arms at side. (C) Arms pressed on hips. (D) Hands pressed together. (E) Leaning forward, arms extended.

INSPECTION (continued)

PROCEDURE	NORMAL FINDINGS	DEVIATIONS FROM NORMAL
Observe **breasts** *for the following:*		
• Size and symmetry	• Relatively equal with slight variation	• Recent change to unequal size. Recent increase in size of one breast may indicate inflammation or abnormal growth.
• Shape	• Round and pendulous	• Retraction or dimpling may be due to fibrosis and may indicate a malignant tumor.
• Color	• Pink; striae with age and pregnancy	• Redness, inflammation, blue hue, increased venous engorgement
• Skin surface	• Smooth	• Retraction, dimpling, enlarged pores, "peau d'orange" (seen in metastatic breast disease due to edema from blocked lymphatic drainage), edema, lumps, lesions, rashes, ulcers
Observe **areolae and nipples** *for the following:*		
• Size	• Relatively the same; slight variation	• Large variation
• Color	• Pink to dark brown (varies with skin and hair color)	• Inflamed

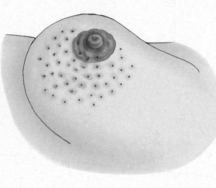

Orange peel (peau d'orange)
appearance of the breast.

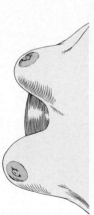

Retracted breast tissue

INSPECTION (continued)

PROCEDURE	NORMAL FINDINGS	DEVIATIONS FROM NORMAL
• Shape	• Round, oval, everted	• Inversion, if it occurs after maturation or changes with movement. Recent retraction of previously everted nipple suggests malignancy.
• Discharge	• None; clear yellow 2 days after childbirth	• Foul, purulent, sanguineous drainage. Any spontaneous discharge needs to be referred for further evaluation.
• Texture	• Small Montgomery tubercles present	• Lesions, rashes, ulcers. Peau d'orange skin is seen with carcinoma. Red, scaly, crusty areas are indicative of Paget disease.

Breast Assessment

PALPATION

Use the flat pads of three fingers to compress tissue against breast wall gently. Palpate with patient sitting. Then have patient lie down and place arm of side being examined over head with small pillow under upper back. Palpate in circular motion starting at the 12-o'clock position and moving in concentric rings inward to areola and nipple (Figure 13–6, *A*). Bimanual palpation may be used in large-breasted clients. A wedge (Figure 13–6, *B*) or vertical (Figure 13–6, *C*) pattern may be used if preferred.

PROCEDURE	NORMAL FINDINGS	DEVIATIONS FROM NORMAL
Palpate **breasts** *for the following:*		
• Temperature	• Warm	• Erythema; heat indicates inflammation if client is not lactating or has not just given birth.
• Elasticity • Tenderness	• Elastic • Nontender; slightly tender (tenderness and fullness may occur before menses)	• Lumpy • Painful
• Masses (note size, shape, mobility, consistency, and location according to quadrant; see Fig. 13–2).	• Bilateral firm inframammary transverse ridge at base of breasts	• Masses or nodules. Malignant tumors are most often found in upper outer quadrant of breast and are usually unilateral with irregular, poorly delineated borders; hard; nontender; and fixed to underlying tissues. Fibroadenomas

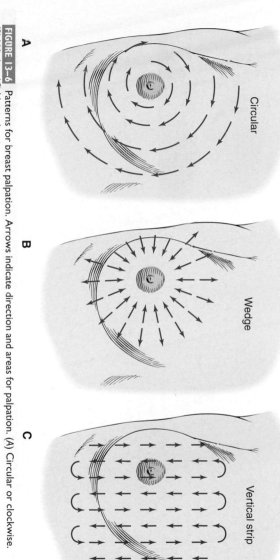

FIGURE 13-6 Patterns for breast palpation. Arrows indicate direction and areas for palpation. (A) Circular or clockwise. (B) Wedge. (C) Vertical strip.

A — Circular

B — Wedge

C — Vertical strip

Breast Assessment

PALPATION (continued)

PROCEDURE	NORMAL FINDINGS	DEVIATIONS FROM NORMAL
		(benign) are usually 1–5 cm, round or oval, mobile, firm, solid, elastic, non-tender, and single or multiple in one or both breasts. Fibrocystic disease (benign) consists of bilateral, multiple, firm, regular, rubbery, mobile nodules with well-demarcated borders (see Fig. 13–7).
Palpate **nipple** gently for discharge.	None; clear yellow 2 days after childbirth.	Unilateral serous, serosanguineous, clear, yellow, dark red. Discharge may be seen in endocrine disorders and with some medications, such as antihypertensives, antidepressants, and estrogen. Discharge from one breast may indicate benign intraductal papilloma, fibrocystic disease, or breast cancer.

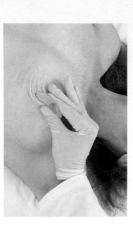

Palpating nipples for masses and discharge.

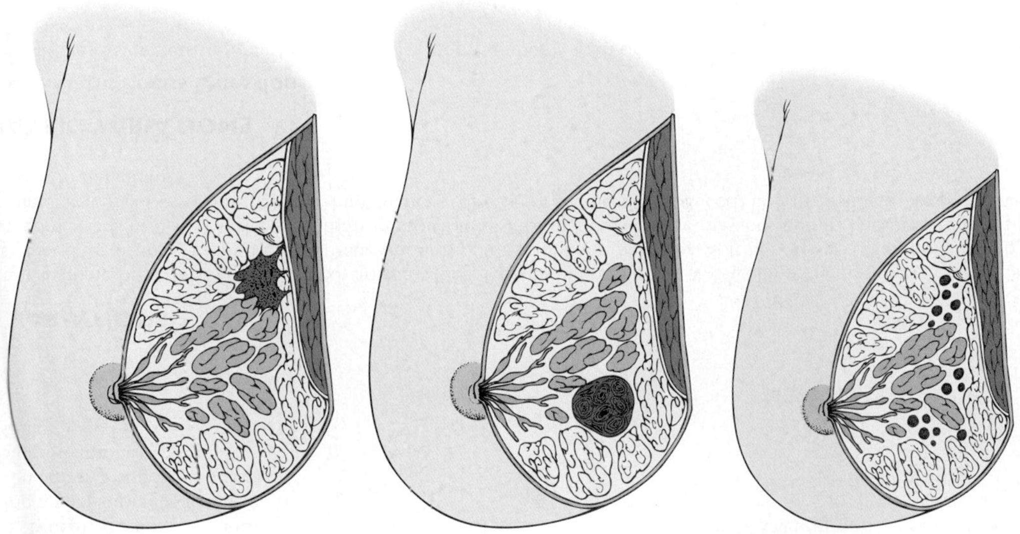

Tumor.

Fibroadenoma.

Benign breast disease (fibrocystic breast disease).

FIGURE 13-7 Breast abnormalities.

Breast Assessment

PALPATION (continued)

PROCEDURE	NORMAL FINDINGS	DEVIATIONS FROM NORMAL
Palpate **lymph nodes** in the following areas: supraclavicular, subclavian, intermediate, brachial, scapular, mammary; internal mammary (see Fig. 13–4).	None palpable (<1 cm)	Palpable lymph nodes (>1 cm)

MALE VARIATIONS

Inspect and palpate breast with client seated, arms at sides. Palpate lymph nodes. No swelling, ulcerations, or nodules should be noted. Flat disk of undeveloped breast tissue under nipple is normally palpated. Soft fatty tissue enlargement seen in obesity. Gynecomastia (Fig. 13–8) and a smooth, firm movable disk of glandular tissue may be seen in one breast during puberty for short time and may be seen in hormonal imbalances (disease or medication induced) and drug abuse. Irregular, hard nodules are seen in malignancy.

PEDIATRIC VARIATIONS

Subjective Data: Focus Questions

Age of menarche? Asymmetrical breast growth? Girls prior to puberty: Pain or discomfort? Boys during adolescence: Abnormal increase in size?

Breast Assessment

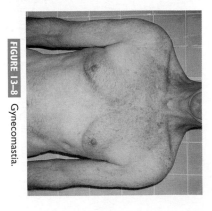

FIGURE 13–8 Gynecomastia.

Objective Data

See normal breast development in Chapter 17, Table 17–1 which varies with age. Adolescent breast development is usually seen between age 10 and 13 years and takes about 3 years for full development.

GERIATRIC VARIATIONS

- Breasts pendulous, atrophied, and less firm owing to a decrease in estrogen levels
- May have smaller, flatter nipples that are less erectile on stimulation. Nipples may retract, but evert with gentle pressure.
- May feel more granular with more fibrotic tissue

CULTURAL VARIATIONS

Breast cancer rates vary between the United States and Europe, with African Americans having the highest age-adjusted death rates. The rates may relate to dry versus wet ear wax also secreted by apocrine glands, active in breast tissue (Overfield, 1995).

Possible Collaborative Problems

Infection (abscess)
Hematoma
Fibrocystic disease
Breast cancer

TEACHING TIPS FOR SELECTED NURSING DIAGNOSES

Adult Client

Nursing Diagnosis: Ineffective Therapeutic Regimen Management related to knowledge deficit of breast self-examination

Women should be told about the benefits and limitations of breast self-examination (BSE) beginning at age 20. Emphasize the importance of reporting any new breast symptoms to a health professional. It is acceptable for women to choose not to do BSE or do it irregularly. If a woman chooses to do BSE, instruct on proper BSE technique (see Appendix 9), allowing time for questions and review of technique (American Cancer Society, 2005). The best time for BSE is right after menstruation or between the fourth and seventh day of the cycle if the cycle is regular. If the client is on cyclic estrogen therapy, she should examine her breasts on the last day that the medicine is not being taken. It is important for women to know their breasts and to report any breast changes promptly to their health care providers. Remember that most of the time breast changes are not cancer, but it is important to detect breast cancer early for effective treatment. Women who have had a breast lumpectomy, augmentation, or breast reconstruction may also perform BSE. Some women may choose not to do BSE even if knowledgeable of the benefits and limitations. This choice needs to be accepted by the examiner.

Reinforce the following American Cancer Society, 2005, recommendations:

- Monthly breast self-examination for women age 20 years or older
- Breast clinical examination for women age 20 to 39 years every 3 years and every year for women age 40 years and older
- Annual mammography for women age 40 years and older as long as a woman is in good health. Women at increased risk should talk to their physician about more frequent exams.

Advise that cancer of the breast can be treated and often cured if detected early.

Encourage breast-feeding, exercise, and maintaining a healthy body weight.

(American Cancer Society. *Cancer prevention and early detection facts and figures*, 2005.)

HEART ASSESSMENT

14

ANATOMY OVERVIEW

Heart and Great Vessels

The heart is a hollow, muscular, four-chambered organ located in the middle of the thoracic cavity between the lungs in the space called the *mediastinum*. It is about the size of a clenched fist and weighs approximately 255 g (9 oz) in women and 310 g (10.9 oz) in men. The heart extends vertically from the second to the fifth intercostal space (ICS) and horizontally from the right edge of the sternum to the left midclavicular line (MCL). The heart can be described as an inverted cone. The upper portion, near the second ICS, is the base, and the lower portion, near the fifth ICS and the left MCL, is the apex. The anterior chest area that overlies the heart and great vessels is called the *precordium* (Fig. 14–1).

The large veins and arteries leading directly to and away from the heart are referred to as the *great vessels*. The *superior and inferior vena cava* return blood to the right atrium from the upper and lower torso, respectively. The *pulmonary artery* exits the right ventricle, bifurcates, and carries blood to the lungs. The *pulmonary veins* (two from each lung) return oxygenated blood to the left atrium. The *aorta* transports oxygenated blood from the ventricle to the body (Fig. 14–2).

The heart consists of four chambers or cavities: two upper chambers, the *right and left atria*, and two lower chambers, the *right and left ventricles*. The entrance and exit of each ventricle are protected by one-way valves that direct the flow of blood through the heart. The *atrioventricular* (AV) valves are located at the entrance into the ventricles. There are two AV valves: the tricuspid valve and the bicuspid, which is also called the *mitral valve*. The tricuspid valve is composed of three cusps or flaps and is located between the right atrium and the right ventricle; the bicuspid (mitral) valve is composed of two cusps or flaps and is located between the left atrium and the left ventricle.

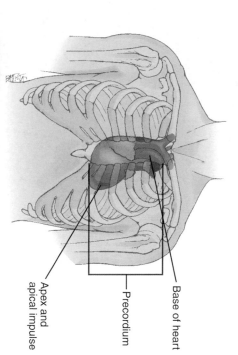

FIGURE 14-1 The heart and major blood vessels lie centrally in the chest behind the protective sternum.

Apex and
apical impulse

Precordium

Base of heart

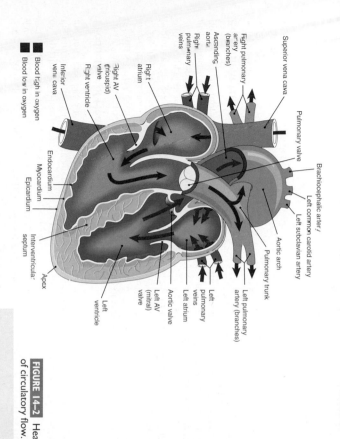

Superior vena cava

Right pulmonary
artery
(branches)

Ascending
aorta

Right
pulmonary
veins

Right
atrium

Right AV
(tricuspid)
valve

Right ventricle

Endocardium

Myocardium

Epicardium

Interventricular
septum

Apex

Pulmonary valve

Brachiocephalic artery
Left common carotid artery
Left subclavian artery

Aortic arch

Pulmonary trunk

Left pulmonary
artery (branches)

Left
pulmonary
veins

Left atrium

Aortic valve

Left AV
(mitral)
valve

Left
ventricle

Inferior
vena cava

■ Blood high in oxygen
■ Blood low in oxygen

FIGURE 14-2 Heart chambers, valves, and direction of circulatory flow.

Open AV valves allow blood to flow from the atria into the ventricles. However, as the ventricles begin to contract, the AV valves snap shut, preventing the regurgitation of blood into the atria.

The *semilunar valves* are located at the exit of each ventricle at the beginning of the great vessels. Each valve has three cusps or flaps that look like half-moons, hence the name "semilunar." There are two semilunar valves: the pulmonic valve is located at the entrance of the pulmonary artery as it exits the right ventricle, and the aortic valve is located at the beginning of the ascending aorta (see Fig. 14–2).

Production of Heart Sounds

Heart sounds are produced by valve closure. The opening of valves is silent. Normal heart sounds, characterized as "lub dubb" (S_1 and S_2), and, occasionally, extra heart sounds and murmurs can be auscultated with a stethoscope over the precordium, the area of the anterior chest overlying the heart and great vessels.

The first heart sound (S_1) is the result of closure of the AV valves—the mitral and tricuspid valves. S_1 correlates with the beginning of systole (Fig. 14–3). If heard as two sounds, the first component represents mitral valve closure (M_1), and the second component represents tricuspid closure (T_1).

The second heart sound (S_2, "dubb") is also usually heard as one sound but may be heard as two sounds. If S_2 is heard as two sounds, the first component represents aortic valve closure (A_2) and the second component represents pulmonic valve closure (P_2).

The second heart sound (S_2) results from closure of the semilunar valves (aortic and pulmonic) and correlates with the beginning of diastole. S_2 ("dubb") is also usually heard as one sound but may be heard as two sounds. If S_2 is heard as two sounds, the first component represents aortic valve closure (A_2) and the second component represents pulmonic valve closure (P_2).

Equipment Needed

- Ruler with centimeters
- Marking pen
- Stethoscope with bell and diaphragm
- Alcohol swab to clean ear and end pieces

Heart Assessment

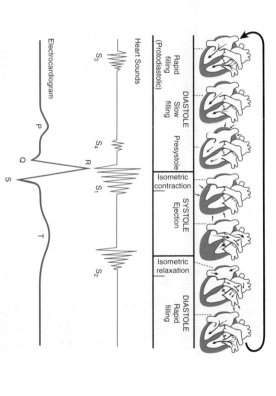

FIGURE 14–3 The cardiac cycle consists of filling and ejection. Heart sounds S_2, S_3, and S_4 are associated with diastole, whereas S_1 is associated with systole. The electrical activity of the heart is measured throughout diastole and systole by electrocardiography.

Subjective Data: Focus Questions

Chest pain—Location? Radiation? Quality? Rating on scale of 1 to 10 (10 being the worst)? Duration? What relieves it? Are there any other associated symptoms, such as nausea, vomiting, sweating? Irregular heartbeat, palpitations? Does your heart pound or beat too fast? Does your heart skip or jump? Dizziness? Swollen ankles? History of heart defect? Murmur? Heart surgery? Smoking? Packs per day? Over how many years? Family history of heart disease? Activities of daily living—Diet? Alcohol consumption? Usual exercise? Daily stressors? Forms of relaxation?

Risk Factors. Risk for coronary heart disease related to hypertension, increased low-density lipoprotein cholesterol and decreased high-density lipoprotein (HDL) cholesterol, diabetes mellitus, minimal exercise, cigarette smoking, diet high in saturated fat and transfatty acids, postmenopausal without estrogen replacement (in females), family history, and upper body obesity.

Objective Data: Assessment Techniques

See Figure 14–2 for a diagram of the heart chambers, valves, and circulation.

INSPECTION

Inspect chest to identify landmarks that aid in assessment of the heart. Check for visibility of point of maximum impulse (PMI) and any abnormal pulsations.

PROCEDURE	NORMAL FINDINGS	DEVIATIONS FROM NORMAL
Inspect the following:		
• Intercostal space (ICS): Locate by finding the sternal angle, which is felt as a ridge in the sternum approximately 2 inches below the	• Small apical impulse (≤2.5 cm) at or medial to left midclavicular line at fourth or fifth ICS. May not be visible in client with large chest.	• Impulses lateral to midclavicular line; pulsations (heaves or lifts) other than the apical pulsation are considered abnormal, and may be seen with an

INSPECTION (continued)

PROCEDURE	NORMAL FINDINGS	DEVIATIONS FROM NORMAL
	sternal notch (Fig. 14-4). The adjacent rib is the second rib with the second ICS directly below it. Other ICSs can be identified by counting from the second ICS. The fifth ICS is at the junction of the sternum and the xiphoid process.	enlarged left ventricle due to work overload; apical impulse on right side of chest. Bulging and/or prominent pulsations (>3 cm) at the PMI.
	• Midsternal line (MSL): Imaginary line extending down the chest through the middle of the sternum. It divides the anterior chest in half (see Fig. 14-4).	
	• Midclavicular line (MCL): Imaginary line extending from the middle of the clavicle down the chest, dividing the left or right anterior chest into two parts (see Fig. 14-4).	• Prominent impulse at right sternal border in pulmonic or aortic area
	• Anterior axillary line (AAL): Imaginary line extending along the lateral wall of the anterior chest and even with the anterior axillary fold (see Fig. 14-4).	

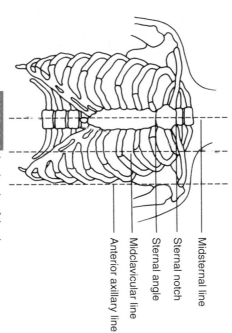

FIGURE 14—4 Landmarks of the chest.

Midsternal line

Sternal notch

Sternal angle

Midclavicular line

Anterior axillary line

PALPATION

The client should be lying down. Palpate using the fingertips and palmar surfaces of fingers in an organized fashion, beginning in the aortic area and moving down the chest toward the tricuspid area (Fig. 14–5).

PROCEDURE	NORMAL FINDINGS	DEVIATIONS FROM NORMAL
Palpate the following:		
• Aortic area: Palpate second ICS at right sternal border (see Fig. 14–5).	• No vibrations or pulsations are palpated in aortic, pulmonic, or tricuspid area.	• Thrill, which feels similar to a purring cat, or pulsation in any of these areas except the mitral area is usually associated with a grade 4 or higher murmur.
• Pulmonic area: Palpate second ICS at left sternal border (see Fig. 14–5).		
• Erb's point: Palpate third ICS at left sternal border (see Fig. 14–5).		
• Tricuspid area: Palpate fifth ICS at lower left sternal border (see Fig. 14–5).		
• Mitral area: Palpate fifth ICS at the left MCL. This is also called the PMI (see Fig. 14–5).	• PMI is felt as a pulsation and is approximately the size of a nickel. May not palpate in large chests.	• No pulsation. If area of pulsation is the size of a quarter or larger, displaced, more forceful, or of longer duration, cardiac enlargement should be suspected.
If this pulsation cannot be palpated, have the client assume a left lateral position. This displaces the heart toward the left chest wall and relocates the apical impulse farther to the left.		

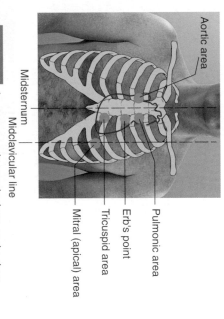

FIGURE 14-5 Areas to auscultate and palpate on the chest.

Aortic area

Pulmonic area

Erb's point

Tricuspid area

Mitral (apical) area

Midsternum

Midclavicular line

PROCEDURE

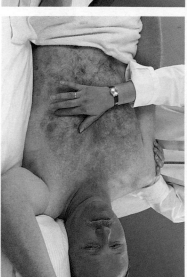

Locate the apical impulse with the palmar surface (left), and then palpate the apical pulse with the fingerpad (right). (© B. Proud.)

PERCUSSION

Percussion may be done to define cardiac borders by identifying areas of dullness, but it is generally unreliable. Size of heart can be more accurately determined by chest x-ray.

AUSCULTATION

Auscultate in an orderly, systematic fashion beginning with the aortic area. Move across and then down the chest. Focus on one sound at a time. Auscultate each area with the stethoscope diaphragm applied firmly to the chest. Repeat the sequence using the stethoscope bell applied lightly to the chest. Auscultate with the client in the supine position. Then listen specifically over the apex with the bell while client is in the left lateral position. Assist client to a sitting position, and auscultate the pericardium with the diaphragm. Then have client lean forward and exhale while you listen over the aortic area with the diaphragm.

PROCEDURE	NORMAL FINDINGS	DEVIATIONS FROM NORMAL
Auscultate to identify the **first heart sound** (S₁), or "lub," and the **second heart sound** (S₂), or "dub" (Fig. 14–6).	S₁ follows the long diastolic pause and precedes the short systolic pause and corresponds to each carotid pulsation. S₂ follows the short systolic phase and precedes the long diastolic phase.	
Auscultate for **rate and rhythm.**	*Rate:* 60–100 bpm *Rhythm* regular	Bradycardia (heart rate <60) tachycardia (heart rate >100) may result in decreased cardiac output; irregular rhythms

Heart Assessment

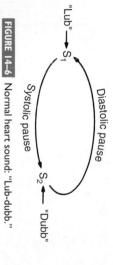

FIGURE 14-6 Normal heart sound: "Lub-dubb."

"Lub" → S₁

Diastolic pause

Systolic pause

S₂

"Dubb"

AUSCULTATION (continued)

PROCEDURE	NORMAL FINDINGS	DEVIATIONS FROM NORMAL
		(eg, premature beats of atrial or ventricular premature contractions, atrial flutter and atrial fibrillation with varying block) need to be referred.
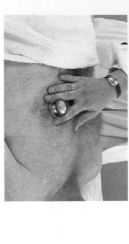\n\nAuscultating S_1. (© B. Proud.)	Radial and apical pulse should be identical.	
If irregular rhythm is detected, auscultate for **pulse rate deficit** by comparing the radial pulse with the apical pulse for a full minute.		A pulse deficit (difference between radial and apical pulses) may indicate atrial fibrillation, atrial flutter, premature ventricular contractions, and varying degrees of heart block.

PROCEDURE

Auscultate and focus on each sound and pause individually:

- Auscultate S₁: Heard best with diaphragm

- Auscultate S₂: Heard best with diaphragm

- Auscultate systolic pause space: Heard between S₁ and S₂ (see Fig. 14–6).

- Auscultate diastolic pause space: Heard between S₂ and the next S₁ (see Fig. 14–6).

NORMAL FINDINGS

Crisp, distinct sound heard in each area but loudest at mitral and tricuspid areas

May become softer with inspiration. Split S₁ is normal in children, young adults, and pregnant women.

Crisp, distinct sound heard loudest at the aortic and pulmonic areas. Split S₂ may be normal in adults if heard only during inspiration.

Silent pause—should hear distinct end of S₁ and beginning of S₂ with nothing in between

Silent pause—should hear distinct end of S₂ and distinct beginning of next S₁

DEVIATIONS FROM NORMAL

Split sound in middle-aged and older adults

Split sound heard equally during inspiration and expiration

- *Murmur:* Swishing sound heard at beginning, middle, or end of systolic pause (note intensity, pitch, and quality—Table 14–1).

- *Murmur:* Swishing sound heard at the middle of the systolic pause

- *Click:* Sharp, high-pitched snapping sound heard immediately after S₁, or in the middle of the systolic pause— Table 14–1

- *Murmur:* Swishing sound heard at beginning, middle, or end of diastolic pause (note intensity, pitch, and quality—Table 14–1).

TABLE 14-1 CLASSIFICATION FOR INTENSITY, PITCH, AND QUALITY OF MURMURS

Intensity

Grade 1—Very faint, heard only after the listener has "tuned in"; may not be heard in all positions

Grade 2—Quiet, but heard immediately upon placing stethoscope on the chest

Grade 3—Moderately loud

Grade 4—Loud with palpable thrill

Grade 5—Very loud, may be heard with stethoscope partly off the chest ⎫
Grade 6—May be heard with stethoscope entirely off the chest ⎬ Associated with thrills

Pitch

High, medium, or low

Quality

Blowing, rumbling, harsh, or musical

Adapted from Bickley,. L. S., & Szilagyi, P. G. (2003). *Bates' guide to physical examination and history taking* (8th ed.). Philadelphia: Lippincott Williams & Wilkins.

PROCEDURE

- Auscultate S_3 with bell of stethoscope: Low, faint sound occurring at the beginning of the diastolic pause (Fig. 14–7).

- Auscultate S_4: Soft, low-pitched sound heard best with client in supine or left lateral position with stethoscope bell (Fig. 14–8).

NORMAL FINDINGS

- S_3 auscultated in children and young adults but disappears upon standing or sitting up; heard in people with a high cardiac output; and in women in the third trimester of pregnancy

- Auscultated in trained athletes and some older clients, especially after exercise

DEVIATIONS FROM NORMAL

Snap: High-pitched snapping sound heard after S_2 during the diastolic pause in the mitral or tricuspid area

- S_3 auscultated in adults or that continues with standing or sitting in children and young adults; also called ventricular gallop (has rhythm of the word "Kentucky"); may be heard with ischemic heart disease, myocardial failure, volume overload of the ventricle from valvular disease; may be earliest sign of heart failure

- Auscultated in adults; also called atrial gallop (has rhythm of the word "Tennessee") and is associated with coronary artery disease, hypertension, aortic and pulmonic stenosis, and acute myocardial infarction

PEDIATRIC VARIATIONS

Subjective Data: Focus Questions

In addition to the focus questions for adults, inquire about the following: Mother's use of therapeutic drugs or drug abuse during pregnancy? Poor weight gain? Signs of delayed development (eg, slowed social development, language development, or motor skills)? Difficulty in feeding (breast, bottle, acceptance of new foods)? Inability to tolerate physical activity or play with peers? Squatting behavior? Excessive irritability or crying? Circumoral cyanosis or central cyanosis?

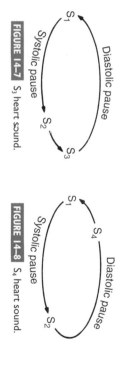

FIGURE 14-7 S_3 heart sound.

FIGURE 14-8 S_4 heart sound.

Objective Data: Assessment Techniques

PROCEDURE	NORMAL FINDINGS AND VARIATIONS
Inspect **chest wall** in semi-Fowler position from an angle for PMI.	PMI easily visible because heart is larger in proportion to chest size (Fig. 14–9). Heart lies more horizontally up to age 5 to 6 years. Thus, the PMI may be lateral to the MCL.
Palpate **peripheral pulse points** in relation to apical pulse and to each other: Femoral, radial, brachial, and carotid.	Symmetrical and equal rate, strength, and rhythm
Percuss **heart size.** (**Note:** This is rarely done owing to inaccuracy of the method.)	Percussion area is slightly larger because of horizontal position and overlying thymus gland.
Auscultate S_1 and S_2 at pulmonic area (Erb's point).	S_1 is louder than S_2, or S_2 is louder than S_1. Splitting of S_2 is heard best at Erb's point (25–33% of all children). This is a frequent site of innocent murmurs (grade 3 or lower), which are common throughout childhood. They are of short duration with no transmission to other areas, are low pitched, musical, or of groaning quality that is variable in intensity in relation to position, respiration, activity, fever, and anemia with no other associated signs of heart disease. Other murmurs may indicate pathology.

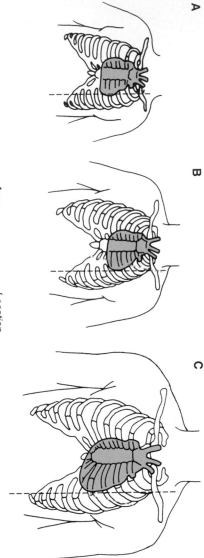

Age	Location
4 years	To left of midclavicular line
4–6 years	At midclavicular line
7–8 years	To right of midclavicular line

FIGURE 14-9 Location of apex of heart in (A) infant, (B) child, and (C) adult.

Objective Data: Assessment Techniques (continued)

PROCEDURE	NORMAL FINDINGS AND VARIATIONS
• Tricuspid area	• S_1 louder, preceding S_2
• Mitral area	• S_1 loudest
• Sinus arrhythmia	• Varies with respiration; very common and disappears with age
• Rate	• See Table 14-2 for normal pediatric pulse rates.

TABLE 14-2	AVERAGE HEART RATE OF INFANTS AND CHILDREN AT REST	
Age	**Average Rate (bpm)**	**±2 Standard Deviations**
Birth	140	90-190
First 6 months	130	80-180
6-12 months	115	75-155
1-2 years	110	70-150
2-6 years	103	68-138
6-10 years	95	65-125
10-14 years	85	55-115

From Bickley, L. S., & Szilagyi, P. G. (2003). *Bates' guide to physical examination and history taking* (8th ed.). Philadelphia: Lippincott Williams & Wilkins.

GERIATRIC VARIATIONS

- Thickening of heart walls
- Decreased elasticity of heart and arteries; reduced pumping ability of heart
- Decreased cardiac output and cardiac reserve
- Apical impulse may be difficult to palpate owing to increase in anteroposterior diameter of chest
- Location of heart sounds and PMI may be varied owing to kyphosis or scoliosis.
- Early and soft systolic murmurs are common.
- Atrial fibrillations often occur.
- Reduced maximum heart rate

CULTURAL VARIATIONS

- African Americans have higher HDL levels, but higher lifestyle risk factors for congenital heart disease (CHD) than white Americans.
- African Americans have higher rates of hypertension, stroke, and CHD than white Americans. Hypertension in U.S. black women has a higher incidence, earlier onset, and higher mortality than in white women (Overfield, 1995; Gillum, 1996).

Possible Collaborative Problems

Decreased cardiac output   Congenital heart disease
Congestive heart failure   Endocarditis
Myocardial ischemia   Angina
Cardiogenic shock   Dysrhythmia

TEACHING TIPS FOR SELECTED NURSING DIAGNOSES

Adult Client

Nursing Diagnosis: **Fear** related to perceived increased risk of heart disease and family history of heart disease

🖐 Explain what you are doing when auscultating so client won't become alarmed by the amount of time you are taking. Explain that vigorous exercise (20–30 minutes three times a week) may decrease serum triglycerides and cholesterol, and therefore may prevent heart disease by increasing the working capabilities of the body and heart capillaries. Advise client to have a complete physical examination prior to starting a new fitness program.

Nursing Diagnosis: **Ineffective Therapeutic Regimen Management** related to knowledge deficit: Taking pulse in order to assess heart rate prior to taking cardiac medications

🖐 Teach client correct method for taking pulse. Instruct on heart rate necessary for taking prescribed medication.

Nursing Diagnosis: **Ineffective Sexuality Patterns** related to fear of injury post myocardial infarction

🖐 Instruct client to discuss limitations on sexual activities as recommended by physician. (Usually, a client can safely engage in sexual intercourse by the time he or she is permitted to walk up a flight of stairs.)

Nursing Diagnosis: **Ineffective Therapeutic Regimen Management** related to knowledge deficit: Optimal diet for preventing coronary heart disease

🖐 Teach client the following dietary and lifestyle guidelines (American Heart Association, 2006):

- Elimination of cigarette smoking
- Appropriate levels of caloric intake and physical activity to prevent obesity and reduce weight if already overweight
- Consumption of 30% or less of the day's total calories from fat

- Limit saturated fat to 10% or less and cholesterol to 300 mg or less.
- Sodium intake should not exceed 6 g/day
- Consumption of 55 to 60% of calories as complex carbohydrates
- Eat a balanced diet including a variety of fruits, vegetables, whole grains, low-fat or nonfat dairy products, fish, legumes, poultry, and lean meat.
- For those who drink and for whom alcohol (ethanol) is not contraindicated, consumption should not exceed two drinks for a man and one drink for a woman per day. "One drink" means no more than 1/2 oz of pure alcohol. (1 oz of 100-proof whisky, 4 oz of wine, or 12 oz of beer contains 1/2 oz of ethanol).

Nursing Diagnosis: Ineffective Cardiopulmonary Tissue Perfusion related to excessive activity and congestive heart failure

🖐 Teach client to follow physician's activity recommendations. Teach client to cluster low-energy tasks (walk to bathroom, brush teeth, gather clothes, return to chair before putting on clothes). Teach client to space higher energy tasks with adequate rest periods. Teach client to take radial pulse and follow physician's recommendations for maximum pulse rate with activity.

Nursing Diagnosis: Readiness for Enhanced activity–exercise pattern

🖐 Teach client to seek physician's recommendation regarding an exercise plan and describe the following guidelines for healthy individuals (American Heart Association, 2005):

- Walk or do other physical activity for at least 30 minutes on most days. To lose weight, do enough activity to use more calories than you eat every day. May need to increase physical activity to 60 minutes most days of the week.
- Exercise only when feeling well. Wait until symptoms and signs of a cold or the flu (including fever) have been absent 2 days or more before resuming activity.
- Do not exercise vigorously soon after eating. Wait at least 2 hours.

- Adjust exercise to the weather. Exercise should be adjusted to environmental conditions. Special precautions are necessary when exercising in hot weather. If air temperature is >70°F (21.1°C), slow pace, be alert for signs of heat injury, and drink adequate fluids to maintain hydration. If air temperature is >80°F (26.6°C), exercise in early morning or late afternoon to avoid the heat. Air-conditioned shopping malls are popular for walking.

- Slow down for hills. When ascending hills, decrease speed to avoid overexertion.

- Wear proper clothing and shoes. Dress in loose-fitting, comfortable clothes made of porous material appropriate for the weather. Use sweat suits only for warmth.

- Understand personal limitations. Everyone should have periodic medical examinations. When under a physician's care, ask if there are activity limitations.

- Select appropriate exercises. Cardiovascular (aerobic) exercises should be a major component of activities. Flexibility and strengthening exercises, however, should also be considered for a well-rounded program.

- Be alert for symptoms. If the following symptoms occur, contact a physician before continuing exercise. Although any symptom should be clarified, these are particularly important: discomfort in upper body, including the chest, arm, neck, or jaw, during exercise; faintness accompanying exercise; shortness of breath during exercise; discomfort in bones and joints either during or after exercise. There may be slight muscle soreness when beginning exercise, but if back or joint pain develops, discontinue exercise until after evaluation by physician.

- Watch for the following signs of overexercising: inability to finish; inability to converse during the activity; faintness or nausea after exercise; chronic fatigue; sleeplessness; aches and pains in joints. Although there may be some muscle discomfort, joints should not hurt or feel stiff.

- Start slowly and progress gradually. Allow time to adapt.

PERIPHERAL VASCULAR ASSESSMENT

15

ANATOMY OVERVIEW

Arteries

Arteries are the blood vessels that carry oxygenated, nutrient-rich blood from the heart to the capillaries. The brachial artery is the major artery that supplies the arm. The brachial artery divides near the elbow to become the radial artery (extending down the thumb side of the arm) and the ulnar artery (extending down the little finger side of the arm). Both of these arteries provide blood to the hand (Fig. 15–1).

The femoral artery is the major supplier of blood to the legs. This artery travels down the front of the thigh and then crosses to the back of the thigh, where it is termed the popliteal artery. The popliteal artery divides below the knee into anterior and posterior branches. The anterior branch descends down the top of the foot, where it becomes the dorsalis pedis artery (see Fig. 15–1).

Veins

Veins are the blood vessels that carry deoxygenated, nutrient-depleted, waste-laden blood from the tissues back to the heart. The veins of the arms, upper trunk, head, and neck carry blood to the superior vena cava, where it passes into the right atrium. Blood from the lower trunk and legs drains upward into the inferior vena cava.

There are three types of veins: deep veins, superficial veins, and perforator (or communicator) veins. The two deep veins in the leg are the femoral vein in the upper thigh and the popliteal vein located behind the knee.

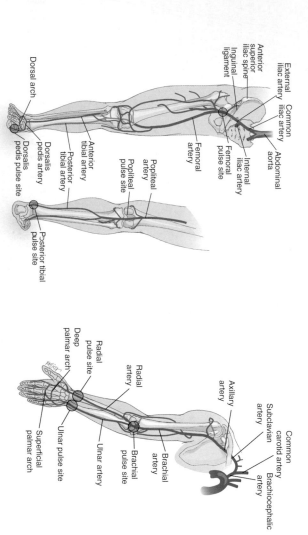

FIGURE 15—1 Major arteries of the arms and legs.

The superficial veins are the great and small saphenous veins. The great saphenous vein is the longest of all veins and it extends from the medial dorsal aspect of the foot, crosses over the medial malleolus, and continues across the thigh to the medial aspect of the groin, where it joins the femoral vein. The small saphenous vein begins at the lateral dorsal aspect of the foot, travels up behind the lateral malleolus on the back of the leg, and joins the popliteal vein. The perforator veins connect the superficial veins with the deep veins (Fig. 15-2).

Equipment Needed

- Stethoscope
- Sphygmomanometer
- Doppler
- Tape measure (paper)
- Cotton (to detect light touch)
- Paper clip (tip used to detect sharp sensation—safer than pin tip)
- Tuning fork (to detect vibratory sensation)

Subjective Data: Focus Questions

Any changes in skin color, texture, or temperature? Pain in calves, feet, buttocks, or legs? What aggravates the pain? Walking? Sitting for long periods? Standing for long periods? Does it awaken you? What relieves the pain? Elevating legs? Rest? Lying down? Is there associated coldness, cyanosis, edema, varicosities, paresthesia, or tingling in legs or feet? Any leg veins that are ropelike, bulging, or contorted? Any sores on legs? Location? Size? Appearance? Length of time? If client is male: Any changes in sexual activity? History of heart or blood vessel surgery? Family history of diabetes, hypertension, coronary artery disease, or elevated cholesterol or triglyceride levels? Is client taking any drugs that may mimic arterial insufficiency? Self-care activities: Does client have well-fitting shoes? Does client wear constricting garments or hosiery? In what type of chair does client usually sit? Does client cross legs frequently? What amount and type of exercise does the client do? Does client smoke? Amount and for how long?

Risk Factors. Risk for arterial peripheral vascular disease related to tobacco smoking, age over 50 years, family history of peripheral vascular disease, hypertension, coronary or peripheral vascular disease, or male sex.

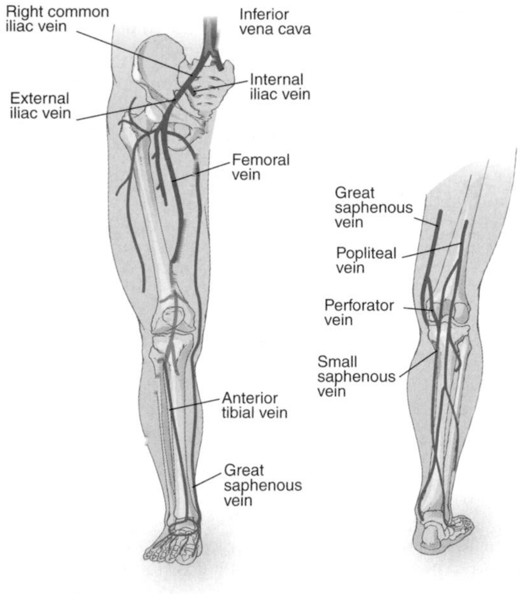

FIGURE 15-2 Major veins of the legs.

Right common
iliac vein

External
iliac vein

Inferior
vena cava

Internal
iliac vein

Femoral
vein

Anterior
tibial vein

Great
saphenous
vein

Great
saphenous
vein

Popliteal
vein

Perforator
vein

Small
saphenous
vein

Risk for venous peripheral vascular disease related to pregnancy, job with prolonged standing, limited physical activity/poor physical fitness, congenital or acquired vein wall weakness, female sex, increasing age, genetics (eg, non–African American), obesity, lack of dietary fiber, use of constricting corsets/clothes.

Objective Data: Assessment Techniques

See Figures 15–1 and 15–2 for diagrams of major arteries and veins.

INSPECTION, PALPATION, AND AUSCULTATION OF CIRCULATION TO ARMS AND NECK

Inspection, palpation, and auscultation are performed together to assess blood pressure and circulation to the upper extremities and neck while the client is in a sitting, then standing, position. A special maneuver (Allen test) is used to detect arterial insufficiency of the hand.

PROCEDURE	NORMAL FINDINGS	DEVIATIONS FROM NORMAL
Palpate brachial artery, and then auscultate arterial blood pressure alternately in both arms with client sitting.	May be difference of 5–10 mm Hg between both arms *Systolic pressure:* <120 mm Hg *Diastolic pressure:* <80 mm Hg* (see Table 4–2)	More than 10 mm Hg difference between both arms *Systolic pressure:* ≥120 mm Hg* *Diastolic pressure:* ≥80 mm Hg* (see Table 4–2)
Palpate brachial artery, and then auscultate arterial blood pressure alternately in both arms with client standing.	*Systolic pressure:* Difference between arms of 15 mm Hg or less *Diastolic pressure:* Difference between arms of 5 mm Hg or less	*Systolic pressure:* Difference between arms of more than 15 mm Hg *Diastolic pressure:* Difference between arms of more than 5 mm Hg

*Values may vary with individuals.

PROCEDURE	NORMAL FINDINGS	DEVIATIONS FROM NORMAL
Palpate each carotid artery alternately for rate, rhythm, symmetry, strength, and elasticity.	60–90 beats per minute; regular, equal, strong, and elastic	<60 or >90 bpm; irregular, unequal, weak and thready; bounding and firm, in-elastic. Pulse inequality may indicate arterial constriction or occlusion in one carotid. Weak pulses occur with hypo-volemia, shock, or decreased cardiac output. Loss of elasticity may indicate arteriosclerosis.

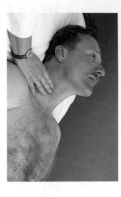

Palpating the carotid artery.
(© B. Proud.)

Caution: Use *light* palpation over carotids (one at a time) because increased pressure may stimulate carotid sinus reflex and lower heart rate and blood pressure.

INSPECTION, PALPATION, AND AUSCULTATION OF CIRCULATION TO ARMS AND NECK (continued)

PROCEDURE	NORMAL FINDINGS	DEVIATIONS FROM NORMAL
Auscultate carotid arteries with stethoscope bell while patient holds breath.	No sound heard	Bruit (swishing sound) is caused by turbulent blood flow through a narrowed vessel and is indicative of occlusive arterial disease.

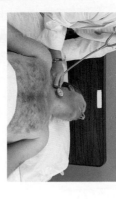

Auscultating the carotid artery.
(© B. Proud.)

Peripheral Vascular Assessment

INSPECTION, PALPATION, AND AUSCULTATION OF CIRCULATION TO ARMS AND NECK (continued)

PROCEDURE	NORMAL FINDINGS	DEVIATIONS FROM NORMAL
Inspect and palpate upper extremities for the following:		
• Color	• Pink; pink or red tones visible under dark pigmentation	• Pallor, cyanosis, rubor; rapid color changes—pallor, cyanosis, and redness seen with Raynaud disease
• Temperature	• Warm	• Cold, cool extremities seen with arterial insufficiency and Raynaud disease • Paresthesia, tenderness, pain; numbness seen in Raynaud disease
• Sensation: Scatter stimuli over trunk and upper extremities with client's eyes closed	• Client can identify light and deep touch; nontender.	
• Mobility • Radial pulses (Fig. 15–3)	• Mobile • Bilateral pulses strong and equal	• Paralysis • Bilateral/unilateral pulses weak, asymmetrical, or absent may indicate partial or complete obstruction; increased radial pulse may indicate hyperkinesis. • Bilateral/unilateral pulses weak, asymmetrical, or absent
• Ulnar pulses (Fig. 15–4)	• Bilateral pulses strong and equal	
If client has weak radial and/or ulnar pulses, perform Allen test, a special maneuver (Fig. 15–5).	Full palm of hand becomes pink with release of ulnar or radial artery.	Only half of palm of hand becomes pink with release of ulnar or radial artery; other half of palm remains whitish. Pallor persists with occlusion of ulnar artery.

Peripheral Vascular Assessment

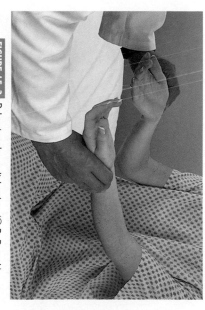

FIGURE 15-3 Palpating the radial pulse. (© B. Proud.)

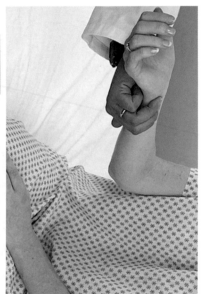

FIGURE 15–4 Palpating the ulnar pulse. (© B. Proud.)

A

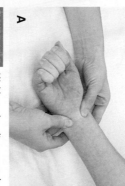

B

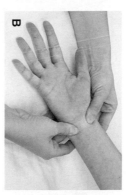

C

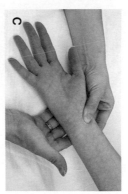

FIGURE 15-5 (A) Have the client rest the hand palm side up on the examination table and then make a fist. Use your thumbs to occlude the radial and ulnar arteries. (B) Continue pressure to keep both arteries occluded, and have the client release the fist. Note that the palm remains pale. (C) Release the pressure on the ulnar artery and watch for color to return to hand. To assess radial patency, repeat the procedure as before, but at the last step, release pressure on the radial artery. (© B. Proud.)

INSPECTION AND PALPATION OF JUGULAR VENOUS PRESSURE AND CIRCULATION OF LOWER EXTREMITIES

Inspection and palpation are performed together to assess the jugular venous pressure and circulation of the lower extremities with the client in a supine position. Finally, special maneuvers are performed to detect venous and arterial insufficiencies of the legs.

PROCEDURE	NORMAL FINDINGS	DEVIATIONS FROM NORMAL
Inspect jugular veins with head elevated 45°. Identify the highest point of venous wave (Fig. 15–6) in relation to the sternal angle. Measure in centimeters or inches.	Pulsation height ≤1 inch (3 cm)	Pulsation height >1 inch (3 cm). Fully distended veins with torso elevated are seen with increased central venous pressure that may be due to right ventricular failure, pulmonary hypertension, pulmonary edema, or cardiac tamponade.
Inspect and palpate legs for the following:		
• Color	• Pink; pink or red tones visible under dark pigmentation	• Pallor, cyanosis, rubor; pallor on elevation and rubor on dependency suggest arterial insufficiency; rusty or brownish pigmentation around ankles indicate venous insufficiency.

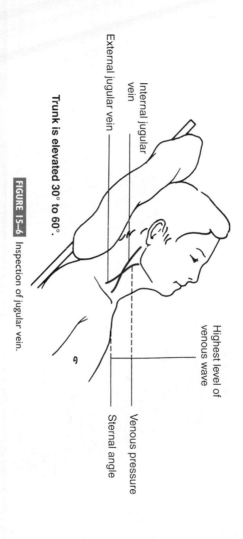

Trunk is elevated 30° to 60°.

Internal jugular vein

External jugular vein

Highest level of venous wave

Venous pressure

Sternal angle

FIGURE 15–6 Inspection of jugular vein.

INSPECTION AND PALPATION OF JUGULAR VENOUS PRESSURE AND CIRCULATION OF LOWER EXTREMITIES (continued)

PROCEDURE	NORMAL FINDINGS	DEVIATIONS FROM NORMAL
• Temperature	• Warm	• Cold; coolness in one leg suggests arterial insufficiency; increased warmth in leg may be due to throm- bophlebitis; bilateral coolness in feet and legs suggests cold room, recent cigarette smoking, or anxiety.
• Sensation: Scatter stimuli with client's eyes closed.	• Client can identify light and deep touch; nontender.	• Paresthesia, tenderness, pain
• Mobility	• Mobile	• Paralysis
• Superficial veins	• Slight venous distention with standing that collapses with elevation	• Severe venous distention and bulging are seen with varicose veins due to incompetent valves, vein wall weakness, or venous obstruction; superficial vein thrombophlebitis is characterized by redness, thickening, and tenderness along the vein.
• Condition of skin	• Intact	• Lesions
• Edema	• Not present	• Present
• Femoral pulse (Fig. 15–7)	• Bilateral pulses strong and equal	• Bilateral/unilateral pulses weak, asym- metrical, or absent in arterial occlusion

Peripheral Vascular Assessment

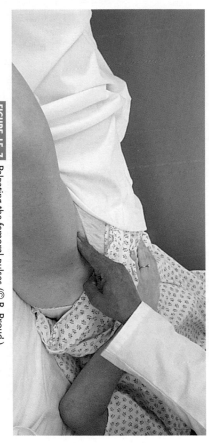

FIGURE 15-7 Palpating the femoral pulses (© B. Proud.)

INSPECTION AND PALPATION OF JUGULAR VENOUS PRESSURE AND CIRCULATION OF LOWER EXTREMITIES (continued)

PROCEDURE	NORMAL FINDINGS	DEVIATIONS FROM NORMAL
• Popliteal pulse: Have client bend knees or, if on table, roll onto stomach and flex leg 90°. Press deeply to feel (Fig. 15–8).	• Bilateral pulses strong and equal, but it is not unusual for popliteal pulse to be difficult or impossible to detect.	• Bilateral/unilateral pulses weak, asymmetrical, or absent may indicate occluded artery.
• Dorsalis pedis pulse: Have client dorsiflex or extend foot (Fig. 15–9).	• Bilateral pulses strong and equal (congenitally absent in 5–10% of population).	• Bilateral/unilateral pulses weak, asymmetrical, or absent may indicate impaired arterial circulation.
• Posterior tibial pulse (located on medial malleolus of ankle; Fig. 15–10).	• Bilateral pulses strong and equal	• Bilateral/unilateral pulses weak or absent may indicate arterial occlusion.

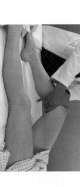
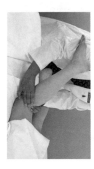

FIGURE 15–8 Palpating the popliteal pulse with the client (*left*) supine and (*right*) prone. If you cannot detect a pulse, try palpating with the client in a prone position. Partially raise the leg and place your fingers deep in the bend of the knee. Repeat palpation in opposite leg and note amplitude bilaterally. (© B. Proud.)

Peripheral Vascular Assessment

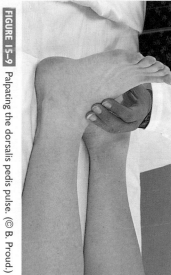

FIGURE 15-9 Palpating the dorsalis pedis pulse. (© B. Proud.)

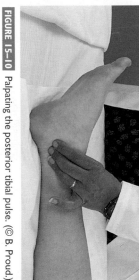

FIGURE 15-10 Palpating the posterior tibial pulse. (© B. Proud.)

INSPECTION AND PALPATION OF JUGULAR VENOUS PRESSURE AND CIRCULATION OF LOWER EXTREMITIES (continued)

PROCEDURE	NORMAL FINDINGS	DEVIATIONS FROM NORMAL
Special maneuvers: • Check for deep phlebitis by quickly squeezing calf muscles against tibia. • Check Homans sign by extending leg and dorsiflexing foot (Fig. 15–11).	• Client verbalizes no calf pain. • Client verbalizes no calf soreness or pain.	• Client verbalizes painful calves with deep phlebitis. • Client reports soreness and pain in calf with deep vein thrombosis or superficial thrombophlebitis; further diagnostic testing, however, is needed to confirm diagnosis.

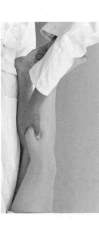 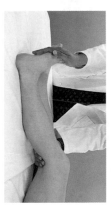

FIGURE 15–11 Elicit Homans sign by (*left*) squeezing the calf muscle and also by (*right*) passive dorsiflexion of the foot. (© B. Proud.)

INSPECTION AND PALPATION OF JUGULAR VENOUS PRESSURE AND CIRCULATION OF LOWER EXTREMITIES *(continued)*

PROCEDURE	NORMAL FINDINGS	DEVIATIONS FROM NORMAL
• Check for arterial insufficiency (Fig. 15–12) if leg pulses are decreased. Have client lie down on back while you support client's legs 12 inches above heart level. Have client flap feet up and down at ankles for 60 seconds, then sit up and dangle legs.	• Feet pink to slight pale color with this maneuver; pink color returns to tips of toes in 10 seconds; veins on top of feet fill in 15 seconds.	Extensive pallor with this maneuver in arterial insufficiency; toes and feet exhibit rubor (dusky red); venous return to feet is delayed 45 seconds or more in arterial insufficiency.

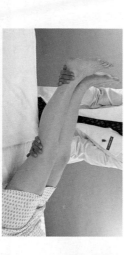 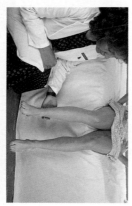

FIGURE 15–12 Testing for arterial insufficiency by *(left)* elevating the legs and then *(right)* having the client dangle the legs. (© B. Proud.)

INSPECTION AND PALPATION OF JUGULAR VENOUS PRESSURE AND CIRCULATION OF LOWER EXTREMITIES (continued)

PROCEDURE	NORMAL FINDINGS	DEVIATIONS FROM NORMAL
• Check for competency of valves (Fig. 15–13) (manual compression test) if client has varicose veins—compress dilated veins with one hand while using the other hand to feel pulsations 6–8 inches above the first hand. Repeat in other leg. Compare venous and arterial insufficiency of lower extremities (Table 15–1).	• No pulsation palpated	• Pulsation felt with incompetent valves **Note:** See Tables 15–1 and 15–2 for characteristics of venous and arterial insufficiencies and differentiation of arterial and venous ulcers.

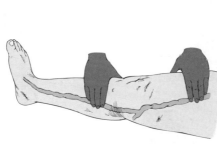

FIGURE 15–13 Performing manual compression to assess competence of venous valves in clients with varicose veins.

TABLE 15–1 COMPARISON OF ARTERIAL AND VENOUS INSUFFICIENCIES

	Arterial Insufficiency	Venous Insufficiency
Pulses	Decreased or absent	Present
Color	Pale on elevation, dusky rubor on dependency	Pink to cyanotic; brown pigment at ankles
Temperature	Cool, cold	Warm
Edema	None	Present
Skin	Shiny skin, thick nails, absence of hair, ulcers on toes, gangrene may develop (Table 15–2)	Ulcers on ankles; discolored, scaly
Sensation	Leg pain aggravated by exercise and relieved with rest; pressure or cramps in buttocks or calves during walking, paresthesias	Leg pain aggravated by prolonged standing or sitting, relieved by elevation of legs, lying down, or walking; also relieved with use of support hose

TABLE 15-2	CHARACTERISTICS OF VENOUS AND ARTERIAL INSUFFICIENCY AND LEG ULCERS

Venous Insufficiency	Arterial Insufficiency
Pain: Aching, cramping	Pain: Intermittent claudication to sharp, unrelenting, constant
Pulses: Present but may be difficult to palpate through edema	Pulses: Diminished or absent
Skin characteristics:	Skin characteristics: Dependent rubor
• Pigmentation in gaitor area (area of medial and lateral malleolus)	• Elevation pallor of foot
• Skin thickened and tough	• Dry, shiny skin
• May be reddish-blue in color	• Cool-to-cold temperature
• Frequently associated with dermatitis	• Loss of hair over toes and dorsum of foot
	• Nails thickened and ridged
Ulcer characteristics:	**Ulcer characteristics:**
• Location: Medial malleolus or anterior tibial area	• Location: Tips of toes, toe webs, heel, or other pressure areas as if confined to bed
• Pain: If superficial, minimal pain, but may be very painful	• Pain: Very painful
• Depth of ulcer: Superficial	• Depth of ulcer: Deep, often involving joint space
• Shape: Irregular border	• Shape: Circular
• Ulcer base: Granulation tissue—beefy red to yellow; fibrinous in chronic long-term ulcer	• Ulcer base: Pale black to dry and gangrene
• Leg edema: Moderate to severe	• Leg edema: Minimal unless extremity kept in dependent position constantly to relieve pain

(Used with permission from Smeltzer, S. C. & Bare, B. G. [2004]. *Brunner and Suddarth's textbook of medical-surgical nursing* [10th ed.]. Philadelphia: Lippincott Williams & Wilkins.)

INSPECTION AND PALPATION OF JUGULAR VENOUS PRESSURE AND CIRCULATION OF LOWER EXTREMITIES (continued)

PROCEDURE	NORMAL FINDINGS	DEVIATIONS FROM NORMAL
Auscultation of Arteries *If arterial insufficiency is found in legs, auscultate over the following areas:*		
• Aorta	• No sound	• Bruits
• Renal arteries	• No sound	• Bruits
• Iliac arteries	• No sound	• Bruits
• Femoral arteries (Fig. 15–14)	• No sound	• Bruits

CULTURAL VARIATIONS

African Americans have fewer valves in the external iliac veins but many more valves lower in the leg than do Caucasians, which may account for a lower prevalence of varicose veins in blacks (1–3%) than in whites (10–18%) [Overfield, 1995].

GERIATRIC VARIATIONS

• Hair loss of lower extremities occurs with aging and may not be an absolute sign of arterial insufficiency.
• Inspect for rigid, tortuous veins and arteries (decreased venous return and competency) because varicosities are common in older adult.

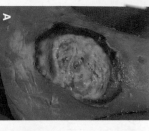

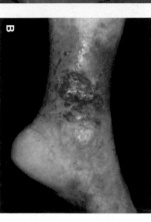

(A) Characteristic ulcer of arterial insufficiency. (© 1994 Michael English, M.D.) (B) Characteristic ulcer of venous insufficiency. (Courtesy of Dermik Laboratories, Inc.)

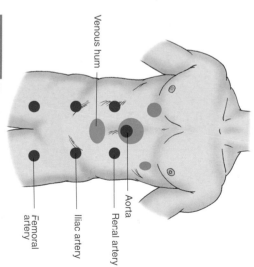

FIGURE 15-14 Vascular sounds and friction rubs can best be heard over these areas.

Venous hum

Aorta

Renal artery

Iliac artery

Femoral artery

- Prominent, bulging veins are common. Varicosities are considered a problem only if ulcerations, signs of thrombophlebitis, or cords are present. Cords are nontender, palpable veins having a rubber tubing consistency.
- Blood pressure increases as elasticity decreases in arteries with proportionately greater increase in systolic pressure resulting in a widening of pulse pressure.

Possible Collaborative Problems

Hypertension
Thrombophlebitis
Arterial insufficiency
Peripheral neuropathy
Thrombosis/emboli
Venous insufficiency

Edema
Gangrene
Vasospasms
Claudication
Stasis ulcers

TEACHING TIPS FOR SELECTED NURSING DIAGNOSES AND COLLABORATIVE PROBLEMS

Adult Client

Nursing Diagnosis: Impaired Skin Integrity related to arterial insufficiency

🕐 Instruct client on importance of exercise and diet (eat foods high in protein, vitamins A and C, and zinc to promote healing, unless contraindicated by other therapies) to aid healing of leg ulcers. Explain importance of keeping area clean and dry.

Nursing Diagnosis: Impaired Skin Integrity related to venous insufficiency

🕐 Instruct client on importance of rest, avoidance of restrictive clothing, elevation of extremities to reduce edema, and proper diet to aid healing of leg ulcers.

Nursing Diagnosis: Ineffective Peripheral Tissue Perfusion related to venous insufficiency

🖐 Teach client how to assess condition of extremities (color, temperature, movement, swelling). Teach client how to use assessment to determine activity level. Teach methods for accomplishing activities of daily living with restricted activity level.

Nursing Diagnosis: Risk for Peripheral Neurovascular Dysfunction related to increasing peripheral vascular disease

🖐 Teach client how to assess condition of extremities (color, temperature, sensation, movement, swelling). Teach client how to modify activities of daily living in order to prevent injury and complications.

Teach client to:

- Stop smoking. Smoking is the single most preventable cause of disease and death in the United States (Healthy People 2010).
- Control hypertension.
- Eat a diet low in saturated and total fat (less than 30% of calories from total fat) (Healthy People 2010).
- Increase dietary fiber intake (vegetables, fruits, and whole grains) (Healthy People 2010).
- Control high blood sugars of diabetes mellitus.
- Limit alcohol intake (Healthy People 2010).
- Get regular exercise (at least 30 minutes of moderate to vigorous exercise most days) (Healthy People 2010).
- Maintain weight within ideal range for height and body structure (Healthy People 2010).
- Avoid prolonged standing or sitting; modify work and leisure habits to vary position (eg, to reduce risk for hemorrhoids, use squatting position when toileting).
- Avoid constrictive clothing, including girdles, garters for stockings or tightly cuffed knee-high hose, or any items that compress vessels.

Collaborative Problem: Potential complication: Hypertension

🖐 Explain the effects of diet (low fat and low cholesterol), reduction of stress, vigorous exercise, not smoking, and decreased use of alcohol on promotion of adequate circulation. Blood pressure checks should be done on a regular basis. Blood pressures of 120–139/80–89 mm Hg are considered prehypertensive and require lifestyle modification (Seventh Report of the Joint National Committee on Prevention, Detection, and Treatment of High Blood Pressure, 2003). Refer any client with a reading ≥140/90 mm Hg for treatment.

ABDOMINAL ASSESSMENT

16

ANATOMY OVERVIEW

Abdominal Quadrants

The abdomen is divided into four quadrants for purposes of physical examination. These are termed the right upper quadrant (RUQ), right lower quadrant (RLQ), left lower quadrant (LLQ), and left upper quadrant (LUQ) (Fig. 16–1). Note which organs are located within each quadrant (Box 16–1).

Internal Anatomy

Within the abdominal cavity are structures of several different body systems—gastrointestinal, reproductive (female), lymphatic, and urinary. These structures are typically referred to as the abdominal viscera and can be divided into two types—solid viscera and hollow viscera. Solid viscera are those organs that maintain their shape consistently—the liver, pancreas, spleen, adrenal glands, kidneys, ovaries, and uterus. The hollow viscera consist of structures that change shape depending on their contents. These include the stomach, gallbladder, small intestine, colon, and bladder.

Solid Viscera

The liver is the largest solid organ in the body. It is located below the diaphragm in the RUQ of the abdomen. (Fig. 16–2). The pancreas, located mostly behind the stomach, deep in the upper abdomen, is normally not palpable (see Fig. 16–2 and 16–3). The spleen is approximately 7 cm wide and is located above the left kidney, just below the diaphragm at the level of

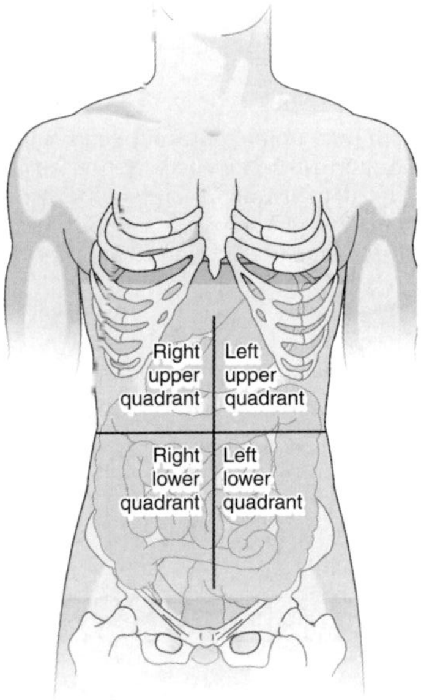

FIGURE 16-1 Abdominal quadrants.

BOX 16-1 ● Locating Abdominal Structures by Quadrants

RIGHT UPPER QUADRANT (RUQ)

Ascending and transverse colon
Duodenum
Gallbladder
Hepatic flexure of colon
Liver
Pancreas (head)
Pylorus (the small bowel—or ileum—traverses all quadrants)
Right adrenal gland
Right kidney (upper pole)
Right ureter

RIGHT LOWER QUADRANT (RLQ)

Appendix
Ascending colon
Cecum
Right kidney (lower pole)
Right ovary and tube
Right ureter
Right spermatic cord

LEFT UPPER QUADRANT (LUQ)

Left adrenal gland
Left kidney (upper pole)
Left ureter
Pancreas (body and tail)
Spleen
Splenic flexure of colon
Stomach
Transverse ascending colon

LEFT LOWER QUADRANT (LLQ)

Left kidney (lower pole)
Left ovary and tube
Left ureter
Left spermatic cord
Sigmoid colon

MIDLINE

Bladder
Uterus
Prostate gland

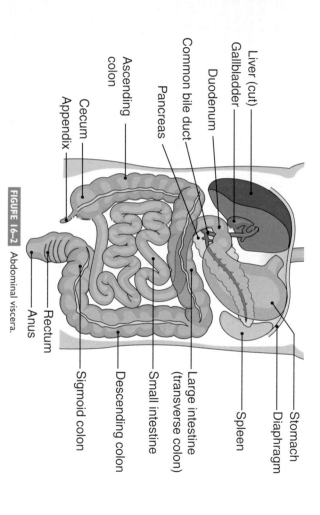

FIGURE 16-2 Abdominal viscera.

Liver (cut)
Gallbladder
Duodenum
Common bile duct
Pancreas
Ascending colon
Cecum
Appendix
Rectum
Anus
Sigmoid colon
Descending colon
Small intestine
Large intestine (transverse colon)
Spleen
Stomach
Diaphragm

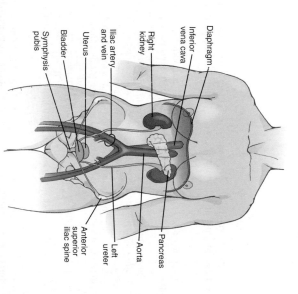

FIGURE 16–3 Abdominal and vascular structures (aorta and iliac artery and vein).

the ninth, 10th, and 11th ribs (see Fig. 16–2). This soft, flat structure is normally not palpable. The kidneys are located high and deep under the diaphragm (see Fig. 16–3).

The pregnant uterus may be palpated above the level of the symphysis pubis in the midline (see Fig. 16–3). The ovaries are located in the RLQ and LLQ and are normally palpated only during a bimanual examination of the internal genitalia.

Hollow Viscera

The stomach is a distensible, flasklike organ located in the LUQ, just below the diaphragm and in between the liver and spleen. The stomach is not usually palpable (see Fig. 16–2).

The gallbladder, a muscular sac approximately 10 cm long, is not normally palpable because it is difficult to distinguish between the gallbladder and the liver (see Fig. 16–2).

The small intestine is actually the longest portion of the digestive tract (approximately 7.0 m long). The small intestine, which lies coiled in all four quadrants of the abdomen, is not normally palpated (see Fig. 16–2).

The colon, or large intestine, has a wider diameter than the small intestine (approximately 6.0 cm) and is approximately 1.4 m long. The colon is composed of three major sections: ascending, transverse, and descending.

The sigmoid colon is often felt as a firm structure on palpation, whereas the cecum and ascending colon may feel softer. The transverse and descending colon may also be felt on palpation (see Fig. 16–2).

The urinary bladder is a distensible muscular sac located behind the pubic bone in the midline of the abdomen. A bladder filled with urine may be palpated in the abdomen above the symphysis pubis (see Fig. 16–3).

Vascular Structures

The abdominal organs are supplied with arterial blood by the abdominal aorta and its major branches. Pulsations of the aorta are frequently visible and palpable midline in the upper abdomen (see Fig. 16–3).

Equipment Needed

- Stethoscope (warm)
- Small ruler
- Marking pencil
- Small pillows

Subjective Data: Focus Questions

Abdominal pain? Character? Onset? Location? Duration? Severity? Relieving and aggravating factors? Associated factors? See Box 16–2. Indigestion? Nausea? Vomiting? Precipitating/relieving factors? Change in appetite? Associated weight loss? Change in bowel elimination? Describe. Constipation? Diarrhea? Associated symptoms? Any past gastrointestinal (GI) disorders (ulcers, reflux, inflammatory, obstructive bowel, pancreatitis, gallbladder or liver disease, diverticulosis, appendicitis, history of viral hepatitis)? Family history of colon, stomach, pancreatic, liver, kidney, or bladder cancer? Use of medications—aspirin, anti-inflammatory drugs, steroids? GI diagnostic tests? Surgeries? Health practices: Usual diet? Exercise? Use of alcohol? Stressors?

Risk Factors. Risk for hepatitis B virus (HBV) exposure related to contact in population of high HBV endemicity, sexual contact with carriers, intravenous drug abusers, heterosexuals who have had more than one sex partner in past 6 months, sexually active homosexual or bisexual males, hemophiliac patients, hemodialysis patients, international travelers in high-risk HBV areas, health care workers, long-term inmates.

Risk for gallbladder cancer related to female sex after menopause, increased parity, obesity, and chronic inflammation.

Risk for colon cancer related to age over 50 years, family history of colorectal cancer, patient history of endometrial, breast, or ovarian cancer, patient history of inflammatory bowel disease, polyps, or colorectal cancer.

Objective Data: Assessment Techniques

Review Figures 16–1 through 16–3 for a diagram of landmarks of the abdomen.

Assessment of the abdomen differs from other assessments in that inspection and auscultation precede percussion and palpation. This sequence allows accurate assessment of bowel sounds and delays more uncomfortable maneuvers until last. The client is placed in the supine position, with small pillows under the head and knees. The abdomen is exposed from the breasts to the symphysis pubis.

Examiner should warm hands and have short fingernails. Stand at the client's right side and carry out assessment systematically, beginning with the LUQ and progressing clockwise through the four abdominal quadrants (see Fig. 16–1). The client's bladder should be empty.

BOX 16-2 • Mechanisms and Sources of Abdominal Pain

Types of Pain

Abdominal pain may be formally described as visceral, parietal, or referred.

- *Visceral pain* occurs when hollow abdominal organs, such as the intestines, become distended or contract forcefully or when the capsules of solid organs such as the liver and spleen are stretched. Poorly defined or localized and intermittently timed, this type of pain is often characterized as dull, aching, burning, cramping, or colicky.

- *Parietal pain* occurs when the parietal peritoneum becomes inflamed, as in appendicitis or peritonitis. This type of pain tends to localize more to the source and is characterized as a more severe and steady pain.

- *Referred pain* occurs at distant sites that are innervated at approximately the same levels as the disrupted abdominal organ. This type of pain travels, or refers, from the primary site and becomes highly localized at the distant site. The accompanying illustrations show common clinical patterns and referents of pain.

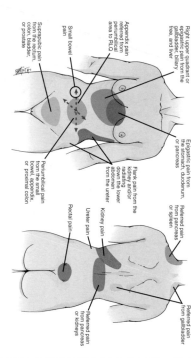

Right upper quadrant or epigastric pain from the gallbladder, biliary tree, and liver

Epigastric pain from the stomach, duodenum, or pancreas

Small bowel pain

Appendix pain referred to periumbilical area to RLQ

Referred pain from pancreas or spleen

Flank pain from the kidney and/or referred radiating down the lower abdomen from the ureter

Referred pain from gallbladder

Suprapubic pain from the rectum, colon, bladder, or prostate

Periumbilical pain from the small bowel, appendix, or proximal colon

Rectal pain

Ureter pain

Kidney pain

Referred pain from pancreas or kidneys

BOX 16-2 • (continued)

Character of Abdominal Pain and Implications

Dull, Aching

Appendicitis
Acute hepatitis
Biliary colic
Cholecystitis
Cystitis
Dyspepsia
Glomerulonephritis
Incarcerated or strangulated hernia
Irritable bowel syndrome
Hepatocellular cancer
Pancreatitis
Pancreatic cancer
Perforated gastric or duodenal ulcer
Peritonitis
Peptic ulcer disease
Prostatitis

Burning, Gnawing

Dyspepsia
Peptic ulcer disease
Cramping ("crampy")
Acute mechanical obstruction
Appendicitis
Colitis
Diverticulitis
Gastroesophageal reflux disease
  (GERD)

Pressure

Benign prostatic hypertrophy
Prostate cancer
Prostatitis
Urinary retention

Colicky

Colon cancer

Sharp, Knifelike

Splenic abscess
Splenic rupture
Renal colic
Renal tumor
Ureteral colic
Vascular liver tumor

Variable

Stomach cancer

INSPECTION

PROCEDURE	NORMAL FINDINGS	DEVIATIONS FROM NORMAL
Inspect the **skin** *for the following:*		
• Color	• Normally paler, with white striae	• Dark bluish striae seen in Cushing syndrome, redness seen in inflammation, pale and taut with ascites, purple flank color (Grey Turner sign) seen with bleeding within the abdominal wall
• Venous pattern	• Fine veins observable	• Engorged, prominent veins seen with cirrhosis of the liver, inferior vena cava obstruction, portal hypertension, or ascites
• Integrity	• No rashes or lesions	• Rashes, lesions
Special maneuver for prominent abdominal veins:		
• Compress a section of vein with two fingers next to each other, remove one finger, and observe for filling; repeat procedure, removing other finger.	• Blood fills from upper to lower abdomen	• Blood fills from lower to upper abdomen (obstructed inferior vena cava)

PROCEDURE	NORMAL FINDINGS	DEVIATIONS FROM NORMAL
Inspect the **umbilicus** for the following:		
• Position	• Sunken, centrally located	• Deviated from midline with mass, hernia, enlarged organs, or fluid; everted with abdominal distention or umbilical hernia
• Color	• Pinkish	• Inflamed, crusted; bluish color (Cullen sign) seen in intra-abdominal hemorrhage
Observe the **abdomen** for the following:		
• Contour	• Rounded or flat	• Generalized distention seen with air or fluid accumulation; distention below umbilicus due to full bladder, uterine enlargement, ovarian tumor or cyst; distention above the umbilicus seen with pancreatic mass or gastric dilation
• Symmetry	• Symmetrical	• Asymmetrical with organ enlargement, large masses, hernia, diastasis recti, or bowel obstruction

INSPECTION (continued)

PROCEDURE	NORMAL FINDINGS	DEVIATIONS FROM NORMAL
• Surface motion	• No movement or slight peristalsis visualized over aorta	• Diminished abdominal movement with peritoneal irritation; bounding peristalsis, bounding pulsations with abdominal aortic aneurysm; peristaltic, ripple waves seen with intestinal obstruction
Observe **color of stools.**	Brown to dark brown	Black, tarry (melena), bright red
Observe **color of emesis.**	Varies	Bloody (hematemesis), coffee grounds (old blood)

AUSCULTATION

Using the diaphragm of a warm stethoscope, apply light pressure to auscultate for bowel sounds for up to 5 minutes in each quadrant. Use the bell to auscultate for vascular sounds.

PROCEDURE	NORMAL FINDINGS	DEVIATIONS FROM NORMAL
Auscultate for **bowel sounds.**	High-pitched, irregular gurgles 5–35 times/min; present equally in all four quadrants	Absent with peritonitis or paralytic ileus; hypoactive in abdominal surgery or late bowel obstruction; hyperactive sounds heard in diarrhea, gastroenteritis, or

AUSCULTATION (continued)

PROCEDURE	NORMAL FINDINGS	DEVIATIONS FROM NORMAL
		early bowel obstruction; high-pitched tinkling and rushes (borborygmus) heard in bowel obstruction
Auscultate for **vascular sounds** (Fig. 16–4).	No bruits, no venous hums, no friction rubs	Bruits heard over aorta, renal arteries, or iliac arteries; venous hum auscultated over epigastric or umbilical area may indicate increased collateral circulation between portal and systemic venous systems as with cirrhosis of the liver.

Caution: If bruits are heard, do *not* palpate abdomen as part of the assessment. (Bruits may be indicative of a narrowed vessel or aneurysm.)

PERCUSSION

Percussion notes will vary from dull to tympanic, with tympany dominating over the hollow organs. The hollow organs include the stomach, intestines, bladder, aorta, and gallbladder. Dull percussion notes will be heard over the liver, spleen, pancreas, kidneys, and uterus. Percuss from areas of tympany to dullness to locate borders of these solid organs.

Abdominal Assessment

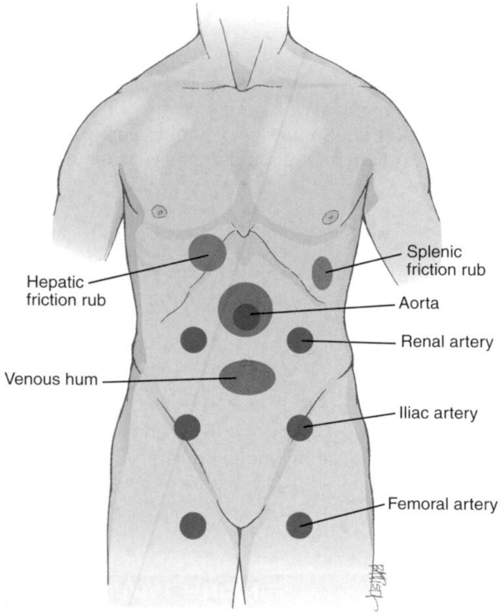

FIGURE 16–4 Vascular sounds and friction rubs can best be heard over these areas.

PROCEDURE

Percuss **all four quadrants** for percussion tones (notes); see Figure 16–5.

Percuss the **liver** *for span (Fig. 16–6) as follows:*

- Percuss starting below umbilicus at client's right midclavicular line (MCL), and percuss upward until you hear dullness; mark this point. Percuss downward from lung resonance in the right MCL to dullness and mark.

- Repeat in midsternal line.

Percuss the **spleen** *(Fig. 16–7) as follows:*

- Percuss for dullness by percussing downward in left midaxillary line, beginning with lung resonance

NORMAL FINDINGS

Generalized tympany over bowels

- Liver span is 6–12 cm (2.5–5 inches) in the right MCL.

Note: Span is greater in men.

- Liver span is 4–8 cm in midsternal line.

- Small area of dullness at sixth to 10th ribs

DEVIATIONS FROM NORMAL

Increased dullness over enlarged organs; hyperresonance over gaseous, distended abdomen

- Liver span is greater than 12 cm in the right MCL with enlarged liver as seen in tumors, cirrhosis, abscess, and vascular engorgement. A liver in a lower position may be caused by emphysema, and a liver in a higher position may be caused by a mass, ascites, or paralyzed diaphragm.
- Liver span is greater than 8 cm in right midsternal line.

- Dullness extends above sixth rib or covers larger area. Enlarged spleen is

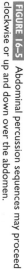

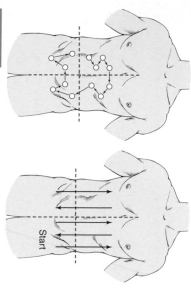

FIGURE 16–5 Abdominal percussion sequences may proceed clockwise or up and down over the abdomen.

Start

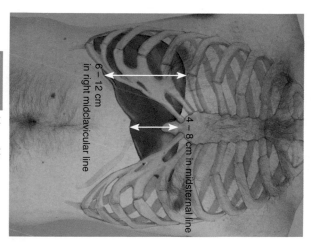

FIGURE 16–6 Normal liver span.

6 – 12 cm in right midclavicular line

4 – 8 cm in midsternal line

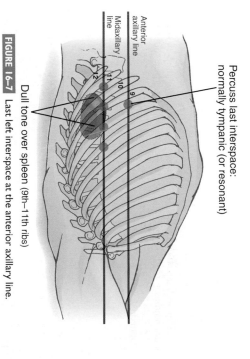

Percuss last interspace:
normally tympanic (or resonant)

Anterior
axillary line

Midaxillary
line

Dull tone over spleen (9th–11th ribs)

FIGURE 16–7 Last left interspace at the anterior axillary line.

PERCUSSION (continued)

PROCEDURE	NORMAL FINDINGS	DEVIATIONS FROM NORMAL
until you hear splenic dullness. (*Note*: Location fluctuates with respiration.)		seen with portal hypertension, mononucleosis, or trauma.
• Splenic percussion sign: Ask client to inhale deeply and hold breath; percuss lowest interspaces at left anterior axillary line.	• Percussion note remains tympanic on inhalation.	• Percussion note becomes dull on inhalation.

PALPATION

Light palpation precedes deep palpation to detect tenderness and superficial masses. Deep palpation is used to detect masses and size of organs.

Watch the client's facial expressions and body posture carefully to help assess pain. Examine tender areas last. Never use deep palpation over tender organs in client with polycystic kidneys, after renal transplant, or after hearing an abnormal bruit. Use deep palpation with caution.

PROCEDURE	NORMAL FINDINGS	DEVIATIONS FROM NORMAL
Lightly palpate all four quadrants for the following (also observe facial expression):		
• Tenderness	• Nontender	• Tender, painful with infection, inflammation, pressure from gaseous distention, tumors, or enlarged organs
• Consistency	• Soft, nontender	• Rigid, boardlike
• Masses	• No masses	• Superficial masses (A superficial mass becomes more prominent against examiner's hand when client lifts head from examination table, whereas a deep abdominal mass does not.)
Deeply palpate all four quadrants for the following:		
• Tenderness	• Mild tenderness over midline at xiphoid, cecum, sigmoid colon	• Tenderness, severe pain seen with tumor, cyst, abscess, enlarged organ, aneurysm, or adhesions
• Guarding	• Voluntary guarding	• Involuntary guarding is seen with peritoneal irritation; right-sided guarding is seen with acute cholecystitis.
• Masses	• No masses; aorta; feces in colon	• Masses

PALPATION (continued)

PROCEDURE	NORMAL FINDINGS	DEVIATIONS FROM NORMAL
Palpate deeply for **liver border** *at right costal margin (Box 16–3) for the following:*		
• Tenderness	• Nontender	• Tenderness seen in trauma or diseased liver
• Consistency	• Smooth, firm sharp edge, no masses	• Hard, firm liver may indicate cancer; nodularity may occur with tumors, metastatic cancer, late cirrhosis, or syphilis.
Palpate deeply for **splenic border,** *using bimanual technique (see Box 16–3). Check for the following:*		
• Size	• Not normally palpable	• Enlarged and palpable with trauma, mononucleosis, blood disorders, and malignancies
• Tenderness	• Nontender	• Tender

BOX 16–3 • Guidelines for Liver and Spleen Palpation

Liver Palpation

1. Stand at client's right side and place your left hand under client's back at the 11th and 12th ribs.
2. Place right hand parallel to right costal margin.
3. Ask client to breathe deeply, and press upward with your right fingers with each inhalation.

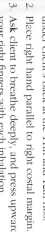

Spleen Palpation

1. Stand at client's right side; reach across client to place your left hand under client's posterior lower ribs, and push up.
2. Place your right hand below client's rib margin.
3. Ask client to breathe deeply.
4. Press hands together to palpate spleen on inhalation.

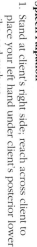

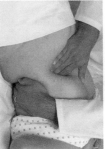

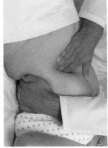

Abdominal Assessment

PROCEDURE	NORMAL FINDINGS	DEVIATIONS FROM NORMAL
Palpate deeply for the **kidneys** by using bimanual technique (Box 16–4). Assess for the following:		
• Size	• Not normally palpable	• Enlarged and palpable owing to cyst, tumor, or hydronephrosis
• Tenderness	• Nontender	• Tender
• Masses	• No masses	• Masses
Special maneuvers for ascites:		
• Measure abdominal girth at same point every day.	• No increase in abdominal girth	• Increase in abdominal girth
• Fluid wave test: Place palmar surfaces of fingers and hand firmly on one side of abdomen. Tap with other hand on opposite abdominal wall side. Have assistant put lateral side of lower arm firmly on center of abdomen (Fig. 16–8).	• No fluid wave transmitted	• Fluid wave palpated with ascites
• Shifting dullness: Place client in supine position and percuss from midline to flank, noting level of dullness. Then assist client to side position and percuss again for level of dullness (Fig. 16–9).	• Level of dullness does not change.	• Level of dullness is higher when client turns on side.

BOX 16-4 ● Guidelines for Kidney Palpation

1. Place one of your hands behind lower edge of rib cage and above iliac crest.
2. Place the other hand over corresponding anterior surface.
3. Instruct client to breathe deeply.
4. Lift up lower hand and push in with upper hand as client exhales.
5. Repeat on other side.

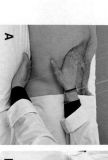

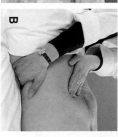

(*Note:* The kidneys are rarely palpable.)

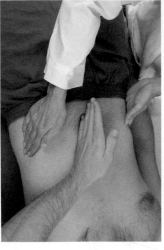

FIGURE 16-8 Performing fluid wave test.

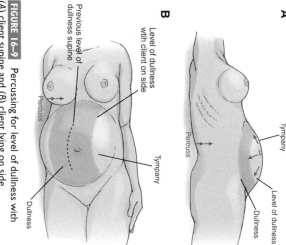

A

Tympany

Percuss

Level of dullness

Dullness

B

Previous level of dullness supine

Level of dullness with client on side

Percuss

Tympany

Dullness

FIGURE 16-9 Percussing for level of dullness with (A) client supine and (B) client lying on side.

PROCEDURE	NORMAL FINDINGS	DEVIATIONS FROM NORMAL
Special tests for appendicitis:		
• Rebound tenderness: Palpate deeply in one of client's four abdominal quadrants, and quickly withdraw palpating hand. Do this at end of abdominal exam.	• No pain present	• Pain is present in peritoneal irritation (as in appendicitis); because of danger of rupture do not repeat if pain is present.
• Psoas sign: Ask client to lie supine and raise right leg. Place pressure on client's thigh.	• No abdominal pain present	• Right lower abdominal pain present with irritation of the iliopsoas muscle due to appendicitis
• Obturator sign: Ask client to flex right leg at hip and knee. Then rotate leg internally and externally.	• No abdominal pain present	• Lower abdominal pain present with irritation of the obturator muscle due to appendicitis
Special test for acute cholecystitis (Murphy sign):		
• Place thumb below right costal margin and ask patient to inhale deeply.	• Client has no increase in pain.	• Client has sharp increase in pain with cholecystitis.
Testing for asterixis (classic sign of hepatic coma):		
• Dorsiflex client's wrist with fingers extended.	• No tremor noted	• Persistent, involuntary flapping tremor

PEDIATRIC VARIATIONS

Subjective Data: Focus Questions

Types of food, fluids, and formula? Bowel patterns? Frequent spitting up? Ability to feed self? Milk intake? Food intolerances? History of eating disorders? History of pica?

Objective Data: Assessment Techniques

INSPECTION

PROCEDURE	NORMAL VARIATIONS
Inspect **contour and size of abdomen.**	Prominent/cylindrical (protuberant) when erect, flat when supine. Superficial veins may be present in infants.
Inspect **abdominal movement** in children younger than 8 years.	Rises with inspiration in synchrony with chest; may have visible pulsations in epigastric region

PALPATION

Palpate **liver border.**	Normal, shortened liver span on percussion. May not extend below costal margin. *Infants and young children:* Liver may be felt 1–3 cm below costal margin; may descend with inspiration.
Palpate **splenic border** (may have child roll on right side).	*Infants and young children:* Spleen may be felt 1–3 cm below costal margin.

PROCEDURE

Palpate for **abdominal tenderness.**

Palpate **kidney borders.**

NORMAL VARIATIONS

Extremely difficult to assess in young children, who may confuse pressure of palpation with pain. Distraction is important.

Difficult to locate except in newborns

GERIATRIC VARIATIONS

- Decline in appetite and at risk for nutritional imbalance
- Dilated superficial capillaries visible
- Abdomen is softer and organs more easily palpated owing to a decrease in tone of abdominal musculature.
- Decreased production of saliva, decreased peristalsis, decreased enzymes, weaker gastric acid
- Gastric mucosa and parietal cell degeneration results in a loss of intrinsic factor, which decreases absorption of vitamin B_{12}.
- Bowel sounds 5–30 sounds/min
- Shortened liver span on percussion due to a decrease in liver size after age 50 years
- Liver border is more easily palpated.
- Decreased nerve sensation to lower bowel contributes to constipation.

Abdominal Assessment

Possible Collaborative Problems

Bowel strangulation	Intestinal obstruction	Peritonitis
Ascites	Paralytic ileus	Malabsorption syndrome
Metabolic acidosis/alkalosis	Diverticulitis	Pancreatitis
GI bleeding	Hepatic failure	Stromal changes
Gastric ulcer	Evisceration	Gallbladder disease (stones and cancer)

TEACHING TIPS FOR SELECTED NURSING DIAGNOSES

Adult Client

Nursing Diagnosis: Imbalanced Nutrition: More or less than body requirements

Discuss essential components of a well-balanced diet in relation to client's level of physical development and energy expenditure (basal metabolic rate). Teach client how to keep a daily food diary in order to assess intake.

Discuss with client the following:

- Decreasing calories
- Increasing carbohydrates (whole grains and vegetables)
- Decreasing saturated fats
- Decreasing refined sugars
- Decreasing intake of cholesterol to 300 mg/day and salt to 5 g/day

Provide information on support groups such as Weight Watchers, TOPS (Take Off Pounds Sensibly).

Nursing Diagnosis: Risk for Constipation

Discuss bowel habits that are "normal" for client. Caution against overuse of laxatives. Discourage overuse of mineral oil as a laxative because it decreases absorption of vitamins A, D, E, and K. Explain the effects of nutrients, bulk, fluids, and exercise on elimination. The American Cancer Society (*Cancer facts and figures*, 2006) recommends a

Pediatric Client

Nursing Diagnosis: Readiness for enhanced nutritional–metabolic pattern of child

⊙ Teach parents nutritional needs of the child at various ages:

Infant: Exclusive breast-feeding is the ideal nutrition for the first 6 months. Gradually introduce iron-enriched solid food at 6 months to complement breast-feeding. When possible, continue breast-feeding for at least 1 year. Introduce finger foods by 1 year. The American Academy of Pediatrics (1999) recommends that formula, if used, be fortified with iron. Breast-fed infants should get oral iron supplements. Fluoride supplements are required only if the water supply is severely deficient in fluoride.

Toddlers: Food fads are common. Accept this as long as child gets balanced diet over period of days versus every day.

Nursing Diagnosis: Fluid Volume Deficit related to vomiting or diarrhea

⊙ Teach parents to give child small amounts of clear liquids (approximately 1 oz every hour for 8 hours) until symptoms subside. May recommend Pedialyte for fluid and electrolyte replacement.

Nursing Diagnosis: Risk for Aspiration related to improper feeding and small size of stomach in newborns

⊙ Explain size of infant's stomach to parents (holds 60 mL), and demonstrate proper burping technique to use after every ½ oz feeding.

high-fiber, low-fat diet that includes a variety of vegetables and fruits to reduce the risk of certain cancers. It also recommends limiting consumption of alcohol. Advise client to eat a varied diet, maintain a desirable weight, eliminate tobacco use, and be physically active. Physical activity is associated with a reduced risk of colon cancer (Healthy People 2010).

Abdominal Assessment

GENITOURINARY ASSESSMENT

17

ASSESSMENT OF FEMALE GENITALIA

Equipment Needed

- Gown and drape
- Pillow
- Movable light source
- Gloves and lubricant
- Private location
- Vaginal speculum of appropriate size
- Vaginal swabs (large cotton-tipped applicators)
- pH paper
- Cotton-tipped applicators
- Mirror

Subjective Data: Focus Questions

Last menstrual period? Length of cycle? Amount of blood flow? Associated symptoms? Age of menarche? Unpleasant odor? Knowledge about toxic shock syndrome? Age of menopause if applicable? Estrogen replacement? Vaginal discharge? Pain, itching, or lumps in inguinal/groin area? Pain with intercourse? Difficulty urinating? Color or odor of urine? Difficulty controlling urine? Stress incontinence? Sexual performance? Activity? Change in libido? Fertility problems/concerns? History of gynecologic problems or sexually transmitted diseases (STDs)? Pregnancies? Number of children? Chance of pregnancy now? History of family reproductive or genital cancer? Self-care: Monthly genital self-examinations? Cotton underwear? Wiping pattern after bowel movement? Douching—how often? Use of contraceptives? Number of sexual partners? Comfort level with talking with sexual partner? Fears related to sex? Tested for HIV (human immunodeficiency virus)?

Risk Factors. Risk for cervical cancer related to sexually active female, human papilloma virus infection, first and frequent intercourse at young age, multiple sexual partners, history of STD, multiple births, history of no prior Pap exams, lower socioeconomic status, low level of education, poor hygiene especially with uncircumcised partner.

Objective Data: Assessment Techniques

See Figure 17–1 for a diagram of the female genitalia.

INSPECTION

Have client empty bladder and lie on her back with head slightly elevated on a pillow. Knees should be bent and separated with feet resting on the bed. Light should be adjusted to provide good visualization of the genitalia.

PROCEDURE	NORMAL FINDINGS	DEVIATIONS FROM NORMAL
*Inspect **labia** for the following:*		
• Lesions, swelling, excoriation	• Equal in size, free of lesions	• Lesions seen in infectious disease; swelling and excoriation seen with scratching or self-treatment of the lesions
• Pubic hair	• Varies with age	• Nits or lice

Genitourinary Assessment

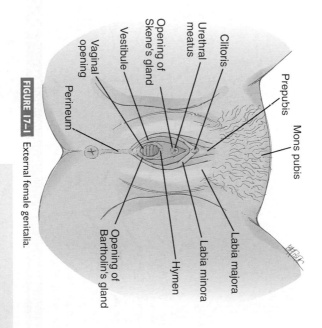

FIGURE 17–1 External female genitalia.

INSPECTION (continued)

PROCEDURE	NORMAL FINDINGS	DEVIATIONS FROM NORMAL
• Skin texture	• Smooth, loose skin	• Vesicles, warts, open sores
• Color	• Pink	• Blue, visible veins, shiny
*Using an examination glove, insert thumb and index or third finger between labia and separate. Inspect **urinary meatus** for the following:*		
• Position	• Small, slitlike, anterior to vaginal orifice and in midline	• Urinary meatus not visible; located within or near anterior surface of vaginal wall
• Color	• Pink	• Red, inflamed with perineal irritation
*Apply labial traction and inspect **vaginal orifice** for the following:*		
• Hymen	• Absent; thin, elastic membrane that partially occludes orifice; varies with estrogen effects, thick in newborn and at puberty, thin in infants, prepubescent patients, and elderly	• Completely occludes orifice
• Discharge	• Clear, milky, serosanguineous with menstrual cycle	• Any purulent, irritating, foul-smelling discharge is abnormal and should be cultured.

INSPECTION (continued)

PROCEDURE	NORMAL FINDINGS	DEVIATIONS FROM NORMAL
Have client strain down, and observe **vaginal wall** for bulging.	Slight movement	Bulging of anterior wall may be a cystocele; bulging of posterior vaginal wall may indicate a rectocele; if cervix or uterus protrudes down, the client may have a uterine prolapse; if urine is produced, stress incontinence may be present.

PALPATION

Don gloves. Using left thumb and index or third finger, gently separate labia and hold apart. Lubricate right index finger and insert into vaginal opening. Push up on anterior wall and "milk" toward opening. Push down on posterior wall and grasp tissue between thumb and index finger. Palpate tissue along entire lower half of vaginal orifice.

PROCEDURE	NORMAL FINDINGS	DEVIATIONS FROM NORMAL
Assess **Skene's glands** (see Fig. 17–1) for the following:		
• Openings	• Not visible	• Visible openings
• Discharge	• None	• Exudate from openings or urethra

Genitourinary Assessment

PALPATION (continued)

PROCEDURE	NORMAL FINDINGS	DEVIATIONS FROM NORMAL
Assess **Bartholin's glands**		
• Palpate posterior aspect of labia majora	• Soft	• Tenderness • Pain • Swelling • Discharge
*Palpate **posterior vaginal orifice** for the following:*		
• Swelling • Lumps or nodules	• None	• Present • Hard, nonpliable tissue
Assess **internal genitalia**	• Smooth, soft tissue	
• Determine size of vaginal opening.	• Size varies with age, sexual history, vaginal deliveries	
• Determine position of cervix. Insert gloved index finger into the vagina.	• Anterior or posterior • Midline • Extends into the vagina 1–3 cm	
• With index finger in vagina, ask client to squeeze around finger to check vaginal musculature.	• Able to squeeze finger	• Inability to squeeze finger indicates decreased muscle tone.
• Separate labia minora and ask client to bear down.	• No bulging • No urinary discharge	• Bulging of anterior wall may indicate cystocele. • Bulging of posterior wall may indicate rectocele.

PALPATION (continued)

PROCEDURE	NORMAL FINDINGS	DEVIATIONS FROM NORMAL
Insert speculum, then inspect		
• Cervix for color, size, position	• Surface of cervix smooth, pink, even	• Asymmetric, reddened area, strawberry spots, white patches
	• Pregnant clients bluish	
	• Older women pale	
• Cervical secretions	• Clear to opaque	• Discolored (gray, yellow, green)
	• Odorless	• Malodorous
	• Nonirritating	• Irritating
• Cervical os	• Small, round if nulliparous	• Lesions
	• Horizontal slit if parous	• Erosions
Rotate speculum and inspect:		
• Vagina for color, surface, consistency, discharge, vaginal pH of secretions, using cotton swab on lateral or anterior (not posterior) vaginal wall. Touch swab to pH paper strip to test secretions.	• Pink, moist, smooth without lesions, irritations, or malodorous discharge	• Reddened area
		• Lesions
		• Malodorous discharge
	• pH: 3.8–4.2	• <3.8
		• >4.2–6.0: consider bacterial vaginosis, sexual intercourse (pH of semen↑).
		• >6.0: consider trichomoniasis.

BIMANUAL EXAMINATION

Tell client you are going to perform a manual examination. Apply water-soluble lubricant to gloved middle and index fingers of your dominant hand. Stand and place nondominant hand or client's lower abdomen. Next insert index and middle fingers into the vagina.

PROCEDURE	NORMAL FINDINGS	DEVIATIONS FROM NORMAL
Apply pressure to the posterior vaginal wall; wait for relaxation of vaginal opening before palpating (Fig. 17–2).	Vaginal wall is smooth without tenderness.	Tenderness may indicate infection.
Palpate the cervix Advance fingers to the cervix; palpate for: • Contour • Consistency • Mobility • Tenderness	• Feels firm and soft like the tip of the nose	• Hardness and immobility may indicate cancer. • Pain with movement (and chandelier sign) may indicate infection.

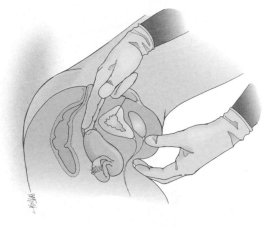

FIGURE 17–2 Palpating the vaginal walls.

PROCEDURE	NORMAL FINDINGS	DEVIATIONS FROM NORMAL
Palpate the uterus Move the fingers intravaginally into the opening above the cervix. Apply pressure with the hand resting on the abdomen. Squeeze the uterus between the two hands. Note uterine		• An enlarged uterus above the level of the pubis is abnormal. • Irregular shape may indicate abnormality.
• Size • Position • Shape • Consistency		
Palpate the ovaries Slide your intravaginal fingers toward the left ovary in the left lateral fornix and place your abdominal hand on the left lower abdominal quadrant. Press your abdominal hand toward your intravaginal fingers and attempt to palpate the ovary.	Ovaries are approximately $3 \times 2 \times 1$ cm (or the size of a walnut) and almond shaped.	Enlarged size, masses, immobility, and extreme tenderness are abnormal and should be evaluated.

BIMANUAL EXAMINATION (continued)

PROCEDURE	NORMAL FINDINGS	DEVIATIONS FROM NORMAL
Slide your intravaginal fingers to the right lateral fornix and attempt to palpate the right ovary. Note size, shape, consistency, mobility, and tenderness.	Ovaries are firm, smooth, mobile, and somewhat tender on palpation.	Ovaries that are palpable 3 – 5 years after menopause are also abnormal.
Withdraw your intravaginal hand and inspect the glove for secretions.	A clear, minimal amount of drainage appearing on the glove from the vagina is normal.	Large amounts of colorful, frothy, or malodorous secretions are abnormal.
Perform the rectovaginal examination.		
• Explain that you will perform a rectovaginal examination. Forewarn the client that she may feel uncomfortable as if she wants to move her bowels, but that she will not. Encourage her to relax. Change the glove on your dominant hand and lubricate your index and middle fingers (Fig. 17–3).	• The rectovaginal septum is normally smooth, thin, movable, and firm. The posterior uterine wall is normally smooth, firm, round, movable, and nontender.	• Masses, thickened structures, immobility, and tenderness are abnormal.
• Ask client to bear down and insert your index finger into the vaginal orifice and your middle		

BIMANUAL EXAMINATION (continued)

PROCEDURE

finger into the rectum. While pushing down on the abdominal wall with your other hand, palpate the internal reproductive structures through the anterior rectal wall. Withdraw your vaginal finger and continue with the rectal examination.

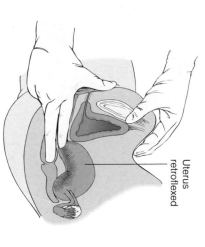

FIGURE 17–3 Hands positioned for rectovaginal examination.

Uterus retroflexed

ASSESSMENT OF MALE GENITALIA

Equipment Needed

- Gloves
- Private location

Subjective Data: Focus Questions

Pain in penis, scrotum, testes, or groin? Lesions in penis or genital area? Discharge from penis? Color? Odor? Lumps, masses, or swelling in scrotum, groin, or genital area? Heavy, draggy feeling in scrotum? Difficulty voiding—hesitancy, frequency, starting or maintaining stream? Change in color, odor, or amount of urine? Pain or burning when urinating? Incontinence or dribbling? Change in sexual activities? Difficulty with maintaining an erection? Problem with ejaculation? Trouble with fertility? Any bulges or pain when straining or lifting heavy objects? History of inguinal or genitalia surgery? History of STD? Self-care: Last testicular exam? Self-examination? Tested for HIV? Result? History of cancer in family? Number of sexual partners? Contraceptive form? Exposure to chemical or radiation? Fertility concerns? Comfort with communicating with sexual partner?

Risk Factors. Risk for HIV/AIDS (acquired immune deficiency syndrome) related to anal intercourse (especially men having sex with men), intravenous drug use, having multiple sexual partners, bisexual partners, or partner who uses intravenous drugs.

Objective Data: Assessment Techniques

See Figure 17–4 for a diagram of the male genitalia.

INSPECTION

The male genitalia should be inspected with the client in a standing position. Privacy should be ensured.

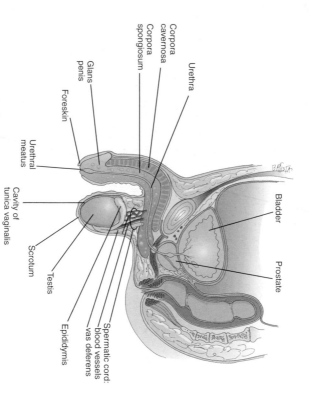

FIGURE 17–4 External and internal male genitalia.

Corpora
cavernosa

Corpora
spongiosum

Urethra

Glans
penis

Foreskin

Urethral
meatus

Cavity of
tunica vaginalis

Scrotum

Testis

Epididymis

Spermatic cord:
blood vessels
vas deferens

Bladder

Prostate

INSPECTION (continued)

PROCEDURE	NORMAL FINDINGS	DEVIATIONS FROM NORMAL
Observe **penis** *for the following:*		
• Urinary meatus	• Located at tip of glans penis	• Displaced to ventral side (hypospadias) or dorsal side (epispadias) of penis
• Discharge	• No discharge	• Any drainage—yellow discharge is seen with gonorrhea; clear or white discharge is seen with urethritis.
• Skin texture	• Wrinkled • Hairless	• Nodules, growths, lesions • Swelling • Phimosis • Paraphimosis
Observe **glans** *for the following:*		
• Size, shape, and lesions	• Size varies; rounded, broad, or pointed; free of lesions.	• Chancres (red, oval ulcerations from syphilis); pimple lesions in herpes; venereal warts
Observe **scrotum** *for the following:*		
• Size	• Left side lower than right	• Unilateral or bilateral enlargement due to presence of blood (hematocele), fluid (hydrocele), bowel (hernia), or tumor (cancer)
• Color	• Pink or normal skin color	• Red, shiny, bruised
• Texture	• Many skin folds	• Lesions, ulcers, taut skin

Genitourinary Assessment

PALPATION

With client standing, gently palpate shaft of penis between gloved thumb and fingers. If foreskin is present, retract from tip of penis, then replace. Grasp each testicle between thumb and fingers. Gently roll testicle so all surfaces are palpated. Client may do self-examination with instructions and report findings (Appendix 10).

PROCEDURE	NORMAL FINDINGS	DEVIATIONS FROM NORMAL
*Palpate **penis** for the following:*		
• Masses	• None	• Nodules, masses, or lesions anywhere on shaft or glans may indicate STDs or cancer.
• Tenderness	• Slightly tender	• Very tender or painful; hardness along central shaft may indicate cancer; tenderness is seen with infection or inflammation.
• Discharge	• None	• Clear or purulent from lesions or urinary meatus
• Foreskin	• May not be present; should retract and return easily with clean, smooth skin underneath	• Unable to retract owing to phimosis or adherence to underlying tissue; any drainage or sores under skin; discoloration of foreskin seen with scarring or infection
*Palpate each **testis** for the following:*		
• Location	• Each should be entirely in sac, left slightly lower than right.	• One or both are absent or cannot be palpated at inguinal border (partially descended).

PALPATION (continued)

PROCEDURE	NORMAL FINDINGS	DEVIATIONS FROM NORMAL
• Shape • Texture • Tenderness	• Oval, symmetrical • Smooth, firm • Very tender	• Enlarged, different sizes • Grainy or coarse; lumps or nodules • Pain; dull ache in lower abdomen or groin with feeling of heaviness

ASSESSMENT OF INGUINAL AREA

Objective Data: Assessment Techniques

See Figure 17-5 for a diagram of the inguinal area.

INSPECTION

Have client stand so inguinal area is visible. Have client strain down.

PROCEDURE	NORMAL FINDINGS	DEVIATIONS FROM NORMAL
Inspect **inguinal area.**	Smooth, symmetrical	Bulging on one or both sides that increases with straining indicates inguinal or femoral hernia.
Inspect **scrotum.**	Varies in size; left side of scrotal sac hangs slightly lower than right side.	Enlarged scrotal sac is seen with presence of fluid (hydrocele), blood (hematocele), bowel (hernia), or tumor (cancer).

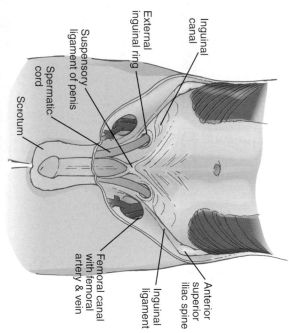

FIGURE 17–5 Inguinal area.

Inguinal canal

External inguinal ring

Suspensory ligament of penis

Spermatic cord

Scrotum

Anterior superior iliac spine

Inguinal ligament

Femoral canal with femoral artery & vein

PALPATION

Palpate inguinal area. Then have client strain down as you palpate inguinal area and scrotum (Fig. 17–6). Use right hand for right side and left hand for left side.

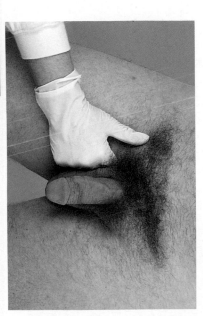

FIGURE 17–6 Palpating for an inguinal hernia. (© B. Proud).

PALPATION (continued)

PROCEDURE	NORMAL FINDINGS	DEVIATIONS FROM NORMAL
Palpate for the following:		
• Lymph nodes	• Nonpalpable	• Palpable, tender
• Masses	• Smooth, no masses	• Bulge of soft tissue that increases with straining indicates hernia.
• Scrotum	• No change	• Enlargement; mass felt increases with straining—bulge may disappear with scrotal hernia when client lies down; if you cannot push the mass back in, suspect an incarcerated hernia; client complains of extreme tenderness and nausea with a strangulated hernia.

ASSESSMENT OF RECTUM

Equipment Needed

- Examination gloves
- Drape
- Pillow

Subjective Data: Focus Questions

Usual bowel pattern? Changes? Diarrhea? Constipation? Color of stools? Mucus in stools? Pain? Itching? Bleeding after stools? History of rectal or anal surgery? Proctosigmoidoscopy? Family history of polyps, colon, rectal, or prostate cancer? Self-care: Use of laxatives? Engage in anal sex? Amount of roughage, fat, and water in diet? Last digital rectal exam by a physician or midlevel provider?

Risk Factors. Risk for colorectal cancer related to age over 40 years, history of rectal or colon polyps, inflammatory bowel disease, history of colorectal cancer, diet high in fat, protein, beef, and low in fiber; risk for prostate cancer related to dietary fat intake, age over 50 years, exposure to cadmium, high-risk occupations (eg, tire and rubber manufacturers, farmers, mechanics, sheet metal workers), lack of circumcision.

Objective Data: Assessment Techniques

See Figure 17–7 for a diagram of the anus and rectum.

INSPECTION

Have client lie on left side with right leg flexed at hip and knee. Support leg on pillow if necessary. Provide a pillow for under the head. With one hand, gently separate buttocks so rectum is exposed.

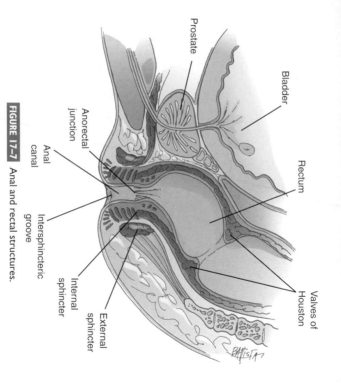

FIGURE 17-7 Anal and rectal structures.

Prostate

Bladder

Rectum

Anorectal
junction

Anal
canal

Intersphincteric
groove

Internal
sphincter

External
sphincter

Valves of
Houston

PROCEDURE	NORMAL FINDINGS	DEVIATIONS FROM NORMAL
*Palpate the **anus.*** Explain to the client what you are going to do. Explain that the client may feel like his bowels will move.		
Lubricate gloved index finger and ask client to bear down. Then place the pad of your index finger on the anal opening (Fig. 17–8).		
Assess sphincter tone.	Sphincter relaxes.	Sphincter tightens, preventing further examination.
Palpate for tenderness, nodules, and hardness.	Can close sphincter around gloved finger	Poor tone may be a result of spinal cord injury, previous surgery, trauma, prolapsed rectum, sexual abuse. Tightened sphincter may be the result of anxiety, scarring, inflammation.
*Palpate **rectum.*** Insert finger farther into rectum. Turn finger clockwise, then counterclockwise. Note tenderness irregularities, nodules, hardness.	Normally smooth, nontender, without nodules or hardness	Tenderness indicates hemorrhoids, fistula, fissure; nodules indicate polyps, cancer; hardness scarring, cancer.

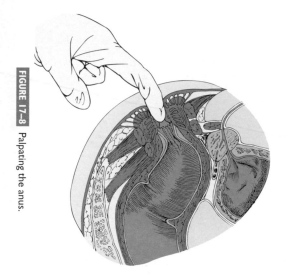

FIGURE 17–8 Palpating the anus.

PROCEDURE	NORMAL FINDINGS	DEVIATIONS FROM NORMAL
*Palpate the **prostate***. On the anterior surface of the rectum, turn the hand fully counterclockwise so the pad of your index finger faces toward the client's umbilicus. Tell the client he may feel an urge to urinate but will not. Move the pad of your index finger over the prostate gland, trying to feel the sulcus between the lateral lobes (Fig. 17–9).	Prostate nontender and rubbery with two lateral lobes that are divided by a median sulcus. The lobes are normally smooth, 2.5 cm long, and heart shaped.	A swollen, tender prostate may indicate acute prostatitis. An enlarged, smooth, firm, slightly elastic prostate that may not have a median sulcus suggests benign prostatic hypertrophy (BPH). A hard area on the prostate or hard, fixed, irregular nodules on the prostate suggest cancer.
Inspect **perianal area** for color, hair, lesions, masses, or drainage.	Hairless, moist, and tightly closed with no redness, lesions, masses, or rashes	Lesions are seen in external hemorrhoids, cancer, and STDs. Painful mass may be an abscess. Shiny blue skin sac suggests thrombosed hemorrhoid.
Inspect **sacrococcygeal area** for color, hair, and texture.	Smooth, free of hair and redness	Red, swollen area covered by a small tuft of hair located in the lower sacrum suggests the presence of a pilonidal cyst.

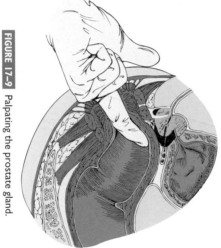

FIGURE 17–9 Palpating the prostate gland.

PEDIATRIC VARIATIONS

Subjective Data: Focus Questions

During puberty: Development of secondary sexual characteristics? Previous education on sexual development and activities? Use of contraceptives? Type?

Females: Age of menarche? Frequency of menstrual periods? Amount of flow? Pain? Irregularities? Attitude toward menstrual cycle?

Objective Data: Assessment Techniques

Inspection and palpation of external male and female genitalia constitute the *total* genitourinary assessment until puberty. Assessment of the level of sexual development of girls and boys usually begins at approximately age 11 years. This determination involves assessment of secondary characteristics associated with sexual maturity. Tables 17–1 and 17–2 summarize the timing of sexual development for boys and girls.

CULTURAL VARIATIONS

Male and female genitalia are mutilated in pubertal rites in some cultures, for example, circumcision, removal of clitoris, or surgical incision along penile shaft and into its base for passage of urine and semen. Female pubic hair is shaved or plucked in some cultures.

GERIATRIC VARIATIONS

- Bladder capacity decreases to 250 mL owing to periurethral atrophy.
- One to two periods of nocturia

Developmental Stage	Pubic Hair	Breast
Stage 1 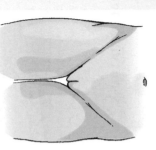	Prepubertal: no pubic hair; fine vellus hair	Prepubertal: elevation of nipple only 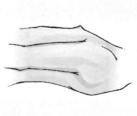

Stage 2

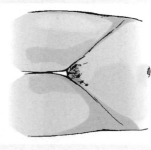

Sparse, long, straight, downy hair

Breast bud stage; elevation of breast and nipple as small mound; enlargement of areolar diameter

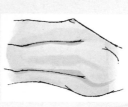

(continued)

Developmental Stage	Pubic Hair	Breast
Stage 3 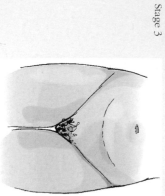	Darker, coarser, curly; sparse over mons pubis	Enlargement of the breasts and areola with no separation of contours 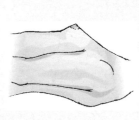

Stage 4

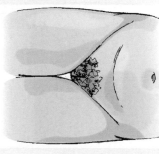

Dark, curly, and
  abundant on
  mons pubis;
  no growth on
  medial thighs

Projection of areola
  and nipple to form
  secondary mound
  above level of
  breast

Genitourinary Assessment

(continued)

Developmental Stage	Pubic Hair	Breast
Stage 5	Adult pattern of inverse triangle; growth on medial thighs	Adult configuration: projection of nipple only, areola re-ceded into contour of breast

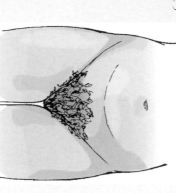
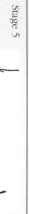
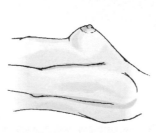

TABLE 17–2	TANNER'S SEXUAL MATURITY RATING: MALE GENITALIA DEVELOPMENT AND PUBIC HAIR GROWTH	
Developmental Stage	**Genitalia**	**Pubic Hair**
Stage 1 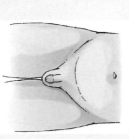	Prepubertal	Prepubertal: no pubic hair; fine vellus hair

(continued)

Developmental Stage		Genitalia	Pubic Hair
Stage 2	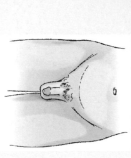	Initial enlargement of scrotum and testes with rugation and reddening of the scrotum	Sparse, long, straight, downy hair

Stage 3

Elongation of the penis; testes and scrotum further enlarge

Darker, coarser, curly; sparse over entire pubis

Genitourinary Assessment

(continued)

Developmental Stage		Genitalia	Pubic Hair
Stage 4	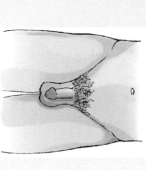	Increase in size and width of penis and the development of the glans; scrotum darkens	Dark, curly, and abundant in pubic area; no growth on thighs or up toward umbilicus

Stage 5

Adult configuration

Adult pattern (growth up toward umbilicus may not be
seen); growth continues until
mid 20s

Female

- Decrease in size and elasticity of labia; constriction of vaginal opening
- Diminished vaginal secretions and decreased elasticity of vaginal walls
- Shortened and narrowed vaginal vault
- Cervix appears paler after menopause.

Male

- Decrease in size and firmness of testicles
- Loss of tone in musculature of scrotum
- Slowed erections and less forceful ejaculations
- Enlargement of medial lobe of prostate

Possible Collaborative Problems

Bladder perforation   Obstruction of urethra   Renal calculi

Urinary tract infection   Hemorrhage   Hypermenorrhea

Pelvic inflammatory disease   Hormonal imbalances   Polymenorrhea

Genitalia ulcers or lesions   Renal failure

TEACHING TIPS FOR SELECTED NURSING DIAGNOSES AND COLLABORATIVE PROBLEMS

Adult Client

Nursing Diagnosis: Readiness for Enhanced Urinary Elimination and Reproductive Pattern

Teach client to drink eight glasses of fluid per day and to limit intake of alcohol, caffeine, and carbonated beverages. Teach client to avoid bubble baths and scented tissue that may irritate urethra. Teach female client to wear cotton underwear and to wipe perineum from front to back when cleansing.

Nursing Diagnosis: Readiness for Enhanced Health-Seeking Behaviors: Testicular Self-Examination

🖐 Instruct client on proper method of testicular self-examination, performed once a month after a warm bath or shower. Instruct client to roll each testicle gently between thumb and fingers of both hands, feeling for lumps or nodules (see Appendix 10). Have client demonstrate. Begin at puberty, because testicular cancer is one of the most common cancers in men 15 to 34 years old.

Nursing Diagnosis: Risk for Infection (STD) related to unprotected intercourse with multiple partners

🖐 Teach early warning signs and symptoms. Discuss methods of prevention (limit to one uninfected partner and use of condoms) and modes of transmission. Routine screening for infection is recommended during pelvic exam (Healthy People 2010).

Nursing Diagnosis: Ineffective Health Maintenance related to a lack of knowledge of birth control methods

🖐 Teach alternate forms of birth control, proper use of methods, and advantages and disadvantages of each. Discuss the importance of increasing vitamin B_6 and folic acid in the diet because of malabsorption of these vitamins while taking birth control pills. Instruct on use of alternate birth control for 3 months after discontinuing the pill to reestablish menstrual cycle before attempting to conceive.

Nursing Diagnosis: Readiness for Enhanced Health Maintenance During Menopause

🖐 Inform client that pregnancy may still occur during early menopausal years. Instruct to consume calcium 1200 mg/day along with a well-balanced diet (The 2004 Surgeon General Report on Bone Health and Osteoporosis). Explain that water-soluble lubricant may be used for vaginal dryness if intercourse is painful. Explain ways to help client cope with hot flashes (eg, use of cool clothing, fans, showers, cool drinks; avoidance of red wine, aged cheeses, and chocolate—these contain tyramine, which can trigger hot flashes.) Teach male clients about the male climacteric period (during the 50s or 60s) when sexual hormones are reduced. Symptoms of hot flashes, sweating, headaches, dizziness, and heart palpitations may be experienced.

Nursing Diagnosis: Ineffective Health Maintenance related to knowledge deficit of need for colorectal and pelvic examinations and Pap smears

Explain procedure. Teach relaxation. Approach sexuality as a normal part of activities of daily living. Prepare adolescent girl for first pelvic examination. The American Cancer Society (*Cancer facts and figures*, 2006) recommends that women who have been sexually active for 3 years or are 21 years old should have an annual Pap test and pelvic examination. For a woman 30 years or older who has had three or more consecutive satisfactory and normal annual examinations, the Pap test may be performed every 2 to 3 years at the physician's discretion. Most women 70 years and older who have had three or more consecutive normal Pap tests and most who have had total hysterectomies do not need continued screening. Women at high risk for endometrial cancer (major risk factors—weak immune system, estrogen replacement therapy, tamoxifen, early menarche, late menopause, never having children, and history of failure to ovulate; other risk factors—infertility, diabetes, gallbladder disease, hypertension, and obesity) should have an endometrial tissue sample at menopause and thereafter at the physician's discretion (*Cancer facts and figures*, 2006).

Men and women age 50 or older should follow one of these three examination schedules:

- A fecal occult blood test or fecal immunochemical test every year
- A flexible sigmoidoscopy every 5 years
- Annual fecal occult blood test or fecal immunochemical test and flexible sigmoidoscopy every 5 years*
- A double-contrast barium enema every 5 years
- A colonoscopy every 10 years

---

*Combined testing is preferred. People who are at moderate or high risk for colorectal cancer should talk with a doctor about a different testing schedule (*Cancer facts and figures*, 2006).

Nursing Diagnosis: Sexual Dysfunction: impotence related to unknown etiology

Explore possible etiologies and alternate forms of sexual satisfaction. Refer to urologist for information on penile implants, surgery, and other alternatives.

Nursing Diagnosis: Sexual Dysfunction related to deficient knowledge of psychological and physical health and sexual performance

Teach effects and benefits of exercise. Explore communication with partner. Refer to counselor (psychiatric, sexual, marriage) as needed. Provide adequate literature on sex and health teaching for client.

Nursing Diagnosis: Sexual Dysfunction related to loss of body part or physiologic limitations (eg, dyspareunia with aging)

Explore prior sexual patterns. Explore alternatives. Provide resource material on self-help groups (eg, Ostomy Association, Reach for Recovery). Suggest use of foreplay and lubricants to increase secretions as necessary. Provide literature and referrals.

Pediatric Client

Nursing Diagnosis: Risk for Impaired Elimination Pattern related to parental knowledge deficit of toilet-training techniques

Teach parents the importance of physiologic and psychological readiness in toilet training. Explain use of "potty chairs" and that bowel control precedes bladder control. Inform parents of the benefits of positive reinforcement and that nocturnal enuresis may persist up to age 4 to 5 years.

Nursing Diagnosis: Readiness for Enhanced Sexual Function

Sexual education is recommended in the early school years. Assess what child already knows and what he or she is ready to know.

Fourth to fifth grade: Interested in conception and birth

Fifth to sixth grade: Interested in their bodies and opposite sex changes. Education on birth control may be appropriate because of early experimentation. Discuss normal development of secondary sexual characteristics and the normal psychological changes associated with puberty.

Genitourinary Assessment

Adolescent: Teach the importance of abstinence or use of condoms if currently sexually active. Explain that there are an estimated 15 million new cases of STDs reported yearly and one half of all new HIV infections in the US are in people under age 25 and most are infected through sexual behavior *(Healthy People* 2010).

Geriatric Client

Nursing Diagnosis: Impaired Urinary Elimination: functional incontinence, reflex urinary incontinence, stress incontinence

- Explain to family how to decrease environmental barriers (offer bedpan frequently; provide proper lighting; ensure availability and proximity of commode) for functional incontinence. Teach client cutaneous triggering mechanisms for reflex incontinence. Teach client Kegel exercises to strengthen pelvic floor muscles (ie, tightening of buttocks and practicing starting and stopping stream) for stress incontinence.

Collaborative problem: Potential complication: prostate hypertrophy

- Teach client about effects of normal enlargement of prostate on urination (frequency, dribbling, and nocturia). Encourage yearly digital rectal exams and prostate-specific antigen (PSA) testing for men 50 years and older *(Cancer facts and figures,* 2006)

MUSCULOSKELETAL ASSESSMENT

18

OVERVIEW OF ANATOMY

The body's bones, muscles, and joints compose the musculoskeletal system. Two hundred and six (206) bones make up the axial skeleton (head and trunk) and the appendicular skeleton (extremities, shoulders, and hips; Fig. 18–1).

The body consists of three types of muscles: skeletal, smooth, and cardiac. The musculoskeletal system is made up of 650 skeletal (voluntary) muscles, which are under conscious control (Fig. 18–2).

The joint (or articulation) is the place where two or more bones meet. Joints provide a variety of range of motion (ROM) for the body parts. Synovial joints (eg, shoulders, wrists, hips, knees, ankles; Fig. 18–3) contain a space between the bones that is filled with synovial fluid, a lubricant that promotes a sliding movement of the ends of the bones. Bones in synovial joints are joined by ligaments, which are strong, dense bands of fibrous connective tissue. Synovial joints are enclosed by a fibrous capsule made of connective tissue and connected to the periosteum of the bone.

Equipment Needed

- Tape measure
- Goniometer (measures angles of joints)
- Marking pen

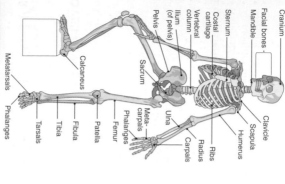

FIGURE 18–1 Major bones of the skeleton. The axial skeleton is shown in yellow; the appendicular, in blue.

Cranium
Facial bones
Mandible
Sternum
Costal cartilage
Vertebral column
Ilium
Pelvis
Sacrum
Calcaneus
Metatarsals
Phalanges
Tarsals
Tibia
Fibula
Patella
Femur
Phalanges
Meta-carpals
Carpals
Radius
Ulna
Humerus
Ribs
Scapula
Clavicle

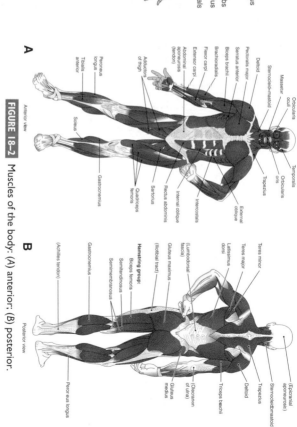

A

Anterior view

Tibialis anterior
Peroneus longus
Adductors of thigh
Abdominal aponeurosis (tendon)
Extensor carpi
Flexor carpi
Brachioradialis
Biceps brachii
Serratus anterior
Pectoralis major
Deltoid
Sternocleido-mastoid
Masseter
Orbicularis oculi
Orbicularis oris
Temporalis
Trapezius
External oblique
Internal oblique
Intercostalis
Rectus abdominis
Sartorius
Quadriceps femoris
Gastrocnemius
Soleus

B

Posterior view

Gastrocnemius
Peroneus longus
Hamstring group:
Biceps femoris
Semitendinosus
Semimembranosus
(Iliotibial tract)
Gluteus maximus
(Lumbodorsal fascia)
Latissimus dorsi
Teres major
Teres minor
(Epicranial aponeurosis)
Sternocleidomastoid
Trapezius
Deltoid
Triceps brachii
(Olecranon of ulna)
Gluteus medius
(Achilles tendon)

FIGURE 18–2 Muscles of the body: (A) anterior; (B) posterior.

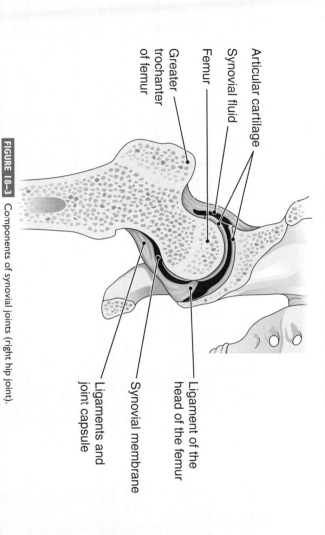

FIGURE 18–3 Components of synovial joints (right hip joint).

Labels:
- Articular cartilage
- Synovial fluid
- Femur
- Greater trochanter of femur
- Ligament of the head of the femur
- Synovial membrane
- Ligaments and joint capsule

Subjective Data: Focus Questions

Pain in joints, muscles, or bones? At rest? With exercise? Changes in shape or size of an extremity? Changes in ability to carry out activities of daily living, sports, work? Stiffness? Time of day? Relation to weight bearing and exercise? Decreased, altered, or absent sensations? Redness or swelling of joints? History of past problems with bones, joints, muscles, fractures? Treatment? Orthopedic surgery? Last tetanus and polio immunizations? History of osteoporosis or osteomyelitis? Family history of rheumatoid arthritis, gout, osteoporosis? Age of menopause if applicable? Occupational and recreational history? Self-care: Exercise, weight lifting, weight reduction, diet, use of tobacco or alcohol?

Risk Factors. Risk for osteoporosis related to lack of exercise, low calcium intake, excessive caffeine or alcohol consumption, smoking, use of steroids, low estrogen levels in women or postmenopausal women not on estrogen replacement therapy. Risk for sports injury related to lack of wearing protective gear, poor physical fitness, lack of warm-up exercises, and overuse of joints.

Objective Data: Assessment Techniques

See Figures 18–1 and 18–2 for diagrams of the bones and muscles of the body.

Inspection and palpation are performed while client is standing, sitting, and supine. ROM can be measured by degrees, using approximation or a goniometer. (Normal trunk ROM is given as an example—see Fig. 18–5.) In assessing muscle weakness or swelling, size is compared bilaterally by measuring circumference with a tape measure. Joints should not be forced into painful positions. Muscle strength can be estimated using a muscle strength scale (Table 18–1).

Inspection: Observe for ROM, swelling, deformity, atrophy, condition of surrounding tissues, and pain.

Palpation: Palpate for heat, strength, tone, tone, edema, crepitus, and nodules. **(Note:** Dominant side is normally stronger in muscle strength and tone.)

TABLE 8–1	SCALE FOR MUSCLE STRENGTH	
Rating	**Explanation**	**Strength Classification**
5	Active motion against full resistance	Normal
4	Active motion against some resistance	Slight weakness
3	Active motion against gravity	Average weakness
2	Passive ROM (gravity removed and assisted by examiner)	Poor ROM
1	Slight flicker of contraction	Severe weakness
0	No muscular contraction	Paralysis

INSPECTION OF STANCE AND GAIT

Observe stance and gait as client enters and walks around the room.

Objective Data: Assessment Techniques

PROCEDURE	NORMAL FINDINGS	DEVIATIONS FROM NORMAL
Inspect the **stance** *for the following:*		
• Base of support	• Weight evenly distributed	• Uneven base, with unequal weight bearing, wide based
• Weight-bearing stability	• Able to stand on right/left heels, toes	• Weakness or inability to use either extremity
• Posture	• Erect	• Stooped
Inspect the **gait** *for the following:*		
• Position of feet	• Toes point straight ahead	• Toes point in or out
• Posture	• Erect	• Stooped
• Stride	• Equal on both sides	• Wide based, propels forward, shuffling, or limping
• Arm swing	• Swing in opposition	• No swing

INSPECTION OF THE SPINE, SHOULDER, AND POSTERIOR ILIAC CREST

With client standing, observe in the erect position and as the client bends forward to touch toes. Stabilize client at the waist, and evaluate ROM of the upper trunk.

Objective Data: Assessment Techniques

PROCEDURE	NORMAL FINDINGS	DEVIATIONS FROM NORMAL
Inspect the **spine** *for the following:*		
• Curves	• Cervical concave; thoracic convex; lumbar concave (Fig. 18–4)	• Kyphosis, scoliosis, lordosis (see Fig. 18–4); a flattened lumbar curve is seen with herniated lumbar disk or ankylosing spondylitis; lateral curvature of spine is seen with scoliosis; and exaggerated lumbar curve (lordosis) is seen with pregnancy or obesity.
• Posture	• Erect	• Stooped
• ROM—flexion, lateral bending, rotation, extension (Fig. 18–5)	• Full ROM	• Limited ROM with pain or crepitation

PALPATION OF THE SPINE, SHOULDER, AND POSTERIOR ILIAC CREST

With client in standing or sitting position, palpate the paravertebral muscles, using both moderate pressure and gentle sweeping motions. Ask client to shrug shoulders against resistance.

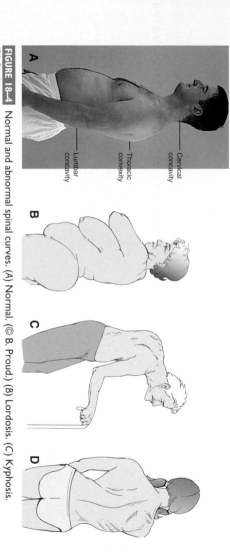

FIGURE 18-4 Normal and abnormal spinal curves. (A) Normal. (© B. Proud.) (B) Lordosis. (C) Kyphosis. (D) Scoliosis.

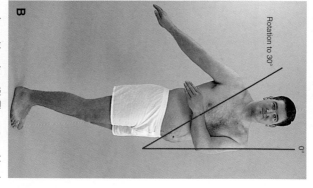

FIGURE 18–5 Range of motion of trunk. (A) Thoracic and lumbar spines: lateral bending; (B) Thoracic and lumbar spines: rotation.

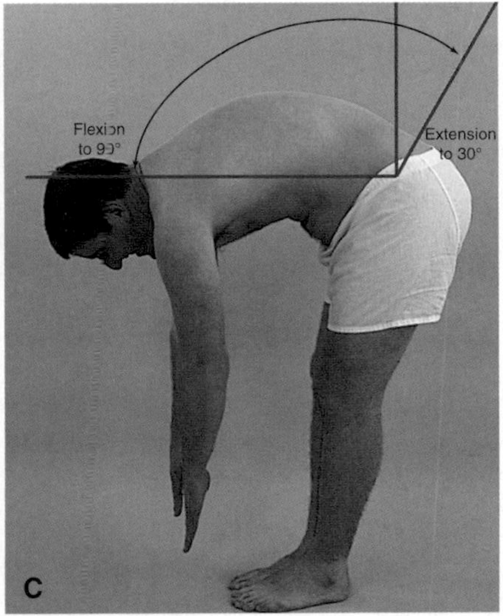

FIGURE 18-5 (continued) (C) Thoracic and lumbar spines: flexion. (© B. Proud.)

Flexion to 90°

Extension to 30°

PROCEDURE	NORMAL FINDINGS	DEVIATIONS FROM NORMAL
*Palpate the **paravertebrals** for the following:*		
• Muscle strength and tone	• Equally strong	• Weak, spasm
• Temperature	• Warm	• Hot and swollen
• Sensation	• Nontender	• Tender, painful
*Palpate the **shoulder** (trapezius muscle) for the following:*		
• Muscle strength and tone	• Able to shrug shoulders against resistance (3–5)	• Weakness with shrugging of shoulders; pain (0–2)
• Sensation	• Nontender	• Tender, painful with shoulder strains, sprains, arthritis, bursitis, and degenerative joint disease
*Palpate the **shoulder, scapula, and posterior hip** for the following:*		
• Bony prominences	• Smooth and nontender, no swelling	• Bony enlargement and tenderness, swelling, pain
• Muscle size, strength, and tone	• Equal in size bilaterally, equally strong (3–5)	• Muscle atrophy, weakness, flabbiness, or swelling (0–2)
• Temperature	• Warm to cool	• Hot

INSPECTION OF THE HEAD, THORAX, AND NECK

With client in sitting position facing you, inspect body parts. Ask client to open and close mouth to assess temporomandibular joint (TMJ) function.

PROCEDURE	NORMAL FINDINGS	DEVIATIONS FROM NORMAL
Observe the **head** *for the following:*		
• Facial structure and muscle development	• Symmetrical structure and development of muscles	• Asymmetrical structure and development of muscles
• TMJ function	• Can open mouth 2 inches	• Limited ROM; audible crepitation, click; trismus (muscle spasms), pain, tenderness, and swelling seen with TMJ syndrome
Observe the **thorax** for posture.	Erect, slight kyphosis	Stooped; abnormal spinal curves
Observe the **neck** for ROM: Flexion, extension, rotation, lateral bending (Fig. 18–6).	Full ROM; no pain	Limited ROM with crepitation or pain; nuchal rigidity; neck pain with radiation to back, shoulder, or arms seen with cervical disk degeneration. Neck pain with weakness or loss of sensation in legs is seen with cervical spine compression.

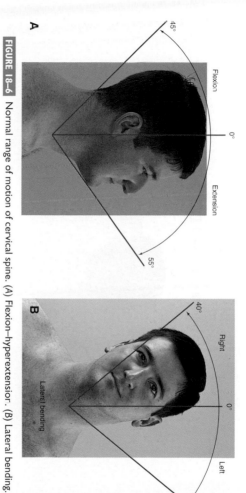

A

45°

Flexion

0°

Extension

55°

B

40°

Right

0°

Left

40°

Lateral bending

FIGURE 18–6 Normal range of motion of cervical spine. (A) Flexion–hyperextension. (B) Lateral bending.

Musculoskeletal Assessment

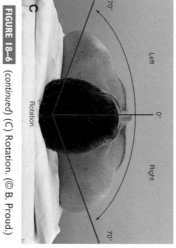

FIGURE 18–6 *(continued)* (C) Rotation. (© B. Proud.)

PALPATION OF THE HEAD, THORAX, AND NECK

While inspecting the TMJ, palpate it bilaterally anterior to the tragus of the ear as client opens mouth and clenches teeth. Ask client to turn head laterally against resistance.

PROCEDURE	NORMAL FINDINGS	DEVIATIONS FROM NORMAL
 Palpating the temporomandibular joint. (© B. Proud.)		
Palpate the **TMJ** *for the following:*		
• Joint function	• Smooth movement bilaterally on opening, with no clicks or pain	• Palpable click, pain
• Joint contour	• Symmetrical	• Asymmetrical
• Temperature	• Warm	• Hot and swollen
Palpate the **neck** (sternocleidomastoid) for muscle strength and tone.	Can turn head laterally against resistance without pain (3–5)	Weakness or pain when turning head against resistance (0–2)

Musculoskeletal Assessment

INSPECTION OF THE UPPER EXTREMITIES

Position client in the sitting position facing you, with the upper extremities exposed. Inspect each joint and determine ROM. Both active and passive ROM may be assessed. It is easier for the client to carry out ROM if you demonstrate movements first.

PROCEDURE	NORMAL FINDINGS	DEVIATIONS FROM NORMAL
Observe the **shoulder, elbow, wrist, hand, and fingers** for bone structure, bony prominences, muscle mass, joint structure, and symmetry.	Bilaterally symmetrical	Bony deformity, muscle atrophy, swelling, deviation, contractures, nodes, tophi. Swelling of wrists, tenderness, and nodules are seen in rheumatoid arthritis; nontender, round, enlarged, swollen cysts may be ganglion of the wrists.
Observe the **shoulder, elbow, wrist, and fingers** for ROM. See Table 18–2 and Figures 18–7 through 18–10 for normal ROM.	Full ROM	Limited ROM with crepitation or pain. Catches of pain with ROM in shoulder are seen with rotator cuff tendinitis; chronic pain and limited ROM seen with calcified tendinitis; pain-limited abduction of shoulder seen with rotator cuff tear; redness and heat of elbows with bursitis; ulnar deviation of wrists and fingers with limited ROM seen in rheumatoid arthritis; inability to extend ring finger seen in Dupuytren contracture; painful extension of finger with tenosynovitis.

TABLE 18-2 NORMAL RANGE OF MOTION FOR JOINTS OF THE UPPER EXTREMITIES

Shoulder	Elbow	Wrist	Fingers
Flexion	Flexion	Flexion	Flexion
Extension	Extension	Hyperextension	Hyperextension
Abduction	Supination	Deviation	Abduction
Adduction	Pronation	Radial	Adduction
Rotation (internal		Ulnar	Thumb away from fingers
and external)			Thumb to base of small finger

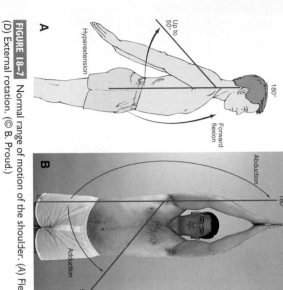

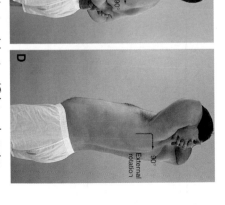

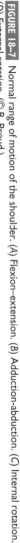

FIGURE 18–7 Normal range of motion of the shoulder. (A) Flexion–extension. (B) Adduction-abduction. (C) Internal rotation. (D) External rotation. (© B. Proud.)

Musculoskeletal Assessment

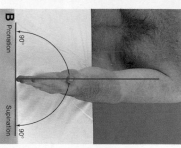

FIGURE 18–8 Normal range of motion of the elbow. (A) Flexion–extension. (B) Pronation–supination. (© B. Proud.)

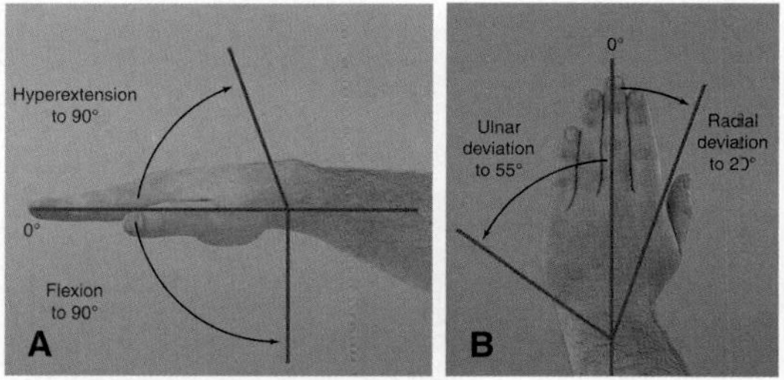

FIGURE 18–9 Range of motion of the wrists. (A) Flexion–hyperextension. (B) Radial–ulnar deviation. (© B. Proud.)

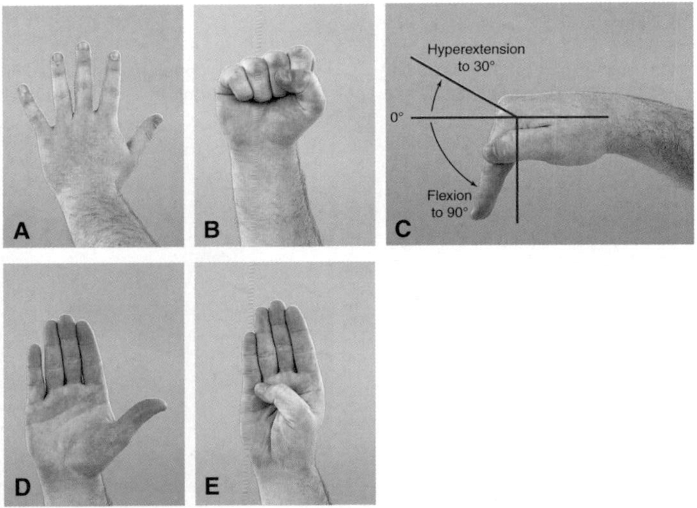

FIGURE 18–10 Normal range of motion of the fingers. (A) Abduction. (B) Adduction. (C) Flexion–hyperextension. (D) Thumb away from fingers. (E) Thumb touching base of small finger. (© B. Proud.)

PALPATION OF THE UPPER EXTREMITIES

As the musculoskeletal structure of the upper extremity is going through active or passive ROM, palpate bones, muscles, tendons, and joints. Assess muscle strength and tone.

PROCEDURE	NORMAL FINDINGS	DEVIATIONS FROM NORMAL
Palpate the **arm** (biceps, triceps) for muscle strength and tone.	Can flex and extend arm against resistance (3–5)	Weakness, paralysis (0–2)
Palpate the **hand** for the following:		
• Muscle strength, tone	• Grip is firm and equal.	• Weakness, paralysis
• Sensation	• Nontender (3–5)	• Tenderness, pain (0–2)
*Palpate the **elbow, wrist, hand, and fingers** for the following:*		
• Bony landmarks	• Nontender, smooth	• Bony enlargement
• Muscle size	• Regular and equal bilaterally	• Muscle atrophy
• Joint structure	• Symmetrical and equal	• Loss of joint structure; joint bogginess; nodules, swelling
• Strength	• Equally strong (3–5)	• Unilateral or bilateral weakness (0–2)
• Temperature	• Warm	• Hot
• Sensation	• Nontender	• Tender, painful
Ask client to close eyes for 20–30 seconds with arms extended in front of body with palms up.	Arms remain up with no drifting.	Arm tends to drift downward and pronate.

INSPECTION OF THE LOWER EXTREMITIES

Position the client in standing or supine position to inspect the hips, and in sitting position with legs hanging freely to inspect the knees, ankles, feet, and toes. If the client is unable to sit or stand, assessments may be made in the supine position. Both active and passive ROM may be assessed.

PROCEDURE	NORMAL FINDINGS	DEVIATIONS FROM NORMAL
Observe the **hip, knee, ankle, foot, and toes** *for the following:*		
• Bone structure and bony landmarks	• Bilaterally symmetrical and equal	• Bony deformity
• Muscle mass	• Muscle symmetrical and equal	• Muscle atrophy
• Joint structure	• Feet maintain straight position.	• Swelling, deviation, or contractures; bunion, deviation, or hammer toe
• Leg length	• Bilateral leg lengths within 1 inch of each other	• Unequal lengths
Observe the **hip, knee, ankle, and toes** for ROM. See Table 18–3 and Figures 18–11 through 18–13 for normal ROM.	Full ROM	Limited ROM with crepitation or pain in joint and muscle disease. Hip pain, decreased ROM, and crepitus in hip inflammation and degenerative joint disease; tenderness and warmth with boggy consistency in synovitis; turned-in knees (genu valgum); knees turned out (genu varum); fluid bulge in knee joint effusion; pain or clicking in torn meniscus.

TABLE 18-3		NORMAL RANGE OF MOTION FOR JOINTS OF THE LOWER EXTREMITIES		
Hip	**Knee**	**Ankle**	**Toes**	
Rotation (internal and external)				
Flexion	Flexion	Dorsiflexion	Flexion	
Extension	Extension	Plantar flexion	Extension	
Abduction		Inversion		
Adduction		Eversion		

PALPATION OF THE LOWER EXTREMITIES

As the musculoskeletal structure of the lower extremity is going through active or passive ROM, palpate bones, bony landmarks, muscles, and joints. Assess muscle strength and tone.

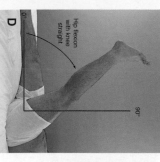

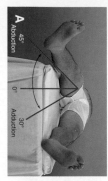

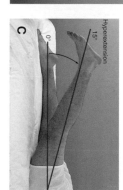

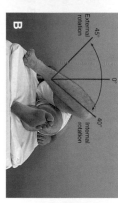

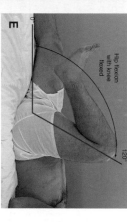

FIGURE 18–11 Normal range of hip motion.
(A) Abduction-adduction. (B) Internal and
external rotation. (C) Hyperextension.
(D) Hip flexion with extended knee straight.
(E) Hip flexion with knee bent. (© B. Proud.)

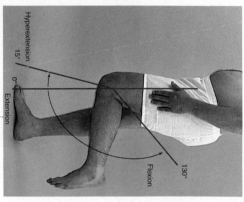

FIGURE 18-12 Normal range of motion of knee. (© B. Proud.)

Hyperextension

15°

0°

Extension

130°

Flexion

Musculoskeletal Assessment

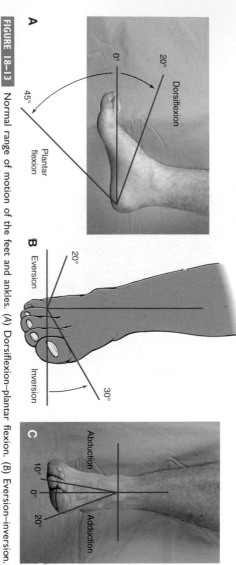

FIGURE 18–13 Normal range of motion of the feet and ankles. (A) Dorsiflexion–plantar flexion. (B) Eversion–inversion. (C) Abduction-adduction. (Photos © B. Proud.)

PALPATION OF THE LOWER EXTREMITIES (continued)

PROCEDURE	NORMAL FINDINGS	DEVIATIONS FROM NORMAL
Palpate the **hip** (quadriceps, gastrocnemius) for the following:		
• Bony landmarks	• Bilaterally symmetrical and equal	• Bony enlargement
• Muscle size and strength	• Smooth, regular, strong (3–5)	• Muscle atrophy and weakness (0–2)
• Joint structure	• Bilaterally symmetrical; strong	• Loss of joint structure; joint bogginess
• Temperature	• Warm	• Hot and swollen
• Sensation	• Nontender	• Tenderness, pain

PEDIATRIC VARIATIONS

Subjective Data: Focus Questions

Birth injuries? Alignment of hips? Trauma? Participation in sports or outdoor activities? Frequent pain in joints?

Musculoskeletal Assessment

Objective Data: Assessment Techniques

PROCEDURE

Infant:
Inspect lower extremities.

NORMAL VARIATIONS

A distinct bowlegged growth pattern persists and begins to disappear at 18 months. At 2 years, a knock-kneed pattern is common (Fig. 18–14), persisting until age 6–10, when legs straighten.

A greater ROM in joints is present in infants. Legs are wide set until the child begins walking; weight is borne on the inside of the feet.

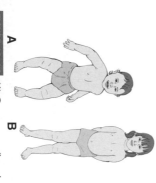

FIGURE 18–14 (A) Genu varum (bow legs).
(B) Genu valgum (knock knees).

A

B

Objective Data: Assessment Techniques *(continued)*

PROCEDURE	NORMAL VARIATIONS
Perform Ortolani maneuver to test for congenital hip dysplasia. With the infant supine, flex the knees while holding your thumbs on midthigh and your fingers over the greater trochanters; abduct the legs, moving the knees outward and down toward the table (Fig. 18-15, A).	Positive Ortolani sign: A click heard along with feeling the head of the femur slip in or out of the hip
Perform Barlow maneuver. With the infant supine, flex the knees while holding your thumbs on midthigh and your fingers over the greater trochanters; adduct legs until thumbs touch (Fig. 18-15, B).	Positive Barlow sign: A feeling of the head of the femur slipping out of the hip socket (acetabulum)
Over age 2 years: Inspect gait. Measure distance between knees with ankles together.	Wide-based gait common until age 2 years Less than 2 inches
3–7 years of age: Measure distance between ankles with knees together. Longitudinal arch of foot is often obscured by adipose until age 3 years, and infant appears flatfooted.	Less than 3 inches
4–13 years of age: See also Appendix 3 for developmental milestones	

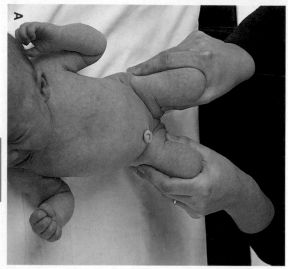

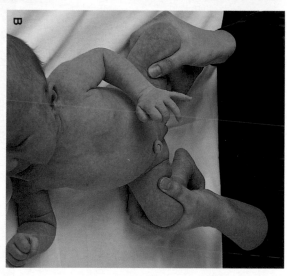

FIGURE 18–15 (A) Barlow maneuver. (B) Ortolani maneuver.

Objective Data: Assessment Techniques (continued)

PROCEDURE

Inspect curvature of spine:

- Stand behind erect child and note asymmetry of shoulders and hips.
- Have child bend forward at waist until back is parallel to floor; observe from side, looking for asymmetry or prominence of rib cage.

Assessing spinal curvature for scoliosis.
(© B. Proud)

NORMAL VARIATIONS

- Shoulders symmetrical, parallel with hips

- Shoulders, scapulae, iliac crests symmetrical

GERIATRIC VARIATIONS

- Decrease in total bone mass due to decreased activity level, change in hormones, and bone resorption; this results in weaker, softer bones.
- Slower gait with wide-based stance and smaller arm swing
- Accentuated dorsal spinal curve (kyphosis)
- Loss of muscle bulk and tone
- Decreased ROM of spine, neck, extremities
- Decrease in height (1.2 cm of height lost every 20 years)
- Shoulder width decreases; chest and pelvis widths increase.
- May have bowlegged appearance due to decreased muscle control

CULTURAL VARIATIONS

- Some variation in muscle size and mass and in bone length and density are seen in different racial/ethnic groups. Overfield (1995) noted that the peroneus tertius in foot or palmaris longus muscles in wrist may be absent in some groups; the number of vertebrae may differ (black women may have 23, Eskimo and Native American men, 25). A large gluteal prominence in some blacks may be mistaken as lordosis, and the ulna and radius may have unequal lengths (eg, Swedes and Chinese). Bone density (and osteoporosis) vary, with men having denser bones, blacks denser than whites, and most East Asians (except Polynesian women) less dense than Caucasians (Overfield, 1995).
- Blacks tend to be advanced in and Asians tend to fall behind in the growth and development norms established for U.S. whites.

Possible Collaborative Problems

Bone fractures
Sprains
Contractures of joints

Osteoporosis
Dislocation of joints
Compartment syndrome

Osteoarthritis
Rheumatoid arthritis

TEACHING TIPS FOR SELECTED NURSING DIAGNOSES

Adult Client

Nursing Diagnosis: Readiness for Enhanced Mobility

🖥 Teach client the importance of maintaining an ideal weight. Explain the importance of doing weight-bearing and muscle-toning exercises at least three times per week. Encourage client to wear seat belts in vehicles, to wear low well-fitted shoes, and to use walking aids (eg, cane) as needed to prevent injury.

Nursing Diagnosis: Chronic Pain (muscles and joints)

🖥 Discuss independent pain management measures the client may find useful (eg, massage, relaxation, distraction). Weight loss may also reduce discomfort if obesity is straining the bones, muscles, and joints. Explain use and side effects of pain medications.

Nursing Diagnosis: Risk for Injury related to excessive exercise/improper body mechanics

🖥 Caution the client against the dangerous effects of excessive exercise. Teach proper body mechanics and correct posture.

Pediatric Client

Nursing Diagnosis: Risk for Injury (child) related to parent's knowledge deficit of correlating musculoskeletal development and home safety

🖥 Caution parents on home safety precautions (eg, gates at stairways, removal of objects that may cause unnecessary falls, avoiding leaving child near water alone) based on child's level of musculoskeletal development. Develop home safety checklist with parents. Teach normal milestones of musculoskeletal development, and advise parent to encourage these skills as appropriate.

Geriatric Client

Nursing Diagnosis: Risk for Injury related to decalcification of bones secondary to sedentary lifestyle and postmenopausal state

Discuss importance of calcium supplements in diet for postmenopausal women. Explain effects of exercise on decreasing bone decalcification.

Nursing Diagnosis: Risk for Injury related to unstable gait secondary to aging process

Explain correct use of aids (eg, crutches, canes, walkers) and other prostheses. Use referrals as necessary. Instruct client on measures to prevent falls (eg, adequate lighting, avoidance of loose board ends and scatter rugs on floor). Discourage use of sleeping pills and suggest alternate methods of promoting sleep (eg, watching TV, reading, warm bath, music, warm milk).

Nursing Diagnosis: Impaired Physical Mobility related to decreased activity secondary to aging process

Instruct client on the hazards of immobility and methods to prevent complications (eg, turning, coughing, deep breathing, repositioning, ROM, adequate diet, plentiful fluid intake, and diversional activities). Encourage mild exercise to loosen joint stiffness.

Nursing Diagnosis: Self-Care Deficit (specify) related to decreased mobility and/or weakness

Assess safe level of activity with client, and teach methods to increase activity gradually to that level. Explore alternate self-help methods of maintaining self-care (eg, feeding aids, wheelchairs, crutches, hygienic aids). Assist client with identifying and utilizing services and groups to assist with activities of daily living (eg, Meals on Wheels). Support and teach family caregivers.

19

NEUROLOGIC ASSESSMENT

ANATOMY OVERVIEW

The very complex neurologic system is responsible for coordinating and regulating all body functions. It consists of two structural components: the central nervous system (CNS) and the peripheral nervous system.

Central Nervous System

The CNS encompasses the brain and spinal cord. Located in the cranial cavity, the brain has four major divisions: the cerebrum, the diencephalon, the brainstem, and the cerebellum (Fig. 19–1).

The cerebrum is divided into the right and left cerebral hemispheres. Located beneath the cerebral hemispheres and consists of the thalamus and hypothalamus. Located between the cerebral cortex and the spinal cord, the brainstem consists of the midbrain, pons, and medulla oblongata. The cerebellum, located behind the brainstem and under the cerebrum, also has two hemispheres.

The spinal cord (Fig. 19–2) is located in the vertebral canal and extends from the medulla oblongata to the first lumbar vertebra.

Peripheral Nervous System

Carrying information to and from the CNS, the peripheral nervous system consists of 12 pairs of cranial nerves and 31 pairs of spinal nerves. The cranial nerves evolve from the brain or brainstem (Table 19–1).

Comprising 8 cervical, 12 thoracic, 5 lumbar, 5 sacral, and 1 coccygeal nerve, the 31 pairs of spinal nerves are named after the vertebrae below each one's exit point along the spinal cord (see Fig. 19–2). Each nerve is attached to the spinal cord by two nerve roots. The sensory (afferent) fiber enters through the dorsal (posterior) roots of the cord, whereas the motor (efferent) fiber

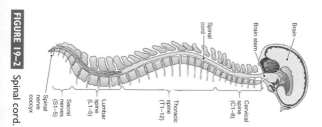

A

■ Frontal lobe ■ Parietal lobe ■ Temporal lobe ■ Occipital lobe

ANTERIOR

Corpus callosum

DIENCEPHALON:
Sagittal plane
Thalamus
Pituitary gland
Hypothalamus

BRAIN STEM:
Midbrain
Pons
Medulla
oblongata
Spinal cord

CEREBRUM

POSTERIOR

CEREBELLUM

B

Pons
Medulla
oblongata
Cerebellum
Spinal cord

FIGURE 19-1 (A) Structures of the brain (sagittal section). (B) Lobes of the brain.

Brain stem

Brain

Spinal
cord

Cervical
spine
(C1–8)

Thoracic
spine
(T1–12)

Lumbar
spine
(L1–5)

Sacral
nerves
(S1–5)

Spinal
nerve
coccyx

FIGURE 19-2 Spinal cord.

TABLE 19–1 CRANIAL NERVES: TYPE AND FUNCTION

Cranial Nerve (Name)	Type of Impulse	Function
I (olfactory)	Sensory	Carries smell impulses from nasal mucous membrane to brain
II (optic)	Sensory	Carries visual impulses from eye to brain
III (oculomotor)	Motor	Contracts eye muscles to control eye movements (inferior lateral, medial, and superior), constricts pupils, and elevates eyelids
IV (trochlear)	Motor	Contracts one eye muscle to control inferomedial eye movement
V (trigeminal)	Sensory	Carries sensory impulses of pain, touch, and temperature from the face to the brain
	Motor	Influences clenching and lateral jaw movements (biting, chewing)
VI (abducens)	Motor	Controls lateral eye movements
VII (facial)	Sensory	Contains sensory fibers for taste on anterior two thirds of tongue and stimulates secretions from salivary glands (submaxillary and sublingual) and tears from lacrimal glands
	Motor	Supplies the facial muscles and affects facial expressions (smiling, frowning, closing eyes)

(continued)

Neurologic Assessment

TABLE 19–1 CRANIAL NERVES: TYPE AND FUNCTION (continued)

Cranial Nerve (Name)	Type of Impulse	Function
VIII (acoustic, vestibulocochlear)	Sensory	Contains sensory fibers for hearing and balance
IX (glossopharyngeal)	Sensory	Contains sensory fibers for taste on posterior third of tongue and sensory fibers of the pharynx that result in the "gag reflex" when stimulated
X (vagus)	Motor	Provides secretory fibers to the parotid salivary glands; promotes swallowing movements
	Sensory	Carries sensations from the throat, larynx, heart, lungs, bronchi, gastrointestinal tract, and abdominal viscera
	Motor	Promotes swallowing, talking, and production of digestive juices
XI (spinal accessory)	Motor	Innervates neck muscles (sternocleidomastoid and trapezius) that promote movement of the shoulders and head rotation. Also promotes some movement of the larynx
XII (hypoglossal)	Motor	Innervates tongue muscles that promote the movement of food and talking

exits through the ventral (anterior) roots of each spinal nerve innervates an area of the skin called a dermatome (Fig. 19-3).

The neurologic assessment is performed last because several of its components may have been integrated into previous parts of the examination. For example, the eighth cranial nerve (CN VIII) may have been tested during the ear examination and therefore will not need to be tested again.

The neurologic assessment consists of six parts: (1) mental status, (2) cranial nerves, (3) sensory function, (4) motor function, (5) cerebellar function, and (6) reflexes.

Equipment Needed

- Penlight
- Tuning fork
- Reflex hammer
- Cotton wisp
- Paper clip (for detection of sharp/dull sensations)

- Salt
- Sugar
- Cotton-tipped applicators
- Glass of water
- Tongue blade
- Ophthalmoscope

Subjective Data: Focus Questions

Numbness? Paralysis? Tingling? Neuralgia? (Timing, duration, associated factors?) Seizures? Auras? Medications taken for seizures? Wear Medicalert identification? Tremors? Headaches? (Frequency, duration, character, precipitating/relieving factors?) Loss of consciousness? Dizziness? Fainting? Loss of memory? Confusion? Visual loss, blurring, pain? Facial pain, weakness, twitching? Speech problems (aphasia—expressive/receptive)? Swallowing problems? Drooling? Neck weakness, spasms? Any muscle weakness or loss of bowel or urinary control? History of head injury? Meningitis? Encephalitis? Treatment? Family history of high blood pressure, stroke, Alzheimer disease, epilepsy, brain cancer, or Huntington chorea?

Self-care: Use of medications? Alcohol intake? Use of drugs such as marijuana, tranquilizers, barbiturates, or cocaine? Smoking? Use of seat belt, head gear for sports? Daily diet and exercise? Prolonged exposure to lead, insecticides, pollutants, or other chemicals?

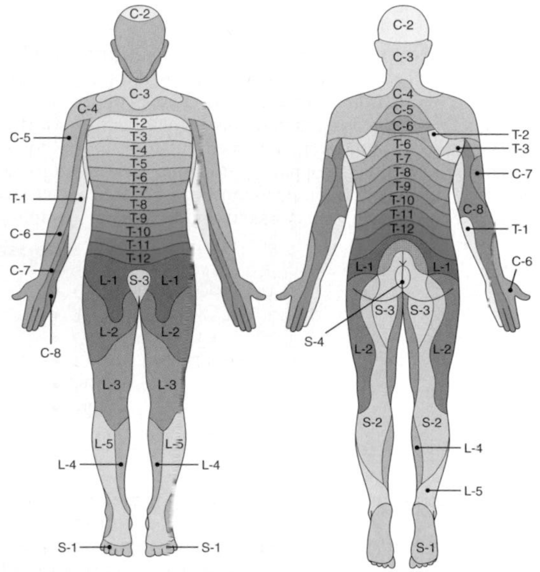

FIGURE 19-3 Anterior and posterior dermatomes (areas of the skin innervated by spinal nerves).

Risk Factors. Risk for cerebrovascular accident (stroke) related to age older than 60 years, male sex (slightly higher risk), hypertension, smoking, chronic alcohol intake, history of cardiovascular disease, sleep apnea, high levels of fibrinogen, diabetes mellitus, drug abuse, oral contraceptives, high estrogen levels, postmenopausal woman not taking estrogen replacement, obesity, African American, and newly industrialized environment.

MENTAL STATUS ASSESSMENT

Assessment of mental status is performed by observing the client and asking questions. Much of this information may have already been assessed during the initial interview and general survey.

Objective Data: Assessment Techniques

See Figure 19-1 for a diagram of the brain.

PROCEDURE	NORMAL FINDINGS	DEVIATIONS FROM NORMAL
Observe level of consciousness. • Response to calling the client's name. If the client does not respond, call the name louder. If necessary, shake the client gently. If the client still does not respond, apply a painful stimulus.	• Alert and awake with eyes open and looking at examiner; client responds appropriately.	• Lethargy: Opens eyes, answers questions, and falls back asleep • Obtunded: Opens eyes to loud voice, responds slowly with confusion, seems unaware of environment • Stupor: Awakens to vigorous shake or painful stimuli, but returns to unresponsive sleep

PROCEDURE	NORMAL FINDINGS	DEVIATIONS FROM NORMAL
		• Coma: Remains unresponsive to all stimuli; eyes stay closed. Client with lesions of the corticospinal tract draws hands up to chest (*decorticate* or abnormal flexor posture) when stimulated.
		• Client with lesions of the diencephalon, midbrain, or pons extends arms and legs, arches neck, and rotates hands and arms internally (*decerebrate* or abnormal extensor posture) when stimulated.
*Observe **appearance and movement.***		
• Posture	• Relaxed, with shoulders back and both feet stable	• Tense, rigid, slumped, asymmetrical posture. Slumped posture is seen with depression or organic brain disease.
• Gait	• Smooth, coordinated movements; client alters position occasionally.	• Uncoordinated—staggering, shuffling, stumbling
• Motor movements	• Same as above	• Jerky, uncoordinated; tremors, tics, fast or slow movements. Bizarre movements are seen with schizophrenia; tense, fidgety, and restless behavior in anxious patients.

MENTAL STATUS ASSESSMENT (continued)

PROCEDURE	NORMAL FINDINGS	DEVIATIONS FROM NORMAL
• Dress	• Clothes fit and are appropriate for occasion and weather.	• Clothes extra large or small and inappropriate for occasion. Inappropriate dress is seen with depression, dementia, Alzheimer disease, and schizophrenia.
• Hygiene	• Skin clean, nails clean and trimmed	• Dirty, unshaven; dirty nails; foul odors. Poor hygiene is seen with depression, dementia, Alzheimer disease, and schizophrenia; meticulous, finicky grooming in obsessive-compulsive disorder.
• Facial expression	• Good eye contact, smiles/frowns appropriately	• Poor eye contact is seen in apathy or depression; masklike expression in Parkinson disease; extreme anger or happiness in anxious clients.
• Speech	• Clear with moderate pace	• High pitched; monotonal; hoarse; very soft or weak. Slow, repetitive speech is present in depression or Parkinson disease; loud and rapid in manic phases; irregular, uncoordinated speech in multiple sclerosis; dysphonia in impairment of CN X; dysarthria in Parkinson or cerebellar disease; aphasia in lesions of dominant hemisphere.

MENTAL STATUS ASSESSMENT (continued)

PROCEDURE	NORMAL FINDINGS	DEVIATIONS FROM NORMAL
*Observe **mood*** by asking, "How are you feeling?" or "What are your plans for the future?"		
• Feelings (vary from joy to anger)	• Responds appropriately to topic discussed; expresses feelings appropriate to situation	• Expresses feelings inappropriate to situation (eg, extreme anger or euphoria)
• Expressions	• Expresses good feelings about self, others, and life; verbalizes positive coping mechanisms (talking, support systems, counseling, exercise, etc.)	• Expresses dissatisfaction with self, others, and life in general; verbalizes negative coping mechanisms (use of alcohol, drugs, etc.); prolonged negative feelings seen with depression; elation and high energy seen with manic phases; excessive worry seen in obsessive–compulsive disorders; eccentric moods not relevant to situation are seen in schizophrenia.

PROCEDURE	NORMAL FINDINGS	DEVIATIONS FROM NORMAL
Observe thought process and perceptions by stating, "Tell me your understanding of your current health situation."		
• Clarity and content	• Expresses full and free-flowing thoughts during interview	• Expressed thoughts are jumbled, confusing, and not reality oriented. Repetition and expression of illogical thoughts are seen with schizophrenia; rapid flight of ideas with manic phases; irrational fears with phobias; delusions seen with psychotic disorders, delirium, and dementia; illusions seen with acute grief, stress reactions, schizophrenia, and delirium; hallucinations with organic brain disease or psychotic illness.
• Perceptions	• Follows directions accurately; perceptions realistic and consistent with yours and others.	• Is unable to follow through with directives; perceptions unrealistic and inconsistent with yours and others
• Judgment	• Answers to questions are based on sound rationale.	• Impaired judgment may be seen in organic brain syndrome, emotional disturbances, mental retardation, or schizophrenia.

MENTAL STATUS ASSESSMENT (continued)

PROCEDURE	NORMAL FINDINGS	DEVIATIONS FROM NORMAL
*Observe **cognitive abilities.***		
• Orientation—Ask client name, hour, date, season, where he or she lives now.	• Aware of self, others, place, time; has address	• Unable to express where he or she is, time, and who others are; does not follow instructions. Reduced level of orientation is seen with organic brain disorders.
• Length of concentration	• Listens to you and responds with full thoughts	• Fidgets; does not listen attentively to you; expresses incomplete thoughts. Distraction and inability to focus are noted with anxiety, fatigue, attention deficit disorders, and altered states due to drug or alcohol intoxication.
• Memory—Ask client, "What did you eat today?" (recent) and "When is your birthday?" (past)	• Correctly answers questions about current day's activities; recalls significant past events	• Unable to recall any recent events with delirium, dementia, depression, and anxiety; unable to recall past events with cerebral cortex disorders.
• Abstract reasoning—Ask client to explain a proverb, eg, "A stitch in time saves nine."	• Explains proverb accurately	• Unable to give abstract meaning of proverb with schizophrenia, mental retardation, delirium, or dementia

MENTAL STATUS ASSESSMENT (continued)

PROCEDURE	NORMAL FINDINGS	DEVIATIONS FROM NORMAL
• Ability to make sound judgments—Ask client question such as "Why did you come to the hospital?" or "What do you do when you have pain?"	• Answers to questions based on sound rationale	• Answers to questions are not based on sound rationale in organic brain syndrome, emotional disturbances, mental retardation, or schizophrenia.
• Ability to identify similarities—Ask client questions such as "How are birds and bees alike?"	• Identifies similarity	• Unable to identify similarity with schizophrenia, mental retardation, delirium, or dementia
• Sensory perception and coordination—Ask client to write name and draw the face of a clock or copy simple figures such as:	• Writes name, draws clock and/or simple figures	• Does not write name or draw clock/figures accurately with mental retardation, dementia, or parietal lobe dysfunction

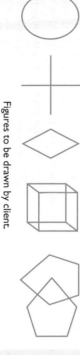

Figures to be drawn by client

The Glasgow Coma Scale

Use the Glasgow Coma Scale (GCS) for clients who are at high risk for rapid deterioration of the nervous system (Table 19–2). A GCS score of 14 points indicates an optimal level of consciousness. A GCS score of less than 14 points indicates some impairment in the level of consciousness. A score of 3 points, the lowest possible score, indicates deep coma.

Mini-Mental State Examination

Perform the Mini-Mental State Examination if time is limited and a quick standard measure is needed to evaluate or reevaluate cognitive function (Box 19–1).

Scores from 24 to 30 points are normal. Scores lower than 21 points may be seen in organic brain disease (delirium or dementia) or affective disorders. Scores of 21 to 24 points are questionable with regard to disease and require further evaluation.

Note that potential harm from labeling or identifying clients with possible dementia must be weighed against benefits of assessment.

PEDIATRIC VARIATIONS

Subjective Data: Focus Questions

Excessive difficulty in relationships with siblings, peers, parents, and teachers? Sudden changes in activities such as play or school activities? Excessive fears? Change in attention span?

NORMAL VARIATIONS

- Abstract reasoning is not possible before ages 10 to 12 years. Judgment ability varies with level of development.
- From birth to 11 years, knowledge of normal development is most important in evaluating cognition. Cues for evaluating cognition in infants and young children are primarily *not* valid. Awareness, attention to mother, and a parent's report on the infant's attentiveness are also important. Play activities or games can be used to elicit many desired responses. For example, a young child can be asked to recall three to four numbers in sequence as a test of memory.
- From birth to 6 years, objective findings can be determined using the Denver Developmental Screening Test.

TABLE 19-2 GLASGOW COMA SCORE

The GCS is scored between 3 and 15, with 3 being the worst and 15 the best. It is composed of three parameters: Best Eye Response, Best Verbal Response, and Best Motor Response, as given below:

Best Eye Response (4)

1. No eye opening
2. Eye opening to pain
3. Eye opening to verbal command
4. Eyes open spontaneously

Best Verbal Response (5)

1. No verbal response
2. Incomprehensible sounds
3. Inappropriate words
4. Confused
5. Oriented

Best Motor Response (6)

1. No motor response
2. Extension to pain
3. Flexion to pain
4. Withdrawal from pain
5. Localizing pain
6. Obeys commands

Note that the phrase "GCS of 11" is essentially meaningless, and it is important to break the figure down into its components, such as E3V3M5 = GCS 11.

A GCS of 13 or higher correlates with a mild brain injury, 9–12 is a moderate injury, and 8 or less is a severe brain injury.

(From Teasdale, G., and Jennett, B. [1974]. *Lancet, ii*: 81–83.)

BOX 19-1 ● Annotated Mini-Mental State Examination

NAME OF SUBJECT _____   Age _____

NAME OF EXAMINER _____   Years of School Completed _____

Approach the patient with respect and encouragement.   Date of Examination _____

Ask: Do you have any trouble with your memory?   ☐ Yes   ☐ No

May I ask you some questions about your memory?   ☐ Yes   ☐ No

SCORE	ITEM
5 ( )	**Time orientation**

Ask:

What is the year _____ (1), season _____ (1),

month of the year _____ (1), date _____ (1).

day of the week _____ (1)?

5 ( )   Place orientation

Ask:

Where are we now? What is the state _____ (1), city _____ (1),

part of the city _____ (1), building _____ (1), floor of the building _____ (1)?

3 ( )   Registration of three words

Say: Listen carefully. I am going to say three words. You say them back after I stop. Ready? Here they are ...
PONY (wait 1 second), QUARTER (wait 1 second), ORANGE (wait 1 second). What were those words?

_____ (1)

_____ (1)

_____ (1)

Give 1 point for each correct answer, then repeat them until the patient learns all three.

Neurologic Assessment

BOX 19-1 ● (continued)

5( ) **Serial 7s as a test of attention and calculation**

Ask: Subtract 7 from 100 and continue to subtract 7 from each subsequent remainder until I tell you to stop. What is 100 take away 7? _____ (1)

Say:

Keep going. _____ (1), _____ (1),

_____ (1), _____ (1).

3( ) **Recall of three words**

Ask:

What were those three words I asked you to remember?

Give 1 point for each correct answer _____ (1),

_____ (1), _____ (1).

2( ) **Naming**

Ask:

What is this? (show pencil) _____ (1). What is this? (show watch) _____ (1).

1( ) **Repetition**

Say:

Now I am going to ask you to repeat what I say. Ready? No ifs ands or buts.

Now you say that _____ (1).

3( ) **Comprehension**

Say:

Listen carefully because I am going to ask you to do something:

Take this paper in your left hand (1), fold it in half (1), and put it on the floor (1).

BOX 19-1 • (continued)

1 ( )   Reading
Say:
Please read the following and do what it says, but do not say it aloud (1).

Close your eyes

1 ( )   Writing
Say:
Please write a sentence. If patient does not respond say: Write about the weather (1).

1 ( )   Drawing
Say: Please copy this design.

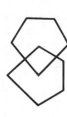

TOTAL SCORE _____ Assess level of consciousness along a continuum

| Alert | Drowsy | Stupor | Coma |

Neurologic Assessment

BOX 19-1 • (continued)

	YES	NO		YES	NO	FUNCTION BY PROXY
Cooperative	☐	☐	Deterioration from previous level of functioning	☐	☐	Please record date when patient was last able to perform the following tasks. Ask caregiver if patient independently handles.
Depressed	☐	☐	Family history of dementia	☐	☐	
Anxious	☐	☐	Head trauma	☐	☐	
Poor vision	☐	☐	Stroke	☐	☐	
Poor hearing	☐	☐	Alcohol abuse	☐	☐	
Native language	☐	☐	Thyroid disease	☐	☐	

	YES	NO	DATE
Money/bills	☐	☐	—
Medication	☐	☐	—
Transportation	☐	☐	—
Telephone	☐	☐	—

CULTURAL VARIATIONS

The stroke rate, although decreasing in industrialized countries, remains high in African Americans, and across the U.S. "Stroke belt" of southern states, Indiana, and Washington, D.C. (Centers for Disease Control and Prevention [CDC], 2005). A changing pattern is expected with decreasing incidence in Alabama and Mississippi and increases in Oregon, Washington, and Arkansas. Stroke rates are also expected to continue to decrease in New York and Florida (Howard et al., 2001). However, the difference in stroke by region or race may be due to differences in education, rates of diabetes and hypertension, smoking, and poor health insurance coverage (CDC, 2005).

GERIATRIC VARIATIONS

- May seem confused in a new or acute care setting owing to slowed thought processes and slowed responses to questions; however, is oriented to person, time, and place
- Decreased ability to recall directions
- Slight decline in short-term memory
- Use the GDS-5/15 Geriatric Depression Scale to screen older adults for depression (Box 19-2).
- Slowed reaction time
- Likes to reminisce and tends to wander from topic at hand
- May have hesitation with short-term memory
- Clients over 80 years should be able to recall two to four words after a 5-minute time period.

Possible Collaborative Problems

Depression	Suicide attempt
Alcohol abuse	Drug abuse

BOX 19-2 • The GDS-5/15 Geriatric Depression Scale

Directions: If the patient scores 0 or 1 point on the GDS-5, the patient is classified as "not depressed" and no further questions are asked. If the patient scores 2 points or more on the GDS-5, the screener continues asking the remaining 10 questions and classifies the patient as "suggesting depressed" or "not depressed" according to the GDS guidelines. Those classified as "suggesting depressed" on the full GDS-5/15 need to be referred for further clinical investigation for symptoms of depression.

1. Are you basically satisfied with your life?[1,3]	Yes	No*
2. Do you often get bored?[3]	Yes*	No
3. Do you often feel helpless?[3]	Yes*	No[3]
4. Do you prefer to stay home rather than going out and doing new things?[2,3]	Yes*	No
5. Do you feel pretty worthless the way you are now?[3]	Yes*	No

Score of 2 or more on GDS-5? Please continue with the remaining 10 questions:

Score GDS-5 = _____

6. Have you dropped many of your activities and interests?[2]	Yes*	No
7. Do you feel that your life is empty?[1]	Yes*	No
8. Are you in good spirits most of the time?	Yes	No*
9. Are you afraid that something bad is going to happen to you?[1]	Yes*	No

BOX 19-2 • (continued)

10. Do you feel happy most of the time?[1,2]	Yes	No*
11. Do you feel you have more problems with memory than most?	Yes*	No
12. Do you think it is wonderful to be alive now?	Yes	No*
13. Do you feel full of energy?	Yes	No*
14. Do you feel your situation is hopeless?	Yes*	No
15. Do you think that most people are better off than you are?	Yes*	No

Circle each answer. Each answer indicated by * counts as 1 point.

Score GDS-15 = _____

Note:
[1] = Included on 4-Item, D'Ath.
[2] = Included on 4-Item, van Marwijk.
[3] = Included on 5-Item, Hoyl.
GDS-5 score of 2 or more indicates possible depression (Hoyl et al., 1999).; ask remaining 10 questions.
GDS-15 score of 5–9 indicates possible depression; scores above 9 usually indicate depression (Sheikh & Yesavage, 1986).
Used with permission from Brink, T., Yesavage, J. A., Lum, O., Heersema, P., Adey, M., & Rose, T. (1982). Screening tests for geriatric depression. *Clinical Gerontologist 1*(1), 37–44.

TEACHING TIPS FOR SELECTED NURSING DIAGNOSES

Adult Client

Nursing Diagnosis: Disturbed Thought Processes related to neurologic changes (aging, head injury, stroke, etc.)

🔘 Inform client of the purpose and benefits of community agencies that offer support. Refer client as necessary. Assist family in coping, and explain how to communicate accurately using short sentences.

Nursing Diagnosis: Ineffective Individual Coping related to inadequate opportunity to prepare for stressor

🔘 Teach client the use of appropriate stress-reducing measures (eg, relaxation techniques, biofeedback, exercise, hobbies). Inform client of beneficial effects of decreasing coffee, sugar, and salt in diet and maintaining adequate B and C vitamins in diet for adequate functioning of the endocrine and nervous systems. Refer client to community agencies and support groups as necessary.

Nursing Diagnosis: Impaired Memory

🔘 Teach client memory-enhancing techniques.

Nursing Diagnosis: Readiness for enhanced critical thinking

🔘 Teach client critical-thinking skills. Assist client to obtain resources to enhance critical thought processes.

Pediatric Client

Nursing Diagnosis: Compromised Family Coping: Compromised related to family developmental crisis adjusting to infant/child development

🔘 Discuss social development of the child. Infant's "stranger anxiety" is normal. Teach parents ways to assist infant to warm up to strangers. Encourage verbalization, reassurance, and cuddling. Help parent assess child's readiness to begin school and to verbalize any school problems with child.

CRANIAL NERVE ASSESSMENT

Various techniques are used to assess cranial nerve (CN) functioning.

Objective Data: Assessment Techniques

Assess CN I through XII.

PROCEDURE	NORMAL FINDINGS	DEVIATIONS FROM NORMAL
CN I—Olfactory: Hold scent (eg, coffee, orange) under one nostril with other occluded while client closes eyes. Repeat with other nostril.	Identifies scent correctly with each nostril	Unable to identify correct odor
CN II—Optic: Assess vision. Assess visual fields. Do funduscopic examination for direct visualization of optic nerve.	See Chapter 9, Eye Assessment.	See Chapter 9, Eye Assessment.
CN III—Oculomotor: ***CN IV—Trochlear:*** ***CN VI—Abducens:*** Assess extraocular movements. Assess PERRLA (pupils equal, round, and reactive to light and accommodation).	See Chapter 9, Eye Assessment.	See Chapter 9, Eye Assessment.

PROCEDURE	NORMAL FINDINGS	DEVIATIONS FROM NORMAL

CN V—Trigeminal:

Assess sensory function by:

- Touching cornea lightly with wisp of cotton (Fig. 19–4)

  - Eyelids blink bilaterally.

  - Absent blink of eyelids with lesion of CN V (trigeminal) or lesions of the motor part of CN VII (facial)

- Testing client's ability to feel light touch, dull, and sharp facial sensations on both sides of face at the forehead, cheek, and chin areas (with client's eyes closed; Fig. 19–5)

  - Identifies light touch, dull, and sharp sensations to forehead, cheeks, and chin

  - Unable to identify or feel facial sensations with lesions of CN V, spinothalamic tract, or posterior columns

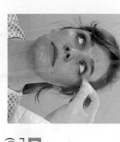

FIGURE 19–4 Testing corneal reflex with wisp of cotton. (© B. Proud.)

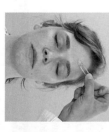

FIGURE 19–5 Testing sensory function of cranial nerve V: dull stimulus using a paper clip. (© B. Proud.)

Neurologic Assessment

CRANIAL NERVE ASSESSMENT (continued)

PROCEDURE	NORMAL FINDINGS	DEVIATIONS FROM NORMAL
Assess motor function by palpating masseter and temporal muscles as client clenches teeth (Fig. 19–6).	Muscles contract bilaterally.	Asymmetrical or no muscle contractions; irregular facial movements; pain or bilateral muscle weakness is seen with peripheral or CNS dysfunction. Unilateral weakness is seen with lesion of CN V.
CN VII—Facial: Assess sensory function by asking client to identify sugar, lemon, salt on anterior two thirds of tongue, with eyes closed and tongue protruded.	Identifies taste correctly	Unable to taste or to identify taste correctly with impaired CN VII

Neurologic Assessment

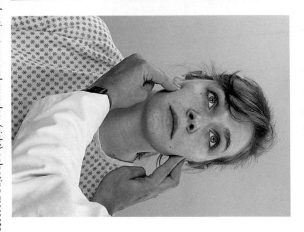

FIGURE 19-6 Testing motor function of cranial nerve V: (left) palpating temporal muscles; (right) palpating masseter muscles.
(© B. Proud.)

CRANIAL NERVE ASSESSMENT (continued)

PROCEDURE	NORMAL FINDINGS	DEVIATIONS FROM NORMAL
Assess motor function by asking client to do the following: • Smile • Frown • Show teeth • Blow out cheeks • Raise eyebrows and tightly close eyes	• Smiles • Frowns • Shows teeth • Blows out cheeks • Raises eyebrows and closes eyes tightly as instructed; facial movements are symmetrical.	• Unable to perform facial movements as instructed, or movements asymmetrical on one side of face. Unable to do facial movements along with paralysis of the lower part of the face seen in Bell palsy; paralysis of lower part of face on opposite side is seen with central lesion affecting upper motor neurons from cerebrovascular accident.
CN VIII—Acoustic: Assess hearing.	See Chapter 10, Ear Assessment.	See Chapter 10, Ear Assessment.
CN IX—Glossopharyngeal Assess taste and gag reflex.	See CN VII for taste and CN X for gag reflex.	See CN VII (taste) and CN IX (gag reflex).
Ask client to identify lemon juice and salt on posterior one third of tongue with eyes closed.	• Identifies taste and gag reflex present	Unable to identify correct taste with lesion of CN IX

PROCEDURE	NORMAL FINDINGS	DEVIATIONS FROM NORMAL
CN X—Vagus: Ask client to open mouth and say "ah."	Bilateral, symmetrical rise of soft palate and uvula	Unequal or absent rise of soft palate and uvula with lesions of CN X
Touch back of tongue or soft palate with tongue blade (Fig. 19–7).	Gag reflex present	Gag reflex absent with lesions of CN IX or X
CN XI—Spinal Accessory: Palpate strength of trapezius muscles by asking client to shrug shoulders against your hands (Fig. 19–8).	Symmetrical, strong contraction of trapezius muscles	Asymmetrical, weak, or absent contraction of trapezius muscles seen with paralysis or muscle weakness
Palpate strength of sternocleidomastoid muscles by asking client to turn head against your hand (Fig. 19–9).	Strong contraction of sternocleidomastoid muscle on opposite side that head is turned	Weak or absent contraction of sternocleidomastoid muscle on opposite side that head is turned seen with peripheral nerve disease
CN XII—Hypoglossal: Ask client to protrude tongue and move it to each side against tongue blade.	Symmetrical tongue with smooth outward movement and bilateral strength	Asymmetrical tongue; deviation to one side seen with unilateral lesion; fasciculations and atrophy of tongue seen with peripheral nerve disease; unequal or no strength

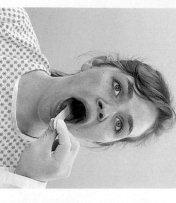

FIGURE 19-7 Testing cranial nerves IX and X: checking uvula rise and gag reflex. (© B. Proud.)

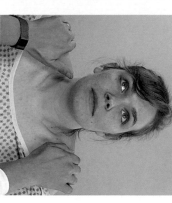

FIGURE 19-8 Testing cranial nerve XI: assessing strength of the trapezius muscle. (© B. Proud.)

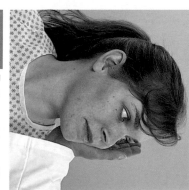

FIGURE 19-9 Testing cranial nerve XI: assessing strength of sternocleidomastoid muscle. (© B. Proud.)

GERIATRIC VARIATIONS

- Decreased ability to see, hear, taste, and smell

Possible Collaborative Problems

Cranial nerve impairment
Corneal ulceration
Increased intraocular pressure

TEACHING TIPS FOR SELECTED NURSING DIAGNOSES

Adult Client

Nursing Diagnosis: Sensory/Perceptual Alterations (specify) related to injury or aging

Explain to family the use and benefits of sensory therapy. Refer for hearing/visual aids as necessary. Teach client slowly and concisely. Speak clearly and demonstrate instructions from client's best side for hearing and seeing. Teach client how to prevent thermal injuries.

SENSORY NERVE ASSESSMENT

To test the client's ability to perceive various sensations over the extremities and abdomen, stimuli must be scattered to cover all dermatomes. The client is asked to close his or her eyes and identify the type of sensation perceived and the body area where it was felt. If a perceptual deficit is identified, the area is mapped out to determine the extent of impaired sensation.

SENSORY NERVE ASSESSMENT (continued)

PROCEDURE	NORMAL FINDINGS	DEVIATIONS FROM NORMAL
Test for **primary sensations** with client's eyes closed by touching client with the following:		
• Piece of cotton	• Identifies area of light touch	• Unable to identify location or light touch sensation
• Alternately with sharp tip and dull tip of paper clip	• Identifies area touched and differentiates between sharp and dull sensations	• Unable to identify location or differentiate touch sensations
• Vibrating tuning fork on major distal bony prominences of wrist, sternum	• Identifies vibratory sensation	• Unable to identify vibratory sensation
Test for **cortical and discriminatory sensation** with client's eyes closed by asking client to identify the following:		
• The number of points touching him or her while you touch client with two points simultaneously (two-point discrimination; Fig. 19–10)	• Identifies two points on forearm at 40 mm apart; back at 40–70 mm apart, dorsal hands at 20–30 mm apart, fingertips at 2–5 mm apart	• Unable to identify two points at normal ranges with lesions of the sensory cortex

SENSORY NERVE ASSESSMENT (continued)

PROCEDURE	NORMAL FINDINGS	DEVIATIONS FROM NORMAL
• The object (eg, a coin) you place in client's hand (stereognosis)	• Identifies correct object	• Unable to identify object with lesions of the sensory cortex
• A number you write on client's palm with a tongue blade (graphesthesia)	• Identifies correct number	• Unable to identify number with lesions of the sensory cortex
• The direction you move a part of client's body (eg, move fingers or toes up or down with eyes closed; kinesthesia; Fig. 19–11)	• Identifies correct direction body part is moved	• Unable to identify direction in which body part is moved with lesions of the sensory cortex

GERIATRIC VARIATIONS

• Touch sensations may diminish normally with aging due to atrophy of peripheral nerve endings
• Decreased light touch and pain perception
• Vibratory sensation at ankles often decreased after age 70 years

Possible Collaborative Problems

Peripheral nerve impairment
Neuropathies

Neurologic Assessment

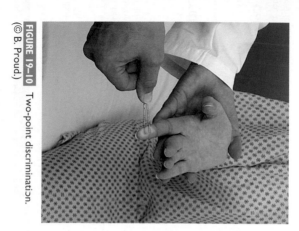

FIGURE 19–10 Two-point discrimination. (© B. Proud.)

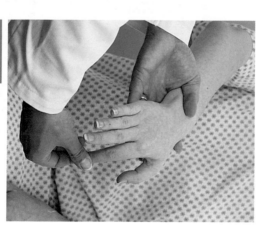

FIGURE 19–11 Testing position sense (kinesthesia). (© B. Proud.)

TEACHING TIPS FOR SELECTED NURSING DIAGNOSES

Adult Client

Nursing Diagnosis: Risk for Injury related to decreased tactile sensations

🖐 Instruct on proper inspection and protective care of extremities. Caution client on dangers of exposure to extreme hot and cold temperatures, contact with sharp objects, and wearing tight-fitting shoes or garments.

MOTOR ASSESSMENT

Assess muscle size, tone, movement, voluntary movements, and strength. See Chapter 18, Musculoskeletal Assessment.

CEREBELLAR ASSESSMENT

Ask the client to perform the following actions, after you demonstrate them, in order to assess coordination.

Objective Data: Assessment Techniques

Ask client to do the following:

CEREBELLAR ASSESSMENT (continued)

PROCEDURE	NORMAL FINDINGS	DEVIATIONS FROM NORMAL
Close eyes, and hold arms over head and straight out in front.	Holds arms over head and straight out steadily for 20 seconds	Downward drift; a flexion of one or both arms
With arms extended to the sides, touch each forefinger alternately to nose, first with eyes open and then with eyes closed (Fig. 19–12).	Smooth accurate movements while touching finger to nose	Uncoordinated jerky movements; inability to touch nose seen with cerebellar disease

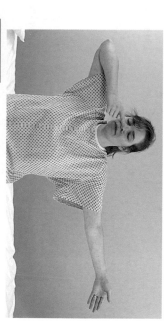

FIGURE 19–12 Testing coordination: finger-to-nose test. (© B. Proud.)

CEREBELLAR ASSESSMENT (continued)

PROCEDURE	NORMAL FINDINGS	DEVIATIONS FROM NORMAL
Put the palms of both hands down on both legs, then turn the palms up, and then turn the palms down again. Ask client to increase speed (Fig. 19–13).	Rapidly turns palms up and down	Uncoordinated movements or tremors are seen with cerebellar disease.
Button and unbutton coat/shirt.	Buttons and unbuttons clothes smoothly	Clumsy attempts to button and unbutton clothes
Run each heel down opposite shin one at a time (Fig. 19–14).	Runs each heel smoothly down each shin	Unable to place heel on shin and move it down shin with coordination with cerebellar disease
Stand erect with feet together and arms at sides, first with eyes open and then with eyes closed. (Put your arms around client to prevent falls—Romberg test.)	Stands straight with minimal swaying	Sways, moves feet out to prevent fall with disease of posterior column, vestibular dysfunction, or cerebellar disorders
Walk naturally.	Steady gait with opposite arm swing	Unsteady gait, uncoordinated arm swing; uses wide foot stance; shuffles or drags feet; lifts feet high off ground; crosses feet when walking. Gait is affected by disorders of the motor, sensory, vestibular, and cerebellar systems.

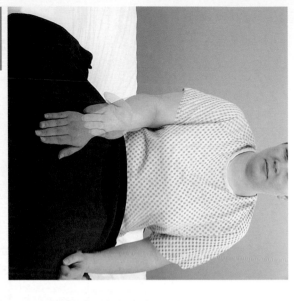

FIGURE 19–13 Testing rapid alternating movements: palms. (© B. Proud.)

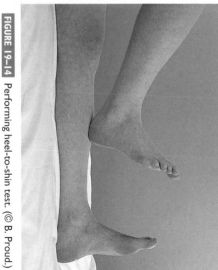

FIGURE 19–14 Performing heel-to-shin test. (© B. Proud.)

CEREBELLAR ASSESSMENT (continued)

PROCEDURE	NORMAL FINDINGS	DEVIATIONS FROM NORMAL
Walk in a heel-to-toe fashion (tandem walk, Fig. 19–15).	Maintains balance with tandem walk	Unsteady tandem walk; unable to walk tandem style
Stand on each foot (one at a time). Hop on each foot (one at a time) (Fig. 19–16).	Stands on one foot at a time Hops on each foot without losing balance	Unable to stand on one foot at a time Inadequate strength or balance to hop on each foot with muscle weakness or disease of the cerebellum
Walk on heels, then toes.	Walks on heels, then toes	Unable to walk on heels or toes

GERIATRIC VARIATIONS

- Slowed coordination and voluntary movements
- Decreased fine motor coordination
- May see tremors of the hand or head, or repetitive movements of the lips, jaw, or tongue
- May have slower and less certain gait; tandem walking may be very difficult for older client.
- Hopping on one foot is often impossible because of decreased flexibility and strength; it is best to avoid this test with the older client because of risk for injury.

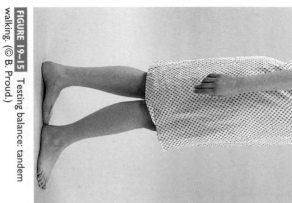

FIGURE 19–15 Testing balance: tandem walking. (© B. Proud.)

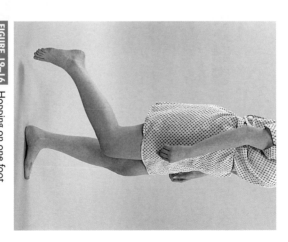

FIGURE 19–16 Hopping on one foot. (© B. Proud.)

REFLEX ASSESSMENT

Objective Data: Assessment Techniques

The reflex (or percussion) hammer is used to elicit deep tendon reflexes. Proceed as follows to elicit a deep tendon reflex:

1. Encourage the client to relax and position the client properly.

2. Hold the handle of the reflex hammer between your thumb and index finger so it swings freely.

3. Palpate the tendon and use a rapid wrist movement to strike the tendon briskly. Observe the response.

4. Compare the response of one side with the other.

5. For arm reflexes, ask the client to clench his or her jaw or to squeeze one thigh with the opposite hand, and then immediately strike the tendon. For leg reflexes, ask the client to lock the fingers of both hands and pull them against each other, and then immediately strike the tendon.

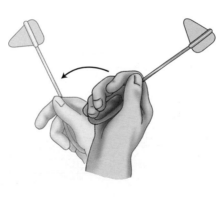

Neurologic Assessment

6. Rate and document reflexes using the following scale and figure:

- Grade 4+ Hyperactive, very brisk, rhythmic oscillations (clonus); abnormal and indicative of disorder
- Grade 3+ More brisk or active than normal, but not indicative of a disorder
- Grade 2+ Normal, usual response
- Grade 1+ Decreased, less active than normal
- Grade 0 No response

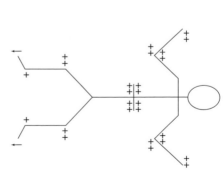

To elicit superficial reflexes, lightly stroke the skin with a moderately sharp instrument (eg, key, tongue blade). Finally, certain maneuvers are performed to elicit any pathologic reflexes.

PROCEDURE	NORMAL FINDINGS	DEVIATIONS FROM NORMAL
*Elicit **deep tendon reflexes** as follows:*		
• Biceps reflex: With reflex hammer, tap your thumb placed over biceps tendon with client's arm flexed (tests nerve roots C5, C6; Fig. 19–17).	• Biceps contract (1+, 2+, 3+ biceps reflex).	• Absent or hyperactive contraction of biceps (0, 4+ biceps reflex)
• Brachioradialis reflex: Tap brachicradialis tendon just above wrist on radial side with client's arm resting midway between supination and pronation (tests nerve roots C5, C6; Fig. 19–18).	• Elbow flexes with pronation of forearm (1+, 2+, 3+ brachioradialis reflex).	• Absent or hyperactive flexion of elbow and forearm pronation (0+, 4+ brachioradialis reflex)
• Triceps reflex: Tap triceps tendon (just above elbow) with client's arm abducted and forearm hanging freely (tests nerve roots C6, C7, C8; Fig. 19–19).	• Elbow extends (1+, 2+, 3+ triceps reflex).	• Absent or hyperactive elbow extension (0, 4+ triceps reflex)

Neurologic Assessment

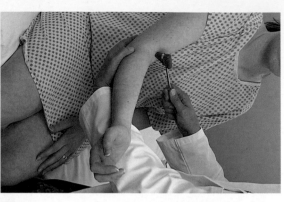

FIGURE 19-17 Eliciting biceps reflex. (© B. Proud.)

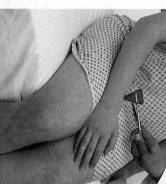

FIGURE 19-18 Eliciting brachioradialis reflex. (© B. Proud.)

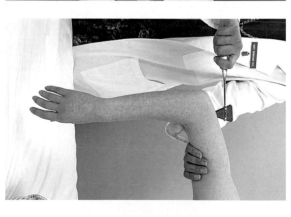

FIGURE 19-19 Eliciting triceps reflex. (© B. Proud.)

REFLEX ASSESSMENT (continued)

PROCEDURE	NORMAL FINDINGS	DEVIATIONS FROM NORMAL
• Patellar reflex: Tap patellar tendon with client's knee flexed and thigh stabilized (tests nerve roots L2, -3; Fig. 19–20).	• Extension of knee (1+, 2+, 3+ patellar reflex)	• Absent or hyperactive extension of knee (0, 4+ patellar reflex)

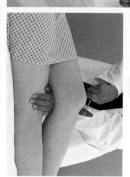

FIGURE 19–20 Eliciting patellar reflex. (*Left*) Sitting position. (*Right*) Supine position. (© B. Proud.)

Neurologic Assessment

REFLEX ASSESSMENT (continued)

PROCEDURE	NORMAL FINDINGS	DEVIATIONS FROM NORMAL
• Achilles reflex: Tap Achilles tendon with client's foot slightly dorsiflexed and stabilized (tests nerve roots S1, S2; Fig. 19–21).	• Plantar flexion of foot (1+, 2+, 3+ Achilles reflex)	• Absent or hyperactive plantar flexion of foot (0, 4+ plantar flexion)

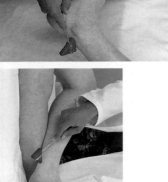 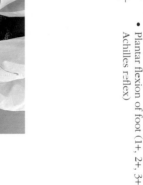

FIGURE 19-21 Eliciting Achilles reflex. (*Left*) Sitting position. (*Right*) Supine position. (© B. Proud.)

PROCEDURE

Elicit superficial reflexes as follows:

- Lightly stroke each side of abdomen above and below umbilicus (umbilicus reflexes; Fig. 19–22).
- Stroke gluteal area.
- Stroke inner upper thigh of males.

NORMAL FINDINGS

- Bilateral upward and downward movements of umbilicus toward stroke abdomen toward stroke; abdomen contracts.
- Anal sphincter contracts.
- Scrotum elevates on side stimulated.

DEVIATIONS FROM NORMAL

- Absent or unilateral movement of umbilicus; no abdominal contraction
- Absent contraction of gluteal reflex
- No elevation of scrotum

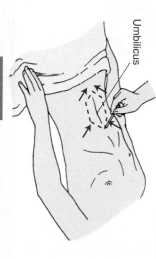

Umbilicus

FIGURE 19–22 Umbilicus reflex.

REFLEX ASSESSMENT (continued)

PROCEDURE	NORMAL FINDINGS	DEVIATIONS FROM NORMAL

*Assess for **pathologic reflexes** as follows:*

- Plantar reflex: Use end of reflex hammer to stroke lateral aspect of sole from heel to ball of foot (Fig. 19-23).

- Flexion of all toes (plantar response) seen in adults (see Fig. 19-23)

- Except in infancy, extension (dorsiflexion) of the big toe and fanning of all toes (positive plantar reflex; Babinski response) are seen with lesions of upper motor neurons. Unconscious states resulting from drug and alcohol intoxication or subsequent to an epileptic seizure may also cause it.

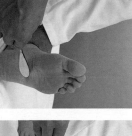
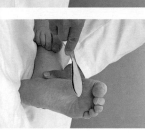

FIGURE 19-23 Eliciting plantar reflex (left). Normal plantar response (right). (© B. Proud.)

PROCEDURE	NORMAL FINDINGS	DEVIATIONS FROM NORMAL
• Ankle clonus: Sharply dorsiflex foot with knee supported and partially flexed, and hold this way (Fig. 19-24).	• Foot stays dorsiflexed with no movement.	• Foot oscillates between dorsiflexion and plantar flexion.
• Brudzinski sign: Ask client to flex the neck; watch the hips and knees in reaction to the maneuver.	• Hips and knees remain relaxed and motionless.	• Flexion of the hips and knees is a positive Brudzinski sign and suggests meningeal inflammation.
• Kernig sign: Flex the client's leg at both the hip and the knee, and then straighten the knee.	• No pain felt. Discomfort behind the knee during full extension occurs in many normal people.	• Pain and increased resistance to extending the knee are a positive Kernig sign. When Kernig sign is bilateral, the examiner suspects meningeal irritation.

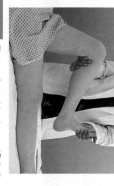

FIGURE 19-24 Testing for ankle clonus. (© B. Proud.)

Neurologic Assessment

PEDIATRIC VARIATIONS: BIRTH TO 1 YEAR

See Appendix 3 for developmental milestones for age 1 to 3 years.

Objective Data: Assessment Techniques

REFLEXES	NORMAL VARIATIONS
Cough	No cough reflex until 1–2 days of age; after 1–2 days, cough should be strong and present even during sleep throughout infancy.
Rooting: Infant turns head toward side of face stroked.	Disappears at about age 3–12 months
Extension: When tongue is pressed or touched, infant forces tongue outward.	Disappears at about age 4 months
Grasp: Touch to palm of hand or soles of feet causes flexion of hands/toes.	Palmar grasp should disappear at about age 3 months.
Plantar reflex: Stroking outer sole of foot from heel to toe causes big toe to rise (dorsiflexion) and other toes to fan out.	Disappears after 1 year
Moro: Sudden jarring or change in equilibrium causes sudden extension and abduction of extremities, with thumb forming "C" shape; crying.	Disappears at about age 3–4 months
Startle: Sudden noise causes abduction of arms, clenched hands.	Disappears at about age 4 months
Crawling: Infant on abdomen will make crawling movements with arms and legs.	Disappears at about age 6 weeks

PEDIATRIC VARIATIONS: BIRTH TO I YEAR (continued)

REFLEXES	NORMAL VARIATIONS
Dance: Infant held so soles of feet touching table will simulate walking movements.	Disappears at about age 3–4 weeks
Neck righting: In supine infant, if head is turned to one side, shoulder and trunk will turn to that side	Disappears around age 10 months
Asymmetrical tonic neck: Infant's head quickly turns to one side, arm and leg on that side will extend, and opposite leg and arm will flex.	Disappears at about age 3–4 months

GERIATRIC VARIATIONS

- Generalized decreased deep tendon reflexes and slowed reflexes
- Decrease in transmission of impulses along with a delay in reaction time

Possible Collaborative Problems

Increased intracranial pressure   Spinal cord compression
Meningitis   Seizures
Paralysis

TEACHING TIPS FOR SELECTED NURSING DIAGNOSIS

Adult Client

Nursing Diagnosis: Risk for Injury related to seizure activity

Teach appropriate precautions and care, including the following:

- Use of padded tongue blade, wallet, or cloth to maintain airway
- Protection of client from harm during seizures
- Positioning on side after seizure
- Significance of drug maintenance

Nursing Diagnosis: Risk for Adult Failure to Thrive

Teach client and family or caregivers to assess behavior patterns that suggest anorexia, fatigue, dehydration, onset of incontinence (bowel or bladder), increase in chronic health problems such as pneumonia and urinary tract infections, cognitive decline, self-neglect, apathy, sadness. Teach client and caregivers to seek appropriate referrals if pattern is detected.

ASSESSMENT OF THE CHILDBEARING WOMAN

20

The body experiences many anatomic/physiologic changes during pregnancy. Findings in a physical assessment that would be considered abnormal in the nonpregnant client may be a result of pregnancy and not an abnormal state. In this chapter, the physical changes that occur in a woman as a result of pregnancy are identified as *normal variations*. Changes that are not a result of pregnancy or that represent an abnormal state during pregnancy are identified as *deviations from normal*.

For the sake of brevity, those systems described previously will not be repeated. Only variations of pregnancy will be noted. For procedures, the reader is referred to sections describing assessment of specific body systems.

During pregnancy, physical assessment should be performed every month for the first 27 weeks, every 2 weeks from week 28 to week 36, and then every week. More frequent examinations may be indicated for pregnancies at risk.

This chapter is divided into four sections: Prenatal Maternal Assessment, Prenatal Fetal Assessment, Intrapartum Maternal Assessment, and Postpartum Maternal Assessment.

PRENATAL MATERNAL ASSESSMENT

Equipment Needed

See Chapters 7 through 19 for the specific body system to be assessed.

Subjective Data: Focus Questions

Past pregnancies: Outcome of each? Number of living children? Complications? Length of labor? Years since last pregnancy?
Current pregnancy: Estimated due date? Confirmed by ultrasound? Problems during pregnancy? Nausea? Vomiting?
Cramping or bleeding? Planned pregnancy? Date of first prenatal visit? Prenatal education?
Concurrent disease? Medications?

Objective Data: Assessment Techniques

Review of Systems

Perform a general physical survey.

PROCEDURE	NORMAL FINDINGS	DEVIATIONS FROM NORMAL
Assess *the following:*		
• Age	• Ideal childbearing years: 16–35	• Younger than 16 or older than 35; advanced maternal age increases risk of genetic abnormalities such as Down syndrome; increased risk to mother and baby with age extremes.
• Weight	• Prenatal weight gain: women of normal weight: 25–35 lbs overweight women: 15–25 lbs obese women: 15 lbs (Fig. 20–1). *First trimester:* 2–4 lb *Second trimester:* 11 lb (1 lb/wk) *Third trimester:* 11 lb (1 lb/wk)	• Prepregnant weight <100 or >200 lb; sudden gain of more than 2 lb/wk may be seen in pregnancy-induced hypertension (PIH); weight loss or failure to gain weight.

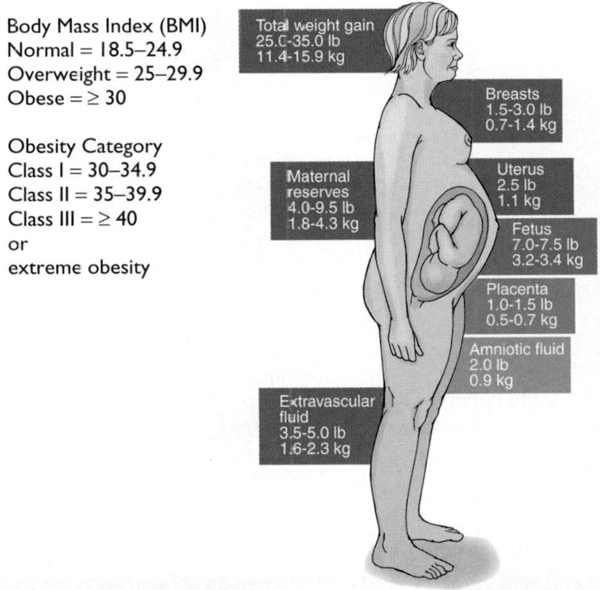

FIGURE 20-1 Distribution of weight gain during pregnancy.

Body Mass Index (BMI)
Normal = 18.5–24.9
Overweight = 25–29.9
Obese = ≥ 30

Obesity Category
Class I = 30–34.9
Class II = 35–39.9
Class III = ≥ 40
or
extreme obesity

Total weight gain
25.0–35.0 lb
11.4–15.9 kg

Maternal
reserves
4.0–9.5 lb
1.8–4.3 kg

Extravascular
fluid
3.5–5.0 lb
1.6–2.3 kg

Breasts
1.5–3.0 lb
0.7–1.4 kg

Uterus
2.5 lb
1.1 kg

Fetus
7.0–7.5 lb
3.2–3.4 kg

Placenta
1.0–1.5 lb
0.5–0.7 kg

Amniotic fluid
2.0 lb
0.9 kg

PRENATAL MATERNAL ASSESSMENT *(continued)*

PROCEDURE	NORMAL FINDINGS	DEVIATIONS FROM NORMAL
• Blood pressure	• Range of 90–139/60–89 mm Hg; falls during second trimester, prepregnant level first and third trimesters	• ≥140/90 mm Hg or increase of 30 mm Hg above baseline systolic or 15 mm Hg above baseline diastolic taken with client in side-lying position; increased levels are seen with PIH.
• Pulse	• 60–90 bpm; may increase 10–15 bpm higher than prepregnant levels	• Irregularities; persistently <60 or >100 bpm at rest
• Behavior	*First trimester:* Tired, ambivalent *Second trimester:* Introspective, energetic *Third trimester:* Restless, preparing for baby, labile moods (the father may experience some of these same behaviors)	• Denial of pregnancy, withdrawal, depression, psychosis
*Observe **skin color.***	Linea nigra (Fig. 20–2), striae gravidarum (see Fig. 20–2); chloasma (Fig. 20–3); spider nevi	Pale, yellowing changes of the skin as seen with liver diseases
*Assess **head and neck.***		Facial edema, headache
• Nose	• Nasal stuffiness, nosebleeds	
• Eyes		• Blurred vision and visual spots are symptoms of PIH.

Assessment of the Childbearing Woman

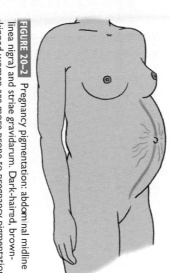

FIGURE 20–2 Pregnancy pigmentation: abdominal midline (linea nigra) and striae gravidarum. Dark-haired, brown-skinned women are more prone to pregnancy pigmentation.

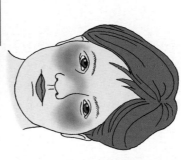

FIGURE 20–3 Marked chloasma of pregnancy.

PRENATAL MATERNAL ASSESSMENT (continued)

PROCEDURE	NORMAL FINDINGS	DEVIATIONS FROM NORMAL
• Neck	• Slight enlargement of thyroid	• Nodules or marked enlargement, asymmetry of thyroid gland as seen with thyroid disease
Assess **cardiovascular system.** • Heart	• Short systolic blowing murmurs	• Progressive dyspnea, palpitations, markedly decreased activity tolerance may be seen with cardiac diseases.
• Blood volume	• Increases throughout pregnancy; peaks at 32–34 weeks, reaching 30–50% above prepregnancy levels	
Assess **peripheral vascular system.**	Late pregnancy: dependent edema, varicose veins; supine hypotension	Perineal varicosities; calf pain may be related to deep vein thrombosis; generalized edema; diminished pedal pulses.
Assess **respiratory system.**	Increased anteroposterior diameter, thoracic breathing, slight hyperventilation, shortness of breath in late pregnancy	Dyspnea may be seen in patients with cardiac disease and/or lung diseases such as asthma.
Assess **breasts.**	Increased size and nodularity, tenderness, prominent vascularization, darkening of nipples and areola, colostrum in third trimester (Fig. 20–4)	Localized redness; localized pain and warmth; erythemic streaks are commonly seen with mastitis; inverted nipples may cause difficulty for breast-feeding infants.

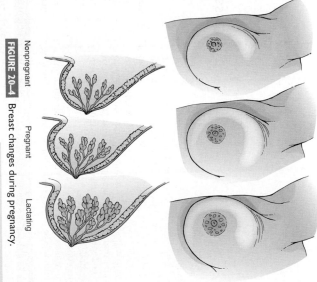

Nonpregnant   Pregnant   Lactating

FIGURE 20–4 Breast changes during pregnancy.

PROCEDURE	NORMAL FINDINGS	DEVIATIONS FROM NORMAL
Assess **gastrointestinal system.**	Nausea and vomiting, increased saliva, heartburn, bloating, constipation	Severe epigastric pain is seen with PIH; severe nausea and vomiting may be seen during the first trimester with hyperemesis gravidarum.
Assess **genitourinary–reproductive systems.**	Urinary frequency in first and third trimesters, increased pigmentation of vulva and vagina, increased vaginal discharge	Flank pain, dysuria, oliguria, proteinuria, purulent vaginal discharge, vaginal bleeding
Assess **musculoskeletal system.**	Relaxation of pelvic joints: "waddling" gait; increased lumbar curve, backache, diastasis recti, leg cramps	
Assess **neurologic system.**		Hyperactive reflexes, positive clonus seen with PIH

PRENATAL FETAL ASSESSMENT

Equipment Needed

- Bed or examination table
- Drape
- Pillow
- Paper centimeter tape measure
- Fetoscope or Doppler

Subjective Data: Focus Questions

Note date of initial fetal movement felt.

Has the fetus been active?

Objective Data: Assessment Techniques

Inspection

With client supine and head slightly elevated on a pillow, inspect abdomen for shape and contour of fetus. (During the second and third trimesters, time spent in the supine position should be minimal. This position puts the weight of the fetus and uterus on the aorta and obstructs blood flow.)

Palpation

Using both hands, gently palpate the outline of the fetus and the top of the uterus (fundus). Using the centimeter tape, measure from the top of the symphysis pubis to the top of the uterine fundus (Fig. 20–5).

PROCEDURE	NORMAL FINDINGS	DEVIATIONS FROM NORMAL
Measure fundal height and multiply by 3/7 (this equals weeks of gestation; Fig. 20–6).	Accurate within 2 weeks until 36 weeks. Obesity or extremes in height may alter findings.	Lag in progression may indicate problems with fetal development and/or oligohydramnios commonly seen with congenital abnormalities. Sudden increase in fundal height size may also indicate fetal abnormalities such as congenital anomalies.

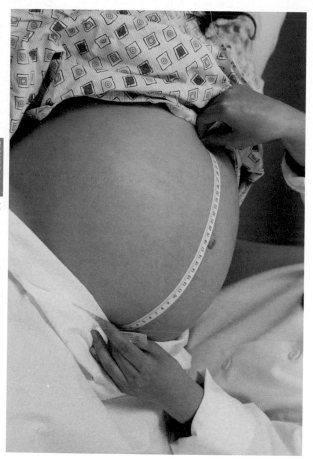

FIGURE 20–5 Measuring the fundal height.

Assessment of the Childbearing Woman

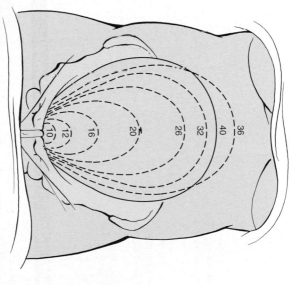

FIGURE 20–6 Approximate height of fundus at various weeks of gestation.

Auscultation

With Doppler or fetoscope, listen for fetal heartbeat. Locate fundus; begin listening halfway between the fundus and the pubis. Work outward in widening circles until a beating sound is heard. Compare with the maternal pulse. If different, count fetal heart rate for 1 full minute.

PROCEDURE	NORMAL FINDINGS	DEVIATIONS FROM NORMAL
Auscultate *fetal heart rate* (FHR) for the following:		
• Presence	• Audible at 10–12 weeks gestation with feta. Doppler; audible at 15–20 weeks gestation with fetoscope	• Absence of fetal heart tones after the 20th week of gestation indicates intra-uterine fetal demise.
• Rate	• Very rapid initially; gradually slows to 120–160 bpm at term; increased rate with fetal movement; during fetal sleep cycle, FHR may be in the 110–120 range.	• <120 bpm; no change or decrease in FHR with movement may indicate fetal distress.
• Rhythm	• Regular	• A marked variance or variance of <5 beats/min may indicate fetal distress.

CULTURAL VARIATIONS

- Rh-negative blood is rare in nonwhite groups
- Dizygote twinning is higher in blacks than whites or Asians.

Possible Collaborative Problems

Bleeding disorder of pregnancy	Hyperemesis gravidarum
Spontaneous abortion	Ectopic pregnancy
Placenta previa	Preexisting medical conditions
Abruptio placentae	Hyperglycemia/hypoglycemia
Pregnancy-induced hypertension	Hypertension
Dehydration	Renal malfunctioning
Gestational diabetes	Cardiac conditions
Preeclampsia	

TEACHING TIPS FOR SELECTED NURSING DIAGNOSES

Nursing Diagnosis: Risk for Ineffective Therapeutic Regimen Management during pregnancy
Inform client of normal variations during the prenatal period. Also inform client of those abnormal symptoms to be reported immediately. Encourage client to write down questions; provide time to discuss them. Instruct client on methods to cope with normal variations (eg, nausea and vomiting). Encourage attendance at prenatal classes and appropriate reading material. Prenatal health care must begin in the first trimester of pregnancy (Healthy People, 2010).

Nursing Diagnosis: Risk for Imbalanced Nutrition: Less Than Body Requirements related to increased metabolism and fetal demands

Diet should be selected from basic five food groups, with an additional 300 calories per day over recommended daily allowances. A balanced diet should provide all essential nutrients during pregnancy except folic acid and iron. These should be supplemented throughout pregnancy, because adequate amounts are closely related to fetal well-being and pregnancy outcome.

Nursing Diagnosis: Disturbed Body Image related to effects of physical changes during pregnancy

An exercise program started early in pregnancy and continued throughout will help maintain muscle tone and facilitate a return to prepregnant size after delivery. Exercise programs should be approved by the obstetrician prior to initiation. In general, those activities practiced prior to pregnancy can be continued unless they have a potential of causing physical harm to mother and baby.

Allow client to express her feelings about body changes, and reassure her that most changes are reversible or minimized after delivery. Emphasize positive changes.

Nursing Diagnosis: Readiness for Enhanced Parenting

Beginning education on growth and development of fetus and infant early in pregnancy can provide an opportunity for prospective parents to anticipate and understand development and expected patterns of developmental skill mastery.

Nursing Diagnosis: Readiness for Enhanced Infant Nutrition

The decision to breast- or bottle-feed the infant is usually made prior to or during pregnancy. Providing factual information with an opportunity for questions and answers early in pregnancy will facilitate a decision best suited to the client's needs and lifestyle.

INTRAPARTUM MATERNAL ASSESSMENT

During the intrapartum period, an initial physical assessment should be done on admission to the labor room, and findings should be compared with those of the prenatal period. The order of the assessment will vary based on presenting signs of labor.

Equipment Needed

- Bed with pillow
- Sterile examination glove
- Lubricant
- Electronic fetal monitor or Doppler
- Nitrazine paper
- Reflex hammer

Subjective Data: Focus Questions

History of prenatal care? Gravida? Para? Age? Estimated date of confinement (EDC)? When did contractions begin? Rupture of membranes? Color of vaginal fluid? Vaginal bleeding and amount? Frequency and duration of contractions? Problems with this pregnancy? Duration and outcome of previous labors? Childbirth preparation? Blood type and Rh status? Concurrent disease?

Objective Data: Assessment Techniques

Abdominal Assessment

INSPECTION

Have client completely undress except for gown. Place in a supine position with head slightly elevated. Knees and hips should be flexed with feet resting on mattress. Examination with the client in this position should be performed as rapidly as possible to prevent supine hypotension or fetal compromise.

INTRAPARTUM MATERNAL ASSESSMENT (continued)

PROCEDURE	NORMAL FINDINGS	DEVIATIONS FROM NORMAL
Inspect **abdomen** for the following: • Uterine size (see Fig. 20–5) • Uterine shape	• Large variation; fundus just below xiphoid process • Fetal outline longitudinal	• Uterus small or large for gestational age may indicate fetal malformations. • Fetal outline horizontal indicates the presentation of the baby may be transverse or breech.

PALPATION

With client on back and head slightly elevated, place fingertips on fundus. During a contraction, the fundus becomes firm. Client should relate when she feels a contraction begin and when it ends. Time seconds from beginning to end of contractions (duration). Calculate elapsed time from beginning of one contraction to beginning of another (frequency). Do this for several contractions in sequence to determine regularity. During contraction, gently push in on uterus with fingertips and note degree to which uterus indents (intensity). A large amount of subcutaneous tissue over the uterus may interfere with accurate assessment of intensity. Palpate several contractions in a row. To palpate bladder, gently push in on abdomen directly above symphysis pubis and release. Note degree of resistance met.

PROCEDURE	NORMAL FINDINGS	DEVIATIONS FROM NORMAL
Palpate uterus for the following: • Frequency of contractions	• As labor progresses, contractions gradually get closer together, in a regular pattern progressing to every 2–3 minutes; may be less frequent during second stage.	• Irregular pattern; more frequent than every 2 minutes may cause placental insufficiency for the fetus to get sufficient oxygenation during labor.

INTRAPARTUM MATERNAL ASSESSMENT (continued)

PROCEDURE	NORMAL FINDINGS	DEVIATIONS FROM NORMAL
• Duration of contractions	• Gradually increases to 60–90 seconds as labor progresses	• No increase; duration >90 seconds may deplete fetal oxygenation reserves.
• Intensity of contractions	• Gradually become stronger, uterus feels firm (rocklike); internal pressure monitor 40–60 mm Hg.	• No increase; pressure > 60 mm Hg is seen with hypertonic contractions.

Note. Contraction frequency and duration may be monitored with an electronic fetal monitor tocodynamometer. Initial assessment of contraction frequency and duration may be performed by palpation. Accurate intensity can only be determined, however, with an intrauterine pressure catheter.

Palpate above symphysis pubis for the bladder.

Soft, spongy

Bouncy, full, distended is seen with overdistention of the bladder.

AUSCULTATION
Locate FHR (see Prenatal section) and apply external fetal monitor ultrasound transducer or Doppler. FHR must be monitored every 5 minutes during the second stage of labor. High-risk pregnancies with ruptured amniotic fluid membranes should be monitored with internal electrodes to assess fetal well-being accurately.

INTRAPARTUM MATERNAL ASSESSMENT (continued)

PROCEDURE	NORMAL FINDINGS	DEVIATIONS FROM NORMAL
Monitor FHR for the following:		
• Baseline rate (must be determined by a 10-minute strip)	• 120–160 bpm	• <120 or >160 bpm for a 10-minute period may indicate fetal distress.
• Baseline variability (measurable only with internal fetal electrode)	• 5–25 bpm	• <5 bpm for longer than 20 minutes and not associated with maternal medication
• Periodic changes	• Periodic acceleration (increased FHR with fetal movement, stimulation, o˜ contractions); early-onset deceleration (mirrors contraction and occurs in late first stage and second stage of labor)	• Periodic deceleration; decreased FHR occurs with contractions; repetitive variable decelerations are seen with cord compression; late decelerations are seen in fetal distress; prolonged or slow return to baseline and associated loss o˜ variability may be seen in fetal distress.

Perineal Assessment

INSPECTION

With client supine, have her rest her feet on the bed with knees and hips flexed. Instruct client to relax and separate knees. If discharge is noted, obtain specimen to assess for ruptured membranes with Nitrazine paper.

INTRAPARTUM MATERNAL ASSESSMENT (continued)

PROCEDURE	NORMAL FINDINGS	DEVIATIONS FROM NORMAL
Observe **perineum** *for the following:*		
• Lesions	• None	• Vesicles could indicate genital herpes; genital warts, open sores may be seen with sexually transmitted infections.
• Discharge	• Bloody mucus; clear or milky fluid amniotic fluid will turn Nitrazine paper blue	• Bright red blood is seen with placenta previa; purulent fluid; green or brown fluid may indicate meconium in utero, which puts the fetus at risk for meconium aspiration at delivery. Lubricant or blood may give a false-positive result with Nitrazine paper.
• Swelling	• May be present in second stage of labor	• Present before second stage of labor
Observe **perineal area** *for the following:*		
• Shape	• As fetal head descends, perineum flattens and bulges.	
• Fetal parts	• Occiput becomes visible during second stage of labor.	• Fetal hand or foot may indicate breech presentation; loop of umbilical cord visible on the perineum puts the fetus at high risk and requires immediate cesarean section.

PALPATION

Have client separate knees, and instruct her to relax perineum. Put on sterile examination glove, and lubricate index and middle fingers. Gently insert fingers into vagina and palpate cervix and fetal presenting part. Insert finger between cervix and presenting part, and rotate entire circumference of cervix. This examination should be performed on admission and thereafter only when behavior and contraction pattern indicate progression of labor.

PROCEDURE	NORMAL FINDINGS	DEVIATIONS FROM NORMAL
Palpate **cervix** *for the following:*		
• Position	• In early labor, cervix may be in posterior vaginal vault; it becomes more anterior as labor progresses.	
• Effacement	• *Primipara:* Effacement before dilatation *Multipara:* Effacement and dilatation simultaneous	• Swelling of part or all of cervix occurs when the patient begins pushing before the cervix is completely dilated.
• Dilatation (in cm)	• *Primipara:* Average 1 cm/hr; may be slower in early phase *Multipara:* Average 1.5 cm/hr	• Failure to progress with active labor longer than 24 hours; complete dilatation in <3 hours of labor
Palpate **presenting part of the** ***fetus*** *for the following:*		
• Amniotic membrane	• If intact, can be felt over presenting part; may rupture prior to or during labor	

INTRAPARTUM MATERNAL ASSESSMENT (continued)

PROCEDURE	NORMAL FINDINGS	DEVIATIONS FROM NORMAL
• Presentation	• Cephalic; should feel skull, suture lines and one or both fontanelles (Fig. 20–7); caput succedaneum may mask landmarks.	• Breech: soft tissue, anus, or testicles; other small parts such as hands, feet seen in breech presentation
• Position	• Cephalic; posterior fontanelle felt in anterior position, anterior fontanelle in posterior position	• Anterior fontanelle in anterior position; fontanelles in transverse position
• Station (Fig. 20–8)	• *Primipara:* 0 station; gradually descends during second stage *Multipara:* May be –1 station or higher at onset of labor	• Failure to descend to 0 station during first stage of labor; failure to descend during second stage with pushing longer than 2 hours is seen in failure to progress, which requires cesarean section.
• Umbilical cord	• Not palpable	• May feel loop or pulsations in the umbilical cord, which requires immediate cesarean section

Note: If painless, bright red vaginal bleeding occurs, vaginal examination should be omitted. If fetal gestational age is less than 34 weeks and membranes have ruptured with no evidence of labor, vaginal examination should be omitted.

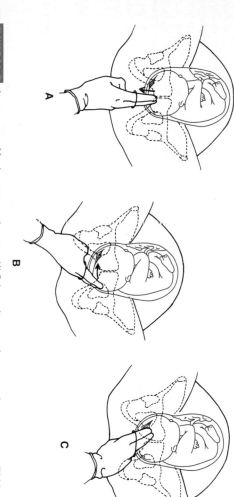

FIGURE 20-7 Assessment of fetal position and station. (A) Palpate the sagittal suture and assess station. (B) Identify posterior fontanelle. (C) Identify anterior fontanelle.

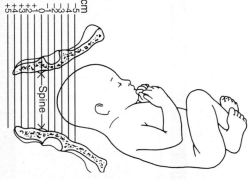

FIGURE 20–8 Measuring station of the fetal head while it is descending.

Peripheral Vascular Assessment

INSPECTION

With client in semi-Fowler position, observe face, hands, legs, and feet.

PROCEDURE	NORMAL FINDINGS	DEVIATIONS FROM NORMAL
Observe **face** *for the following:*		
• Color	• Pink	• Red, pale
• Edema	• None	• Periorbital edema
Observe **extremities** *for the following:*		
• Color	• Pink	• Pale, blue seen with cyanosis
• Swelling	• Dependent in ankles	• Swelling in the tibia or hands, not relieved by elevating

AUSCULTATION

With client in a sidelying position, auscultate blood pressure (BP) between contractions.

PROCEDURE	NORMAL FINDINGS	DEVIATIONS FROM NORMAL
Auscultate BP every hour or more often as indicated.	BP <140/50 mm Hg. May see BP increase during contractions.	BP ≥140/90 mm Hg or increase of 30 mm Hg systolic or 15 mm Hg diastolic over prenatal baseline seen in PIH

PROCEDURE	NORMAL FINDINGS	DEVIATIONS FROM NORMAL
Percuss extremities for reflexes and clonus.	See Chapter 19 for normal findings.	Hyperreflexia or clonus seen in PIH

Behavioral Assessment

PROCEDURE	NORMAL FINDINGS	DEVIATIONS FROM NORMAL
Observe for behavior changes:		
• Early labor (1–4 cm)	• Excited, happy	• Irrational
• Active labor (4–7 cm)	• Cooperative; increased dependence on support person	• Uncooperative, psychotic
• Transition (7–10 cm)	• Irritable, inner focused, hopeless	• Confused

Possible Collaborative Problems

Preeclampsia/eclampsia   Hypertension
Bleeding disorders   Fetal distress
Placenta previa   Labor dystocia
Abruptio placentae   Cephalopelvic disproportion
Uterine rupture   Premature labor
Fetal malpresentation   Fetal malposition

Assessment of the Childbearing Woman

TEACHING TIPS FOR SELECTED NURSING DIAGNOSES

Nursing Diagnosis: Acute pain related to uterine contractions

Instruct and demonstrate relaxation techniques. Provide feedback on muscle relaxation. Offer encouragement and support. Provide comfort measures such as gentle massage; temperature control; clean, dry, and wrinkle-free liners; ice chips or lip lubricant. The laboring woman should be encouraged to assume varying positions of comfort and to ambulate unless complications contraindicate this. Provide analgesics as needed.

Nursing Diagnosis: Fear related to unfamiliar environment, pain, and concern for fetal well-being

Orient to surroundings. Provide short and simple explanation for all procedures and encourage questions. Provide evidence of fetal well-being (monitor data). Encourage support person to stay with client. Client should not be left alone during active labor.

Nursing Diagnosis: Risk for Fluid Volume Deficit related to increased muscle activity, increased respiratory rate, nausea and vomiting, and decreased gastric motility or absorption

Offer small amounts of fluids such as ice chips or popsicles. Avoid solid foods, which are difficult to digest and often promote vomiting. Consider antiemetics for persistent vomiting. Monitor for dehydration or decreased placental perfusion. Administer intravenous fluids as indicated.

POSTPARTUM MATERNAL ASSESSMENT

The postpartum period begins with the delivery of the placenta and lasts an average of 6 weeks, during which time all body systems return to prepregnant levels. Some changes are rapid and others occur over time. During the first 24 hours many changes occur and frequent assessment is essential.

Changes occurring as an expected part of postpartum recovery are identified as *normal findings*. The reader is referred to Chapter 3 for a more detailed description of technique for assessing various body systems.

Subjective Data: Focus Questions

Problems during pregnancy? Labor—induction, augmentation, length of labor? Gravida, para? Method of delivery? Size of baby? Anesthesia/analgesia? Concurrent disease?

Objective Data: Assessment Techniques

PROCEDURE	NORMAL FINDINGS	DEVIATIONS FROM NORMAL
Monitor the following:		
• Temperature	• 100.4°F (38°C) in first 24 hours	• Higher than 100.4°F (38°C) in first 24 hours or 100.4°F (38°C) and above on any 2 of the first 10 days postpartum seen in puerperal infection
• Blood pressure	• No change from prepregnant levels	• PIH can occur up to 48 hours postpartum; persistent elevation of blood pressure from PIH beyond 48 hours
• Pulse	• Bradycardia (50–70 bpm) for 6–10 days	• Tachycardia; preexisting hypertension may be difficult to control; postural hypotension may occur when assuming the upright position after delivery.
• Weight	• Initial 10- to 12-lb loss; 10- to 20-lb loss in next 6–8 weeks	
• Behavior	• *First 2–3 days postpartum:* Preoccupied with food and sleep; passive and dependent	• Psychosis is noted when patient is unable to care for herself and newborn.

POSTPARTUM MATERNAL ASSESSMENT (continued)

PROCEDURE	NORMAL FINDINGS	DEVIATIONS FROM NORMAL
	After 2–3 days postpartum: Increased interest in control of body functions, mothering skills; gradually includes others in social circle; transient depression, let down feeling, cries easily	Failure to assume maternal role; prolonged depression; unrealistic expectations of newborn

Breast Assessment

INSPECTION
With client in supine or semi-Fowler position, inspect breasts.

PROCEDURE	NORMAL FINDINGS	DEVIATIONS FROM NORMAL
Inspect the following in **nonnursing mother:**		
• Size	• May be enlarged initially; will gradually return to prepregnant size	• Full, engorged breasts
• Shape	• May sag	

POSTPARTUM MATERNAL ASSESSMENT (continued)

PROCEDURE	NORMAL FINDINGS	DEVIATIONS FROM NORMAL
• Color	• May have striae	• Localized redness, tenderness may be seen with mastitis.

Inspect the following in *nursing mother:*
- Size
- Texture
- Nipples
- Discharge

	NORMAL FINDINGS	DEVIATIONS FROM NORMAL
	• Enlarged	• Heat, localized pain
	• Increased nodularity	• Blisters, cracked, bleeding
	• Everted, tender	
	• Colostrum, thin milk, may leak between feedings	• Purulent, bloody discharge may indicate infection.

PALPATION
Gently palpate all quadrants of each breast.

PROCEDURE	NORMAL FINDINGS	DEVIATIONS FROM NORMAL
Palpate **nonnursing mother** *for:*		
• Tenderness	• Soft	• Full, tender
• Texture	• Nodular	• Lumps, masses may be seen with clogged breast ducts.

POSTPARTUM MATERNAL ASSESSMENT (continued)

PROCEDURE	NORMAL FINDINGS	DEVIATIONS FROM NORMAL
*Palpate in **nursing mother** for:* • Tenderness • Texture	• Full, slightly tender • Small lumps	• Painful breasts are seen with mastitis. • Hardened area, most often in upper, outer quadrant, indicates clogged milk ducts and/or mastitis.

Abdominal Assessment

INSPECTION

Place client in a supine position with knees extended and head slightly elevated on a pillow.

PROCEDURE	NORMAL FINDINGS	DEVIATIONS FROM NORMAL
Inspect abdomen for the following: • Size	• Uterus visible, outlined unless obese; gradually recedes to prepregnant size with exercise	• Distention seen when patient is unable to void and bladder becomes distended
• Color	• Striae dark red or purple; recede to silvery or white and become smaller	• Yellow, pale
• Texture	• Loose and flabby	• Dry, cracked

PALPATION

Have client empty bladder and assume supine position. Place one hand over lower abdomen above symphysis pubis to support uterus. With the fingertips of the other hand, locate the fundus. Start in the midline, slightly above the umbilicus, and press in and down. Work fingers gradually down toward the symphysis pubis until the fundus of the uterus is located. It should feel like a firm, round ball, similar to a grapefruit. Measure the distance above or below the umbilicus in finger breadths (Figs. 20-9 and 20-10). If the uterus is not firm, gently massage until firm, and then gently push down on fundus and observe for expression of clots from the vagina.

PROCEDURE	NORMAL FINDINGS	DEVIATIONS FROM NORMAL
Palpate fundus for the following:		
• Location	• Midline	• Deviated to left or right could indicate a distended bladder
• Consistency	• Firm; boggy to firm with massage; smooth surface	• Boggy; does not stay firm after massage may indicate uterine atony and/or retained placental fragments
• Height	• Halfway between umbilicus and symphysis immediately after delivery; within 12 hours, at the umbilicus or 1 cm above; descends 1 cm/day	• More than 1 cm above umbilicus; failure to descend
• Expression of clots	• Small clots or increased flow with massage	• Large clots; continuous trickle of bright red blood with firm fundus indicates an unrepaired laceration.

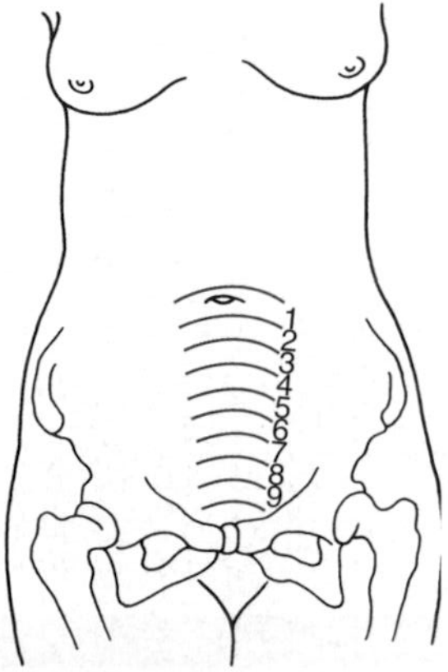

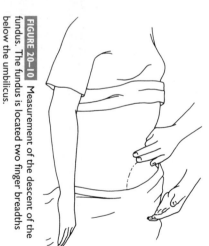

FIGURE 20–9 Involution of the uterus. The height of the fundus decreases about one finger breadth (approximately 1 cm) each day.

FIGURE 20–10 Measurement of the descent of the fundus. The fundus is located two finger breadths below the umbilicus.

Face and Extremities Assessment

INSPECTION

To inspect the face and extremities, the supine position is preferred. Adequate light must be available.

PROCEDURE	NORMAL FINDINGS	DEVIATIONS FROM NORMAL
Inspect *face* for the following:		
• Color	• Petechiae after prolonged second stage of labor	• Paleness may be seen with anemia.
• Edema	• None	• Periorbital
Inspect *extremities* for the following:		
• Color	• Pink red tones visible under dark pigmentation	• Dusky, mottled color indicates decreased oxygenation.
• Edema	• Slight pedal edema	• Pitting edema, edema of hands seen with PIH

PALPATION

With legs extended, gently palpate calves. Place one hand on knee, and gently dorsiflex each foot.

PROCEDURE	NORMAL FINDINGS	DEVIATIONS FROM NORMAL
Palpate calves for the following:		
• Tenderness	• Calves may have generalized muscle tenderness.	• Calf with localized tenderness or pain seen with deep vein thrombosis

POSTPARTUM MATERNAL ASSESSMENT (continued)

PROCEDURE	NORMAL FINDINGS	DEVIATIONS FROM NORMAL
• Texture	• Smooth	• Knots or lumps in calf
• Homans sign	• Negative (no pain)	• Positive (pain in calf) may indicate deep vein thrombosis.

PERCUSSION

Pregnancy-related seizures can occur for up to 48 hours postpartum. Reflexes should be assessed for hyperreflexia and clonus during this time. See Chapter 19 for technique.

Bladder Assessment

INSPECTION

Have client void within 4 hours after delivery or sooner if there are bleeding problems during the immediate postpartum period.

PROCEDURE	NORMAL FINDINGS	DEVIATIONS FROM NORMAL
Inspect voiding for the following:		
• Amount	• 200 mL or more each voiding; diuresis of greater than 2000 mL in first 24 hours	• Less than 100 mL per voiding; unable to void
• Color	• Yellow, clear; may be mixed with lochia	• Dark, cloudy, bloody urine may indicate urinary tract infection.

PALPATION

Have client empty bladder and assume supine position. Palpate for bladder above the symphysis pubis. If unable to void within 4 hours after delivery or if bladder is full, empty bladder with a catheter.

PROCEDURE	NORMAL FINDINGS	DEVIATIONS FROM NORMAL
Palpate bladder.	Nonpalpable	Spongy mass in lower abdomen

Perineum Assessment

INSPECTION

Have client turn to side and flex upper leg. Place one hand on upper buttock and gently separate so perineum is visible.

PROCEDURE	NORMAL FINDINGS	DEVIATIONS FROM NORMAL
Inspect perineum for the following:		
• Approximation of episiotomy	• Skin edges meet.	• Skin edges gape.
• Color	• Pink to red	• Purple, mottled
• Swelling	• Generalized swelling for 12–24 hours	• Localized swelling with increased pain indicates hematoma.
• Lochia	• Color: *days 1–3:* rubra (dark red); small clots may also be expelled. *Days 4–10:* Serosa (pinkish red) *Days 11–20:* Alba (creamy yellow) *Amount: days 1–10:* Vaginal discharge requires 6–10 pads per day (moderate flow).	• More than 8 peri pads per day or saturated pad in 1 hour seen in postpartum hemorrhage; purulent, large clots; return to dark red after several days

POSTPARTUM MATERNAL ASSESSMENT (continued)

PROCEDURE	NORMAL FINDINGS	DEVIATIONS FROM NORMAL
	Days 11–20: Decreased amount of vaginal discharge still requires pad change (less than 6–8 pads per day).	
• Odor	• None; musky scent	• Foul odor with bacterial infections
• Hemorrhoids	• Small, nontender	• Swollen, painful

Possible Collaborative Problems

Urinary retention   Retained placenta
Breast engorgement/abscess   Infections
Preeclampsia/eclampsia   Exacerbation of preexisting medical conditions
Hemorrhage   Heart conditions
Uterine atony   Hypertension
Hematoma   Hyperglycemia
Cervical/vaginal lacerations   Hypoglycemia

TEACHING TIPS FOR SELECTED NURSING DIAGNOSES

Nursing Diagnosis: Disturbed Sleep Pattern related to fatigue and increased need for sleep

🖉 All teaching sessions should be brief and reinforced with written information about infant care and self-care (eg, care of breasts). Encourage mother to sleep when baby sleeps. Advise mother to avoid strenuous activities until 6-week postpartum physical examination. Enlist help of other family members.

Nursing Diagnosis: Readiness for Enhanced Infant Care and Self-Care

Demonstrate infant care and allow time for mother to practice. A follow-up phone call or home visit can assist in evaluation and reinforcement of information taught. Include father whenever possible.

Nursing Diagnosis: Readiness for Enhanced Family Coping related to addition of family member and role changes

Discuss plans for incorporating new member into family. Offer suggestions to decrease sibling jealousy. Explore plans for infant care, division of labor, and changes in activities of daily living.

Nursing Diagnosis: Risk for Impaired Parent/Infant Attachment related to unrealistic expectations of self

Discuss normal growth and development of infant; emphasize things infant can do. Provide early and continued contact of infant and parents to maximize bonding. Teach parents skills needed to meet infant's physical and psychological needs.

Nursing Diagnosis: Impaired Parenting related to inadequate skills, unrealistic expectation of infant, stress, lack of adequate support

Be aware of risk factors for child abuse/neglect that may be evident during postpartal period. Explore resources available to parents, and make appropriate referrals for follow-up or support groups.

Nursing Diagnosis: Ineffective Breast-feeding related to lack of knowledge

Clarify misconceptions, and provide instructions or proper technique. Assist with first feedings and problems such as soreness or difficulty latching on to breasts, etc.

Nursing Diagnosis: Ineffective Infant Feeding Pattern

May use nipple with larger hole. Hold infant in upright position during feeding. Burp infant often (after every ½–1 oz). Infant needs frequent feedings with careful monitoring of intake and weight gain. May need to teach parents gavage feedings. If so, infant will attempt to nurse at each feeding and be gavage-fed remaining formula/breast milk.

Nursing Diagnosis: Interrupted Breast-feeding related to change in daily routine lifestyle

To continue breast milk supply, mother should pump breasts at intervals similar to infant feeding patterns. Milk letdown is optimal immediately after infant contact. Mother should be relaxed and have privacy. If possible, both breasts should be emptied at each feeding. Increased fluid consumption is needed for milk production. Discuss methods to enhance milk production if deficient. To terminate breast-feeding, mother should avoid any stimulation of breasts. Encourage use of good support bra. Painful engorgement may be alleviated with analgesics and intermittent ice packs to breasts.

21

ASSESSMENT OF NEWBORNS AND INFANTS

Equipment Needed

- Gloves
- Stethoscope
- Tape measure

Subjective Data: Focus Questions

Prenatal history: Gravida? Para? Estimated date of confinement (EDC)? Gestational age? Maternal history? Risk factors? Prenatal exposure to drugs? Complications? Blood type? Maternal testing?

Labor and delivery history: Date, time, type of delivery? Prolonged labor? Narcotics? Time of rupture of membranes? Intrapartum complications? Shoulder dystocia?

Delivery history: Apgar scores? Respiratory effort? Resuscitation efforts? Medications? Procedures performed? Evidence of injury? Void? Stool?

Social history: Parent interaction? Significant others? Cultural variations? Type of infant feeding? Male circumcision requested?

Objective Data: Assessment Techniques

Immediately after delivery the general state of the newborn should be evaluated while the infant is supine under a radiant warmer with the temperature probe attached to the abdomen. Apgar scores (Table 21–1) are assigned at 1 and 5 minutes after delivery.

APGAR SCORE ASSESSMENT

PROCEDURE	NORMAL FINDINGS	DEVIATIONS FROM NORMAL
Auscultate apical pulse.	>100 bpm	<100 bpm indicates bradycardia; absent heart beat indicates fetal demise.
Inspect chest and abdomen for respiratory effort.	Crying	Absent, slow, irregular respirations
Stroke back or soles of feet.	Crying	Delayed neurologic function may be seen in grimace, no response.
Inspect muscle tone by extending legs and arms. Observe degree of flexion and resistance in extremities.	Extremities flexed, active movement	Moderate degree of flexion, limp may indicate neurologic deficits.
Inspect body and extremities for skin color.	Full body pink, acrocyanosis	Cyanosis, pale
Determine total Apgar score at 1 and 5 minutes after birth (see Table 21–1).	8–10 points	<8 points may indicate poor transition from intrauterine into extrauterine life.

Assessment of Newborns and Infants

TABLE 21–1 APGAR SCORE

	Scores 0	Scores 1	Scores 2
Heart rate	Absent	<100 bpm	>100 bpm
Respiratory rate	Absent	Slow, irregular	Good lusty cry
Reflex irritability	No response	Grimace, some motion	Cry, cough
Muscle tone	Flaccid, limp	Flexion of extremities	Active flexion
Color	Cyanotic, pale	Pink body, acrocyanosis	Pink body, pink extremities

ASSESSMENT OF VITAL SIGNS AND MEASUREMENTS

After the Apgar score has been assigned, a thorough assessment including vital signs, measurements, and gestational age assessment is performed.

PROCEDURE	NORMAL FINDINGS	DEVIATIONS FROM NORMAL
Monitor axillary temperature.	97.5–99°F (36.4–37.2°C)	<97.5°F (<36.4°C): hypothermia, which may indicate sepsis >99°F (>37.2°C): hyperthermia (Consider infection or improper monitoring of temperature probe.)
Inspect and auscultate lung sounds.	Easy, nonlabored, clear lungs bilaterally	Labored breathing, nasal flaring, rhonchi, rales, retractions, grunting
Monitor respiratory rate.	Rate: 30–60 breaths/min	Rate <30 or >60 breaths/min is seen with respiratory distress.
Auscultate apical pulse.	Regular 120–160 bpm (100 sleeping, 180 crying)	Irregular <100 or >180 bpm may indicate cardiac abnormalities.
Weigh newborn unclothed using a newborn scale (Fig. 21-1).	2500–4000 g	<2500 g >4000 g
Measure length.	44–55 cm	<44 cm >55 cm

Assessment of Newborns and Infants

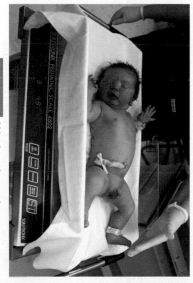

FIGURE 21–1 Weighing the newborn.

ASSESSMENT OF VITAL SIGNS AND MEASUREMENTS (continued)

PROCEDURE	NORMAL FINDINGS	DEVIATIONS FROM NORMAL
Measure head circumference (see Fig. 4–1).	33–35.5 cm	<33 cm >35.5 cm
Measure chest circumference.	30–33 cm (1–2 cm < head)	<29 cm >34 cm

ASSESSMENT OF GESTATIONAL AGE

The newborn's gestational age is examined within 4 hours after birth to identify any potential age-related problems that may occur within the next few hours. The newborn's neuromuscular and physical maturity are examined. After examination, boxes on the New Ballard Scale (Figs. 21–2 and 21–3) that most closely describe and depict the newborn's neuromuscular and physical maturity are marked, and scores are assigned to assess gestational age.

PROCEDURE	NORMAL FINDINGS	DEVIATIONS FROM NORMAL
Assess *neuromuscular maturity (see Fig. 21–2) by performing each of the following with the newborn in the supine position:*		
• Posture (with newborn undisturbed)	• Arms and legs flexed	• Arms and legs limp, extended away from body seen with premature infants

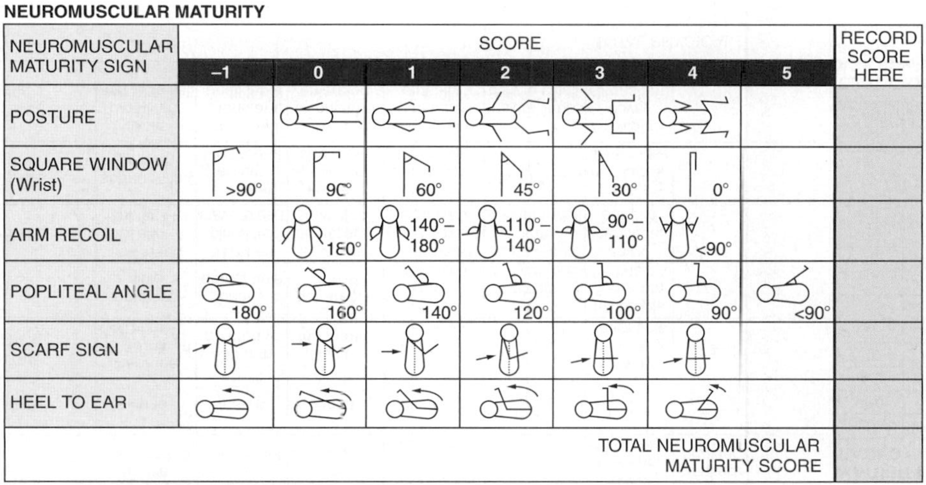

FIGURE 21-2 New Ballard Scale. Used to rate neuromuscular maturity of gestational age.

Assessment of Newborns and Infants

PHYSICAL MATURITY

PHYSICAL MATURITY SIGN	-1	0	1	2	3	4	5	RECORD SCORE HERE
SKIN	sticky, friable, transparent	gelatinous, red, translucent	smooth, pink, visible veins	superficial peeling and/or rash, few veins	cracking, pale areas, rare veins	parchment, deep cracking, no vessels	leathery, cracked, wrinkled	
LANUGO	none	sparse	abundant	thinning	bald areas	mostly bald		
PLANTAR SURFACE	heel-toe 40-50 mm:-1 <40 mm:-2	>50 mm no crease	faint red marks	anterior transverse crease only	creases ant. 2/3	creases over entire sole		
BREAST	imperceptible	barely perceptible	flat areola no bud	stippled areola 1-2 mm bud	raised areola 3-4 mm bud	full areola 5-10 mm bud		
EYE-EAR	lids fused loosely: -1 tightly: -2	lids open pinna flat stays folded	sl. curved pinna; soft; slow recoil	well-curved pinna, soft but ready recoil	formed and firm instant recoil	thick cartilage, ear stiff		
GENITALS (Male)	scrotum flat, smooth	scrotum empty, faint rugae	testes in upper canal, rare rugae	testes descending, few rugae	testes down, good rugae	testes pendulous, deep rugae		
GENITALS (Female)	clitoris prominent and labia flat	prominent clitoris and small labia minora	prominent clitoris and enlarging minora	majora and minora equally prominent	majora large, minora small	majora cover clitoris and minora		
						TOTAL PHYSICAL MATURITY SCORE		

SCORE

Neuromuscular	___
Physical	___
Total	___

MATURITY RATING

Score	Weeks
-10	20
-5	22
0	24
5	26
10	28
15	30
20	32
25	34
30	36
35	38
40	40
45	42
50	44

GESTATIONAL AGE (weeks)

By dates ___
By ultrasound ___
By exam ___

FIGURE 21-3 New Ballard Scale. Used to rate physical maturity of gestational age.

ASSESSMENT OF GESTATIONAL AGE (continued)

PROCEDURE	NORMAL FINDINGS	DEVIATIONS FROM NORMAL
• Square window: bend wrist toward ventral forearm until resistance is met. Measure angle (see Fig. 21–4).	• 0–30°	• Premature infants may have square window measurement of >30°.

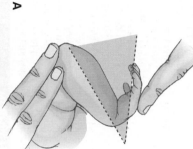

A

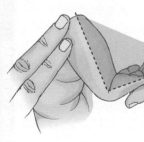

B

FIGURE 21–4 Square window sign. (A) Term infant. (B) Preterm infant.

ASSESSMENT OF GESTATIONAL AGE (continued)

PROCEDURE	NORMAL FINDINGS	DEVIATIONS FROM NORMAL
• Arm recoil: bilaterally flex elbows up with hands next to shoulders and hold approximately 5 seconds; extend arms down next to side; release; observe elbow angle and recoil.	• Elbow angle <90°, rapid recoil to flexed state	• Elbow angle >110°, delayed recoil seen in premature infants
• Popliteal angle: flex thigh on top of abdomen; push behind ankle and extend lower leg up toward head until resistance is met; measure angle behind knee.	• <100°	• >100°
• Scarf sign: Lift arm across chest toward opposite shoulder until resistance is met; note location of elbow in relation to middle of chest (Fig. 21–5).	• Elbow position less than midline of chest	• Elbow position midline of chest or greater, toward opposite shoulder seen in premature infants

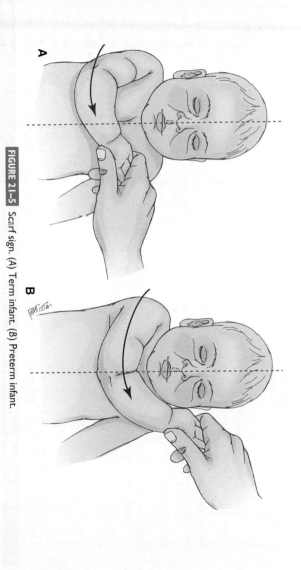

FIGURE 21–5 Scarf sign. (A) Term infant. (B) Preterm infant.

ASSESSMENT OF GESTATIONAL AGE (continued)

PROCEDURE	NORMAL FINDINGS	DEVIATIONS FROM NORMAL
• Heel to ear: pull leg toward ear on same side, keeping buttocks flat on bed; inspect popliteal angle and proximity of heel to ear.	• Poplitea, angle <90°, heel distal from ear	• Popliteal angle >90°, heel proximal to ear seen in premature infants
*Assess **physical maturity** (see Fig. 21–3) by performing the following:*		
• Observe skin.	• Parchment, few or no vessels on abdomen, cracking in ankle area especially	• Translucent, visible veins; rash; leathery, wrinkled skin seen in postmature infants
• Inspect for lanugo.	• Thinning, balding on back, shoulders, knees	• Abundant amount of fine hair on face seen in premature infants
• Inspect plantar surface of feet for creases.	• Creases on anterior two thirds or entire sole	• Anterior transverse crease on sole only, no creases; fewer creases indicate prematurity.
• Inspect and palpate breast bud tissue with middle finger and forefinger; measure bud in millimeters.	• Raised areola, full areola	• Absence of bud tissue, bud <3 mm seen in premature infants
• Observe ear cartilage in upper pinna for curving. Fold pinna down toward side of head and release; observe recoil of ear.	• Pinna well curved, cartilage formed, instant recoil	• Pinna slightly curved, slow recoil seen in premature infants

ASSESSMENT OF GESTATIONAL AGE (continued)

PROCEDURE	NORMAL FINDINGS	DEVIATIONS FROM NORMAL
• Inspect genitals. *Male:* Observe scrotum for rugae and palpate position of testes. *Female:* Observe labia majora, labia minora, and clitoris.	• *Male:* Deep rugae; testes positioned down in scrotal sac *Female:* Labia majora cover labia minora and clitoris.	• *Male:* Decreased presence of rugae; testes positioned in upper inguinal canal *Female:* Labia majora and labia minora equally prominent, clitoris prominent seen with premature infants
Determine **score rating:** On Figure 21-2 and 21-3, mark the boxes that most closely represent each observation.		
• Add the total scores from both tables.	• Total score: 35–45 points	• Total score: <35 points or >45 points
• Using Figure 21-2, plot total score in column on right-hand side of page; this score corresponds to the number in weeks on the maturity rating scale; circle the number of weeks.	• Gestational age: 38–42 weeks	• Gestational age: <38 or >42 weeks
• Using gestational weeks assessed, plo weight, length, and head circumference on Figures 21-6 through 21-9.	• 10th through 90th percentile is appropriate for gestational age (AGA).	• Less than the 10th percentile (small for gestational age), greater than the 90th percentile (large for gestational age)

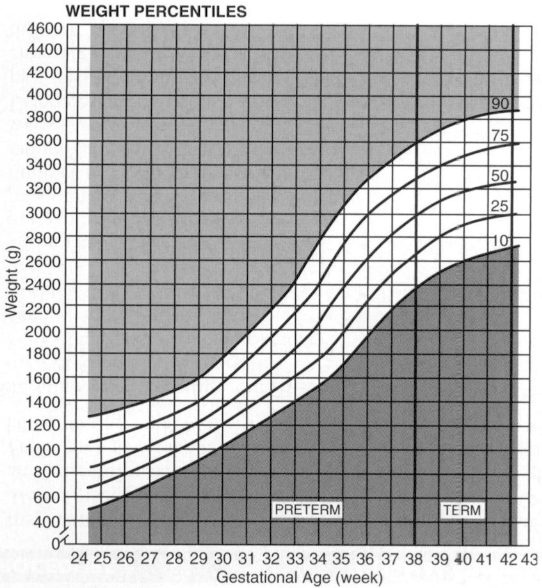

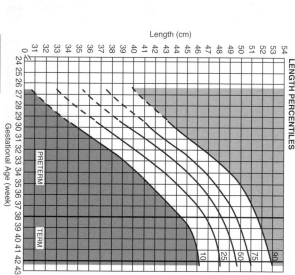

FIGURE 21–6 Weight percentiles for newborn infants.

FIGURE 21–7 Length percentiles for newborn infants.

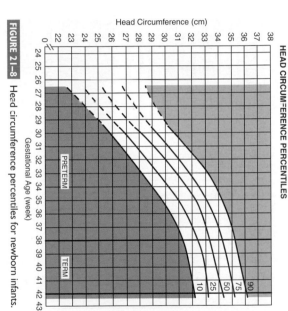

FIGURE 21–8 Head circumference percentiles for newborn infants.

CLASSIFICATION OF INFANT*

	Weight	Length	Head Circ.
Large for Gestational Age (LGA) (>90th percentile)			
Appropriate for Gestational Age (AGA) (10th to 90th percentile)			
Small for Gestational Age (SGA) (<10th percentile)			

*Place an "X" in the appropriate box (LGA, AGA, or SGA) for weight, for length, and for head circumference.

FIGURE 21-9 Classification of infant for gestational age.

PHYSICAL ASSESSMENT

In addition to the Apgar assessment and the gestational age assessment, the nurse also performs a thorough head-to-toe physical assessment. The head-to-toe assessment is reviewed at the end of each chapter under Pediatric Variations.

PROCEDURE	NORMAL FINDINGS	DEVIATIONS FROM NORMAL
Assess **respiratory system.**	30–60 breaths/min. Unlabored, chest/abdominal movement synchronized, lung sounds clear bilaterally, transient rales, nose appears normal with patent nares bilaterally, nose breathers.	<30 or >60 breaths/min. Retractions, nasal flaring, grunting, tachypnea, see-saw movement of chest, apnea, ↓decreased breath sounds indicate respiratory distress.
Assess **cardiovascular system.**	120–160 bpm: regular rhythm; color pink, acrocyanosis; capillary refill <2 seconds; brachial/femoral pulses present, equal bilaterally	<110 or >180 bpm. Weak pulse, tachycardia, bradycardia, persistent murmur, cyanosis indicates congenital heart defects. Unequal pulses may be seen with coarctation of the aorta.
Assess **neurologic system.**	Alert when awake; normal, lusty cry Reflexes: see Neurologic Assessment Chapter 19.	Asymmetrical, weak, or absent response to stimulation seen with neurologic deficits
Assess **sensory system.** • Ear—	• Symmetrical, well formed, parallel to outer canthus of eye, infant responds to sound.	• Preauricle dimple or tag, low-set ears often seen in infants with Down syndrome

PHYSICAL ASSESSMENT (continued)

PROCEDURE	NORMAL FINDINGS	DEVIATIONS FROM NORMAL
• Eyes	• Symmetrical, alert, clear sclera; iris slate gray or brown, infant follows objects to midline; eyelids have transient edema, absence of tears.	• Unequal pupils, purulent discharge seen with sexually transmitted infections (gonorrhea, *Chlamydia*)
*Assess **musculoskeletal system.***	Tone flexed, extremities resist when extended and return to flexed state when released.	Limp, flaccid, poor tone may be seen in infants with neurologic deficits.
• Head	• Anterior fontanelle (Fig. 21–10) has diamond shape, 3–4 cm × 2–3 cm, soft, flat. Posterior fontanelle (Fig. 21–1) has triangular shape, 1–2 cm. Head is round with mild to moderate molding. Sutures are palpable, overriding. A common variation is *caput succedaneum* (Fig. 21-12, A). Face is symmetrical.	• Cephalhematoma (Fig. 21-12, B). Hydrocephalus may be caused by metabolic disturbances or by intrauterine infections. Bulging fontanelle represents increased cranial pressure. Microcephaly may be seen in newborns who have been exposed to congenital infections.

Assessment of Newborns and Infants

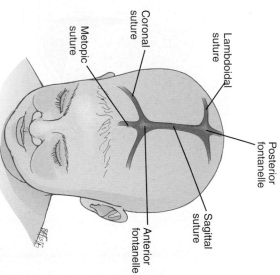

FIGURE 21–10 Palpating the anterior fontanelle. (© B. Proud.)

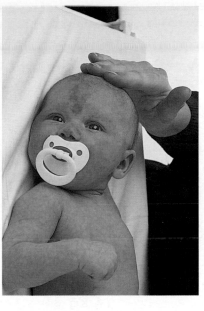

FIGURE 21–11 The infant head.

Coronal
suture

Metopic
suture

Lambdoidal
suture

Posterior
fontanelle

Sagittal
suture

Anterior
fontanelle

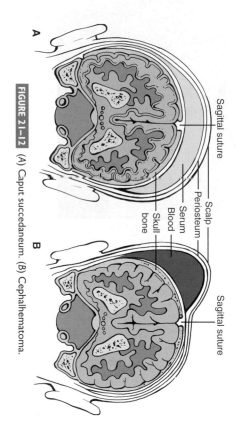

FIGURE 21–12 (A) Caput succedaneum. (B) Cephalhematoma.

A

Sagittal suture

Scalp
Periosteum
Serum
Blood
Skull
bone

B

Sagittal suture

PHYSICAL ASSESSMENT (continued)

PROCEDURE	NORMAL FINDINGS	DEVIATIONS FROM NORMAL
• Neck and clavicles	• Neck moves freely; Infant attempts to control head when hyperextended, holds head midline position. Clavicles are symmetrical and intact.	• Webbing of neck, abnormal masses, limp. Crepitus when clavicle palpated, along with decreased movement in arm of that side, may indicate fractured clavicle.
• Extremities	• Five fingers and toes on each extremity, no webbing, normal palmar creases, bilateral movement with full ROM in arms and legs. Legs have equal length, symmetrical bilateral gluteal/thigh creases, no hip click, normal position of feet.	• Polydactyly, syndactyly, absent digits could indicate genetic abnormality; polydactyly without bone, however, is commonly seen. Positive Ortolani maneuver indicates congenital dislocation of the hip (see Fig. 18–15). Unequal thigh/gluteal creases may indicate unequal leg length or dislocation of the hip.
• Spine	• No openings; spine flexible and rounded in infants younger than 3 months old (Fig. 21-13)	• Opening in spinal column, pilonidal dimple could indicate spina bifida or other spinal abnormalities.
Assess **GI system.** • Mouth	• Oral mucosa and lips pink, palate intact. Epstein pearls, retains feedings	• Cyanosis, white patches on oral mucosa is thrush. Abnormal fusion of lip/palate is seen with cleft lip/palate. Excessive salivation, unable to tolerate feedings may indicate esophageal atresia.

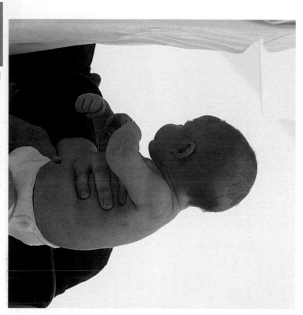

FIGURE 21–13 The spine is rounded in infants under the age of 3 months.

PHYSICAL ASSESSMENT (continued)

PROCEDURE	NORMAL FINDINGS	DEVIATIONS FROM NORMAL
• Anus	• Patent anus, meconium passed within 24–48 hours after birth	• No passage of meconium stool within 24–48 hours after birth could indicate no patency of anus and/or cystic fibrosis.
• Abdomen	• Abdomen shape cylindrical, round, soft; bowel sounds present 30–60 minutes after birth, liver palpable 1–2 cm below costal margin	• Abdomen sunken. Distended abdomen could indicate pyloric stenosis. Hirschsprung disease could also be considered, especially with suprapubic mass palpable.
• Umbilical cord	• Umbilical cord white, drying; three vessels present in cord (two arteries and one vein)	• Abnormal insertion of umbilical cord, discolored cord. Bulge at umbilicus suggests umbilical hernia—may disappear by 1 year of age (Fig. 21–14). Two vessels present in cord could indicate genetic abnormalities; however, is seen in newborns who have no abnormalities.
Assess genitourinary system.		No urinary output beyond 48 hours after birth may indicate kidney problems.
• Male	Void within first 24 hours after birth	• Testes found in inguinal canal, scrotal sac edematous with fluid (hydrocele), meatus positioned above (epispadias) or below (hypospadias) tip of penis; bright red active bleeding at circumcision site
	• Testes descended within scrotal sac, meatus at tip of penis; circumcision site dry, minimal swelling and drainage	

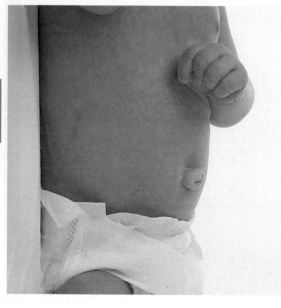

FIGURE 21–14 Umbilical hernia.

PHYSICAL ASSESSMENT (continued)

PROCEDURE	NORMAL FINDINGS	DEVIATIONS FROM NORMAL
• Female	• Labia majora cover labia minora, vaginal discharge.	• Edema, tags present
Assess **skin.**	Pink, warm, dry, smooth, soft, good turgor, peeling hands and feet. Nails extend to end of fingers or beyond, well formed. Common variations: Acrocyanosis, harlequin color change, *vernix caseosa* in creases or absent, lanugo sparse, veins rarely visible, milia over nose/chin Pigmentation: *erythema toxicum*, mongolian spots (Fig. 21–15) common in dark-skinned newborns over dorsal area and buttocks. Stork bites (*nevus flammeus*) (Fig. 21–16)	Minimal adipose tissue indicates fetal wasting; poor turgor, generalized cracking or peeling of skin can be seen in postmature infants. Lacerations, lesions. Yellowish green-stained skin is seen in newborns who have passed meconium in utero secondary to fetal distress. Jaundice within 24 hours after birth is pathologic jaundice caused from blood disorders such as hemolytic disease of the newborn. Cyanosis, generalized edema, pallor, hemangiomas, *nevus vascularis*, café-au-lait spots, skin tags and fibrous tumors may suggest neurofibromatosis.

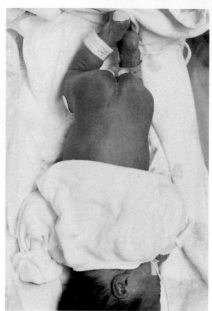

FIGURE 21-15 Mongolian spots.

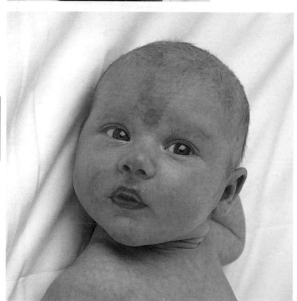

FIGURE 21-16 Stork bites.

Possible Collaborative Problems

Elevated bilirubin levels
Infection
   Circumcision
   Nosocomial
   Bacterial

TEACHING TIPS FOR SELECTED NURSING DIAGNOSES

Nursing Diagnosis: Ineffective Breathing Pattern (transient alteration in lung expansion)

Monitor respiratory status every 30 minutes × 4 until stable, then per protocol. Auscultate breath sounds per protocol. Promote oxygenation and fluid drainage by placing infant on side; use postural drainage with head of bed slightly lower than body. Have suction equipment ready for use.

Nursing Diagnosis: Risk for Suffocation, Sudden Infant Death Syndrome (SIDS)

Healthy infants should be placed on their back when putting them to sleep. Side positioning is an alternative but does carry a slightly higher risk of SIDS (American Academy of Pediatrics, 2000).

Nursing Diagnosis: Ineffective Thermoregulation (cool environment, decrease in body fat)

Assess temperature every 30 minutes × 4, then per protocol. Maintain temperature at 97.6–99.2°F (~36.4–37.3°C). Keep infant temperature probe attached properly to skin to ensure reading probe accurately. Monitor for signs and symptoms of cold stress. Keep infant warm and dry. Postpone bath until temperature is stable. Apply cap to head and extra blankets to infant if temperature <97.6°F (36.4°C). Teach parents mechanisms of heat loss: radiation, convection, conduction, evaporation. Teach techniques used to prevent cold stress and to maintain or increase infant temperature (eg, dress, cap, blanket wrap, cuddle). Teach parents correct procedure in taking newborn axillary temperature, reading thermometer, interpreting results.

Nursing Diagnosis: Imbalanced Nutrition: less than body requirements

Review prenatal history, looking for maternal risk factors such as gestational diabetes. Assess for hypoglycemia, checking blood glucose values at birth and at 1 hour of age or per hospital protocol. Weigh infant on admission and daily. Auscultate bowel sounds every shift. Assess for rooting/sucking behaviors. Initiate breast-bottle-feeding at birth and on demand for breast-feeding and per hospital protocol for bottle-feeding. Record frequency, amount, and length of feeding. If regurgitation occurs, note frequency and amount. Monitor newborn stools/voids and record per shift. Observe for feeding problems (refusal to eat, regurgitation, gagging, difficulty swallowing, difficulty with latching onto breast, etc.). Evaluate neonate after feeding for satisfaction of feeding. Observe parents/newborn for feeding problems; encourage questions and problem solving for parents regarding feeding difficulties or concerns.

ASSESSMENT OF FAMILIES USING VIOLENCE

22

OVERVIEW OF FAMILY VIOLENCE

Family violence can be defined as controlling, coercive behavior evident from intentional acts of violence inflicted on those in familial or intimate relationships, and includes intimate partner violence, child abuse, and elder mistreatment. Family violence affects people of all ages, sexes, religions, ethnicities, and socioeconomic levels.

The categories of family violence include intimate partner violence, child abuse, and elder mistreatment. Intimate partner violence (IPV) includes a range of behaviors including physical abuse, emotional abuse, economic abuse, psychological abuse, and sexual assault. The Child Abuse Prevention and Treatment Act (CAPTA) defines child abuse as "any recent act or failure to act, resulting in imminent risk of serious harm, death, serious physical or emotional harm, sexual abuse, or exploitation of a child (a person under the age of 18, unless the child protection law of the State in which the child resides specifies a younger age for cases not involving sexual abuse) by a parent or caretaker (including any employee of a residential facility or any staff person providing out-of-home care) who is responsible for the child's welfare" (Child Abuse Prevention and Treatment Act, Public Law 104-235, §111-42 U.S.C. 510g, 2003). Elder mistreatment includes physical abuse, neglect, exploitation, abandonment, or prejudicial attitudes that decrease the quality of life of and are demeaning to those over the age of 65 years.

Types of family violence include physical abuse, psychological abuse, economic abuse, and sexual abuse. Physical abuse includes pushing, shoving, slapping, kicking, choking, punching, and burning. It may also involve holding, tying, or other methods of restraint. It may also involve attacking the victim with household items (lamps, radios, ashtrays, irons, etc.) or with common weapons (knives or guns). Psychological abuse involves the constant use of insults or criticism, blaming the victim for things that are not the victim's fault, threats to hurt children or pets, isolation from supporters (family, friends, or coworkers), deprivation, humiliation, and intimidation. Economic abuse may be evidenced by preventing the victim from getting or keeping a job, controlling money and limiting access to funds, and controlling knowledge of family finances. Sexual abuse involves forcing the victim to perform sexual acts against his or her will, pursuing sexual activity after the victim has said no, using violence during sex, and using weapons vaginally, orally, or anally.

Equipment Needed

- All equipment for a complete head-to-toe physical examination
- Safe and secure private screening area (Do not screen in an area that poses any safety concerns for the client or yourself.)

Preparing Yourself for the Examination

To assess for the presence of family violence effectively, first examine your feelings, beliefs, and biases regarding violence. No one under any circumstances should be physically, sexually, or emotionally abused. It is imperative that you become active in interrupting or ending cycles of violence. Be aware of "red flags" that may indicate the presence of family violence.

Risk Factors. Physical abuse may start at any time during a relationship. Consistent risk factors for women at risk have not been identified. The Family Violence Prevention Fund (1999) recommends that all female clients, aged 14 and older, be screened for abuse when seen in emergency departments, urgent care centers, or primary health care clinics. Screen for a history of current and past abuse at initial and annual visits regardless of the presence or absence of abuse indicators. Screen at each visit if there is a history of abuse. Screen all pregnant women at least once per trimester and once postpartum (Washington State Department of Health, May 2004). Screen mothers during well-child visits to the pediatrician. Also screen for abuse if the client is in a new relationship or if there are signs or symptoms indicating the presence of abuse. Refer to Box 22–1.

Subjective Data: Focus Questions

Assessment for family violence mostly consists of the collection of adequate subjective data followed by a physical assessment. Prior to screening, discuss any legal, mandatory reporting requirements or other limits to confidentiality. Convey a concerned and nonjudgmental attitude. Show appropriate empathy.

BOX 22-1 • Danger Assessment

Several risk factors have been associated with increased risk of homicides (murders) of women and men in violent relationships. We cannot predict what will happen in your case, but we would like you to be aware of the danger of homicide in situations of abuse and for you to see how many of the risk factors apply to your situation.

Using the calendar, please mark the approximate dates during the past year when you were abused by your partner or ex-partner. Write on that date how bad the incident was according to the following scale:

1. Slapping, pushing; no injuries and/or lasting pain

2. Punching, kicking; bruises, cuts, and/or continuing pain

3. "Beating up"; severe contusions, burns, broken bones

4. Threat to use weapon; head injury, internal injury, permanent injury

5. Use of weapon; wounds from weapon

(If any of the descriptions for the higher number apply, use the higher number.)

Mark Yes or No for each of the following. ("He" refers to your husband, partner, ex-husband, ex-partner, or whoever is currently physically hurting you.)

_____ 1. Has the physical violence increased in severity or frequency over the past year?

_____ 2. Does he own a gun?

_____ 3. Have you left him after living together during the past year?

_____ 3a. (If you have *never* lived with him, check here_____)

Assessment of Families Using Violence

(continued)

BOX 22-1 • (Continued)

___ 4. Is he unemployed?

___ 5. Has he ever used a weapon against you or threatened you with a lethal weapon? (If yes, was the weapon a gun? ___)

___ 6. Does he threaten to kill you?

___ 7. Has he avoided being arrested for domestic violence?

___ 8. Do you have a child that is not his?

___ 9. Has he ever forced you to have sex when you did not wish to do so?

___ 10. Does he ever try to choke you?

___ 11. Does he use illegal drugs? By drugs, I mean "uppers" or amphetamines, speed, angel dust, cocaine, "crack," street drugs, or mixtures.

___ 12. Is he an alcoholic or problem drinker?

___ 13. Does he control most or all of your daily activities? For instance: does he tell you who you can be friends with, when you can see your family, how much money you can use, or when you can take the car? (If he tries, but you do not let him, check here: ___)

_____ 14. Is he violently and constantly jealous of you? (For instance, does he say "If I can't have you, no one can?")

_____ 15. Have you ever been beaten by him while you were pregnant? (If you have never been pregnant by him, check here: _____)

_____ 16. Have you ever threatened or tried to commit suicide?

_____ 17. Has he ever threatened or tried to commit suicide?

_____ 18. Does he threaten to harm your children?

_____ 19. Do you believe he is capable of killing you?

_____ 20. Does he follow or spy on you, leave threatening notes or messages on your answering machine, destroy your property, or call you when you don't want him to?

_____ Total "Yes" Answers

Thank you. Please talk to your nurse, advocate, or counselor about what the Danger Assessment means in terms of your situation.

Jacquelyn C. Campbell, PhD, RN. Copyright, 2003. In Humphreys, J. & Campbell, J. C. (2004). *Family violence and nursing practice.* Philadelphia: Lippincott Williams & Wilkins.

OVERVIEW OF FAMILY VIOLENCE (continued)

PROCEDURE	NORMAL FINDINGS	DEVIATIONS FROM NORMAL
Ask all clients: Has anyone in your home ever hurt you? Do you feel safe in your home? Are you afraid of anyone in your home? Has anyone made you do anything you didn't want to do? Has anyone ever touched you without your permission? Has anyone ever threatened you? *For intimate partner violence,* begin the screening by telling the woman that it is important to screen all women routinely for intimate partner violence because it affects so many women and men in our society. Make statements that build trust such as: If your situation ever changes, please call me to talk about it.	Client answers no to all questions. Client answers "no" to all three questions (see Box 22-2). If the client replies "no" to screening questions and is not being abused, it is important for the client to know that you are available if she ever experiences abuse in the future. ***Clinical Tip:*** Sometimes no matter how carefully you prepare the	"Yes" to any of the questions indicates abuse. "Yes" to any of the questions strongly indicates initial disclosure of abuse. You should do the following: • Acknowledge the abuse and her courage. • Use supportive statements such as "I'm sorry this is happening to you. This is not your fault. You are not responsible for his behavior. You are not alone.

OVERVIEW OF FAMILY VIOLENCE (continued)

PROCEDURE	NORMAL FINDINGS	DEVIATIONS FROM NORMAL
I am happy to hear that you are not being abused. If that should ever change, this is a safe place to talk. Ask the client to fill out or help the client fill out the Abuse Assessment Screen in Box 22–2.	client and ask the questions, she may not disclose abuse.	You don't deserve to be treated this way. Help is available to you." • Acknowledge her autonomy and right to self-determination. • Reiterate confidentiality of disclosure.

BOX 22–2 • Abuse Assessment Screen

1. WITHIN THE LAST YEAR, have you been hit, slapped, kicked, or otherwise physically hurt by someone?   YES   NO

   IF YES, by whom? _____

   Total number of times _____

2. SINCE YOU'VE BEEN PREGNANT, have you been hit, slapped, kicked, or otherwise physically hurt by someone?   YES   NO

   IF YES, by whom? _____

   Total number of times _____

(continued)

Assessment of Families Using Violence

BOX 22-2 • (Continued)

MARK THE AREA OF INJURY ON THE BODY MAP. SCORE EACH
INCIDENT ACCORDING TO THE FOLLOWING SCALE:

SCORE

1 = Threats of abuse including use of a weapon

2 = Slapping, pushing; no injuries and/or lasting pain

3 = Punching, kicking, bruises, cuts, and/or continuing pain

4 = Beating up, severe contusions, burns, broken bones

5 = Head injury, internal injury, permanent injury

6 = Use of weapon; wound from weapon

If any of the descriptions for the higher number apply, use the higher number.

3. WITHIN THE LAST YEAR, has anyone forced you to have sexual activities?   YES   NO

   If YES, who? _____

   Total number of times _____

Developed by the Nursing Research Consortium on Violence and Abuse. Readers are encouraged to reproduce and use this
assessment tool.

Objective Data: Assessment Techniques

PROCEDURE	NORMAL FINDINGS	DEVIATIONS FROM NORMAL
Perform a general survey. Observe general appearance and body build.	Client appears stated age and well-developed.	Abused children may appear younger than stated age due to developmental delays or malnourishment. Older clients may appear thin and frail due to malnourishment.
Note dress and hygiene.	Client is well groomed and dressed appropriately for season and occasion.	Poor hygiene and soiled clothing may indicate neglect. Long sleeves and pants in warm weather may be an attempt to cover bruising or other injuries. Victims of sexual abuse may dress provocatively.
Assess the following: • Mental status	Client is coherent and relaxed. A child shows proper developmental level for age.	Client is anxious, depressed, suicidal, or withdrawn, or has difficulty concentrating. Client has poor eye contact or soft, passive speech. Client is unable to recall recent or past events. Child does not meet developmental expectations.
• Vital signs	Vital signs are within normal limits.	Hypertension may be seen in victims of abuse.

Objective Data: Assessment Techniques (continued)

PROCEDURE	NORMAL FINDINGS	DEVIATIONS FROM NORMAL
• Skin	Skin is clean, dry, and free of lesions or bruises. Skin fragility increases with age; bruising may occur with pressure and may mimic bruising associated with abuse. Be careful to distinguish between normal and abnormal findings.	Client has scars, bruises, burns, welts, or swelling on face, breasts, arms, chest, abdomen, or genitalia.
• Head and neck	Head and neck are free of injuries.	Client has hair missing in clumps, subdural hematomas, or rope marks or finger/hand strangulation marks on neck.
• Eyes	Eyes are free of injury.	Client has bruising or swelling around eyes, unilateral ptosis of upper eyelids (due to repeated blows causing nerve damage to eyelids), or a subconjunctival hemorrhage.
• Ears • Abdomen	Ears are clean and free of injuries. Abdomen 's free of bruises and other injuries and is nontender.	Client has external or internal ear injuries. Client has bruising in various stages of healing. Assessment reveals intra-abdominal injuries.

Objective Data: Assessment Techniques (continued)

PROCEDURE	NORMAL FINDINGS	DEVIATIONS FROM NORMAL
• Genitalia and rectal area	Client is free of injury.	A pregnant client has received blows to abdomen. Client has irritation, tenderness, bruising, bleeding, or swelling of genitals or rectal area. Discharge, redness, or lacerations may indicate abuse in young children. Hemorrhoids are unusual in children and may be caused by sexual abuse. Extreme apprehension during examination may indicate physical or sexual abuse
• Musculoskeletal system	Client shows full range of motion and has no evidence of injuries.	Dislocation of shoulder; old or new fractures of face, arms, or ribs; and poor range of motion of joints are indicators of abuse.
• Neurologic system	Client demonstrates normal neurologic function.	Abnormal findings include tremors, hyperactive reflexes, and decreased sensations to areas of old injuries secondary to neurologic damage.

Assessment of Families Using Violence

Additional Tools for Victims of Intimate Partner Violence

PROCEDURE	NORMAL FINDINGS	DEVIATIONS FROM NORMAL
If screening for IPV is positive, ask the client if she has a safety plan and where she would like to go when she leaves your agency. Assess her for safety issues in her home using Box 22-3. Make a follow-up appointment and/or referral as appropriate.	Client has a safety plan to prevent further abuse and injury.	If the client says she prefers to return home, ask her if it is safe for her to do so and have her complete the Danger Assessment Tool in Box 22-1. Provide the client with contact information for shelters and groups. Encourage her to call with any concerns.

ASSESSMENT PROCEDURE

PROCEDURE	NORMAL FINDINGS	ABNORMAL FINDINGS
Review past health history and physical examination records.	No indicators of abuse are present.	(Indicators of Violence or Potential Violence) Documentation of past assaults. Unexplained injuries, symptoms of pain, nausea and vomiting, or choking. Repeated visits to emergency department. Signs and symptoms of anxiety. Use of sedatives or tranquilizers. Injuries dur-

BOX 22-3 • Assessing a Safety Plan

Ask the client, do you:

- Have a packed bag ready? Keep it hidden but make it easy to grab quickly?
- Tell your neighbors about your abuse and ask them to call the police when they hear a disturbance?
- Have a code word to use with your kids, family, and friends so they will know to call the police and get you help?
- Know where you are going to go, if you ever have to leave?
- Remove weapons from the home?
- Have the following gathered:
  - Social Security cards/numbers for you and your children?
  - Cash?
  - Birth certificates for you and your children?
  - Driver's license?
  - Rent and utility receipts?
  - Bank account numbers?
  - Insurance policies and numbers?
  - Marriage license?
  - Jewelry?

- Important phone numbers?
- Copy of protection order?

Ask children, do you:

- Know a safe place to go?
- Know who is safe to tell you are unsafe?
- Know how and when to call 911? Know how to make a collect call?

Inform children that it is their job to keep themselves safe; they should not interject themselves into adult conflict.

If the client is planning to leave:

- Remind the client this is a dangerous time that requires awareness and planning.
- Review where the client is planning to go, shelter options, and the need to be around others to curtail violence.
- Review the client's right to possessions and list of possessions to take.

Adapted from material by Jacquelyn C. Campbell.

Assessment of Families Using Violence

ASSESSMENT PROCEDURE (continued)

PROCEDURE	NORMAL FINDINGS	DEVIATIONS FROM NORMAL
		ing pregnancy. History of drug or alcohol abuse, depression, and/or suicide attempts.
If partner/parent/caregiver is present at the visit, observe client's interactions with partner.	Client is not afraid of partner. Client answers questions independently. Partner appears supportive.	Partner criticizes client about appearance, feelings, and/or actions and is not sensitive to client's needs. Partner refuses to leave client's presence and speaks for client. Client is anxious and afraid of partner; is submissive to negative comments from partner.
Perform the rest of the examination without the partner, parent, or caregiver present.		

PEDIATRIC VARIATIONS

Subjective Data: Focus Questions

- For any client over the age of 3 years, ask any screening questions in a secure, private setting with no one else present in the room.
- Receive any information the child may disclose to you in an interested, calm, and accepting manner. Avoid showing surprise or distaste.
- Do not coerce the child to answer questions by offering rewards.

- Establish the child's level of understanding by asking simple questions (name, how to spell name, age, birth date, how many eyes do you have, etc.). Then formulate questions the child can comprehend.
- The majority of children disclose to questions specific to the person suspected of abuse or related to the type of abuse (Hegar, Emans, & Muram, 2000).
- Use multiple-choice or open-ended questions and avoid "yes or no" questions.
- The less information you supply in your questions and the more information the child gives in answering the questions increases the credibility of the collected data.
- Children raised in homes with IPV are more likely to use violence as adults (Lamberg, 2000).

PROCEDURE	NORMAL FINDINGS	ABNORMAL FINDINGS
For child abuse, question the child about safety including physical abuse, sexual abuse, emotional abuse, and neglect. *Tip:* Today more than 3,000,000 children are referred to child protective services yearly. Forty-six out of every 1000 child abuse cases are substantiated. Four children die daily as a result of child abuse (Peddle, Wang, Diaz, & Reid, 2002).	Client shows no signs of abuse.	Client indicates someone has hurt him or her (physically, sexually, or emotionally). Child appears neglected. The majority of children who suffer from psychological abuse often use effective coping mechanisms and will not exhibit any pathologic behaviors.

GERIATRIC VARIATIONS

- It is estimated that 1.2% of persons aged 60 and older suffer elder abuse (National Center on Elder Abuse, 1998).
- The medical consequences of elder abuse include (1) inability of the frail elderly to handle the trauma, (2) inability to get food or medication because of neglect, (3) inability to pay for food or medication because of financial abuse, and (4) inability to deal with illness/malnutrition/problems because of depression associated with abuse.
- Statistics of economic abuse are difficult to find due to underreporting by abused elders.

PROCEDURE	NORMAL FINDINGS	ABNORMAL FINDINGS
For elder mistreatment, start out by asking the client to tell you about a typical day in his or her life. Be alert for indicators placing the older client at a high risk for abuse or neglect. Then ask the following:	Client answers no to all questions.	"Yes" to any of the questions indicates abuse.
Has anyone ever made you sign papers that you did not understand?		
Are you alone often?		
Has anyone ever refused to help you when you needed help?		
Has anyone ever refused to give you or let you take your medications?		
Has anyone ever taken your medications from you? Explain.		

CULTURAL VARIATIONS

Conducting a cultural assessment using assessment guidelines is necessary before attempting to understand family violence. Health care providers are more likely to report child abuse in minority populations or in lower socioeconomic levels (American Nurses Association, 1998). Studies show little difference in rates of abuse among racial groups when income levels are included (Hawkins, 1993).

Possible Collaborative Problems

Fractures
Bruises
Concussion
Subdural hematoma
Subconjunctival hemorrhage
Intra-abdominal injury
Depression
Suicide
Death

TEACHING TIPS FOR SELECTED NURSING DIAGNOSES

Adult Client

Nursing Diagnosis: Risk for Altered Family Processes related to the presence of family violence

Teach the family about the availability of safe community resources.

Avoid giving family print resources that may be accessed by partner, who may respond in a violent manner to this information. Direct client to online Internet resources as available.

Nursing Diagnosis: Health-Seeking Behavior: Requests information related to safety from domestic violence

🔲 Teach the client that he or she is a victim and that no one deserves to be treated with violence in any situation or circumstance.

Teach the client ways to become empowered through healthy lifestyle practices including exercise, diet, and adequate rest and sleep.

Pediatric Client

Nursing Diagnosis: Risk for Sexual Abuse

🔲 Explain to children that their body is theirs and it is appropriate to say "no" to anyone who tries to do any activity that makes them feel uncomfortable.

Geriatric Client

Nursing Diagnosis: Risk for Powerlessness related to control of relationships, control of children, and control of finances by abusive significant other

🔲 Teach the older client about the hazards of myths (eg, teach that this is not the client's fault and that he or she has a right to feel safe).

Give the client simple choices to make him or her feel empowered.

Teach problem-solving and decision-making skills to empower the older client.

Appendices

Nursing Assessment Form Based on Functional Health Patterns

Client Profile

Name _____ Birthdate _____ Sex _____
Ethnic origin _____ Religion _____
Medical diagnoses _____
Present treatment _____
Past treatments _____
Past hospitalizations _____
Allergies _____

Current Medications

Name	Dose	Purpose	Problems

Subjective

Objective

HEALTH PERCEPTION-HEALTH MANAGEMENT PATTERN

Reason for seeking health care _____

Health rating

   1   2   3

Poor   Fair   Excellent

Perception of illness _____

Effect of illness on ADLs _____

Use of alcohol _____

   tobacco _____

   drugs _____

Special health habits _____

Last immunizations _____

Compliance with treatments _____

Appearance _____

Grooming _____

Posture _____

Expressions _____

Ht _____ Wt _____

P _____ R _____ T _____

(oral, axillary, rectal)

BP sitting   R _____ L _____

   standing   R _____ L _____

NUTRITIONAL–METABOLIC PATTERN

Daily Food and Fluid Intake

Breakfast _____

Lunch _____

Supper _____

Snacks _____

Food intolerances _____

Difficulty chewing _____

Dysphagia _____

Sore gums _____

Sore tongue _____

N and V _____

Abdominal pains _____

Antacids _____

Laxatives _____

Skin condition _____

Hair condition _____

Nail condition _____

Ideal wt. _____ Difficulty gaining _____

losing _____

Cold/heat intolerances _____

Voice changes _____

Difficulty with nervousness _____

Skin: Color _____ Texture _____

Lesions _____

Temp _____ Moisture _____

Turgor _____

Hair: Color _____

Amt _____ Texture _____

Scalp lesions _____ Dry _____

Nails: Color _____

Shape _____ Condition _____

Texture _____ Tenderness _____

Oral Mucosa: Number of teeth _____

Condition _____

Lesions _____

Gums _____ Tongue _____

ELIMINATION PATTERN

Bowel habits

Frequency _____ Color _____ Pain _____
Consistency _____
Enemas _____ Laxatives _____ Suppositories _____
Ileostomy _____ Colostomy _____

Bladder habits

Frequency _____ Amt _____ Color _____
Pain _____ Hematuria _____
Incontinence _____ Nocturia _____
Retention _____ Infections _____
Catheter _____ Type _____

Abdomen

Contour _____
Lesions _____ Umbilicus _____
Striae _____ Veins _____
Bowel sounds char. _____
Frequency _____
Size of liver dullness _____
Masses palpated _____
Liver palpated _____
Spleen palpated _____

Rectum

Rashes _____
Lesions _____ Tenderness _____

ACTIVITY–EXERCISE PATTERN

Daily Activities

Hygiene _____

Cooking _____

Shopping _____

Housework _____

Yard work _____

Eating times _____

Dyspnea _____ Palpitations _____

Chest pain _____ Stiffness _____

Weakness _____ Aching _____

Leisure activities _____

Exercise routine _____

Occupation _____

Effect of illness on activities _____

Musculoskeletal

Gait _____ Posture _____

Extremity swelling _____

Symmetry _____ ROM _____

Crepitus _____ Tone _____

Strength _____

Respiratory

Thorax shape _____

Symmetry _____ Retractions _____

Tenderness _____

Diaphragmatic level _____

Breath sounds _____

Adventitious sounds _____

Cardiovascular

Jugular venous pressure _____

Pulsations _____ Heaves _____

Lifts _____

PMI _____ S_1 _____ S_2 _____

S_3 _____ S_4 _____ Murmurs _____

Peripheral Vascular Pulses

Carotid	R ___ L ___	Radial	R ___ L ___
Ulnar	R ___ L ___	Brachial	R ___ L ___
Popliteal	R ___ L ___	Femoral	R ___ L ___
Pedal	R ___ L ___	Posterior tibial	R ___ L ___
Bruits	R ___ L ___		

Nursing Assessment Form Based on Functional Health Patterns

SLEEP–REST PATTERN

Sleep time _____ Quality _____

Difficulty falling asleep _____	Appearance _____	
Difficulty remaining asleep _____	Yawning _____ Irritability _____	
Sleep aids _____	Short attention span _____	
Sleep medications _____		

SEXUALITY–REPRODUCTION PATTERN

Female Menstruation

Age of onset _____ Last menstrual period _____

Length _____

Problems _____

Gravida _____ Para _____ Abortions _____

Current pregnancy _____

Infertility _____

Breasts

BSE _____ When _____

Shape _____ Symmetry _____

Nipples _____ Discharge _____

Masses _____ Lymph nodes _____

Male Genitalia

Testicular exam _____ When _____

Masses _____ Swelling _____

Texture _____

Male–Female

Contraception used _____

Uncesirable side effects _____

Problems with sexual activities _____

Sexually transmitted diseases _____

Effect of illness on sexuality _____

Pain _____ Burning _____

Discomfort during intercourse _____

	Penile exam _____	
	Masses _____	Growths _____
	Lesions _____	Discharge _____
	Foreskin retraction _____	
	Urethral opening _____	
	Lymph nodes _____	
	Inguinal masses _____	

Female Genitalia

	Labia _____	Color _____
	Swelling _____	Symmetry _____
	Urethral opening _____	
	Discharge _____	
	Vaginal opening _____	
	Lesions _____	Discharge _____
	Hymen _____	Inflammation _____

SENSORY-PERCEPTUAL PATTERN

Perceptions of: Vision _____

Hearing _____	Taste _____
Smell _____	Sensation _____
Pain _____	

Vision aids _____

Hearing aids _____

Visual Acuity: OD _____ OS _____

OU _____	Visual fields _____
EOMs _____	
PERRLA _____	

Funduscopic Exam: Red reflex _____

| Optic disc _____ | Macula _____ |
| Arterioles/venules _____ | |

Hearing: Weber _____ Rinne _____
External canal _____
Tympanic membrane _____

Sensations: Superficial _____ Deep pressure _____
2-point discrimination _____

Cranial Nerves
I. Olfactory _____
II. Optic _____
V. Trigeminal _____
III, IV, VI. Oculomotor, trochlear, abducens _____
VII. Facial _____ Acoustic _____

COGNITIVE PATTERN

Understanding of illness _____
Understanding of treatments _____
Ability to express self _____
Ability to recall:
    Remote _____
    Recent _____
Ability to make decisions _____
Expression of feelings _____

Behavior _____
Speech _____ Vocabulary _____
Mood _____
Thought processes _____
Orientation: Person _____
    Time _____ Place _____
Attention _____ Information _____
Vocabulary _____
Abstract reasoning _____
Similarities _____ Judgment _____
Sensory perception and coordination _____

ROLE–RELATIONSHIP PATTERN

Role in family _____

Responsibility _____

Work role _____

Social role _____

Level of satisfaction _____

Effect of illness on roles _____

_____

Communication between family members _____

Family visits _____ Length _____

Draw family genogram:

SELF-PERCEPTION–SELF-CONCEPT PATTERN

Identity _____

Perception of abilities _____

Body image _____

COPING–STRESS TOLERANCE PATTERN

Stressors _____

Coping methods _____

Support systems _____

VALUE–BELIEF PATTERN

Values _____

Goals _____

Source of hope/strength _____

Significant religious person _____

Religious practices _____

Relationship with God _____

Presence of religious articles _____

Religious activities _____

Visits from clergy _____

Physical Assessment Guide

Following is an outline guide for performing a head-to-toe physical assessment. This guide will help you pull together all your assessment skills to complete an integrated and comprehensive physical examination efficiently.

EQUIPMENT FOR A HEAD-TO-TOE ASSESSMENT

- Assessment documentation forms
- Coin or key
- Cotton ball
- Cover card (for eye assessment)
- Gloves
- Goniometer
- Gown for client
- Lubricating jelly
- Magnifying glass
- Marking pencil
- Mini-Menta Status Examination (MMSE) Form
- Newspaper print or Rosenbaum pocket screener
- Notepad and pencil
- Ophthalmoscope
- Otoscope

- Paper clip
- Penlight
- Pillows (two small pillows)
- Platform scale with height attachment
- Reflex hammer
- Ruler with centimeter markings
- Skinfold calibers, flexible tape measure
- Small cup of water for client to drink
- Snellen chart
- Stethoscope and sphygmomanometer
- Substances for testing smell (eg, soap, coffee)
- Substances for testing taste (eg, salt, lemon, sugar, pickle juice)
- Supplies for collecting vaginal specimen (slides, spatula, cotton-tip applicator)
- Thermometer
- Tongue depressor
- Tuning fork
- Vaginal speculum
- Watch

PREPARING THE CLIENT

Discuss the purpose of the physical assessment with your client and acquire his or her permission to perform the various examinations. Ensure privacy and confidentiality. Respect the client's right to refuse any part of the assessment. Ask him or her to change into a gown for the examination.

GENERAL SURVEY

- **Observe appearance including:**
  - Overall physical and sexual development
  - Apparent age (compare with stated age)
  - Overall skin coloring
  - Dress, grooming, and hygiene
  - Body build, as well as muscle mass and fat distribution
  - Behavior (compare with developmental stage)
- **Assess the client's vital signs:**
  - Temperature
  - Pulse
  - Respiration
  - Blood pressure
  - Pain (as the fifth vital sign)
- **Take body measurements:**
  - Height
  - Weight
  - Waist and hip circumference; mid-arm circumference
  - Triceps skinfold thickness (TSF)
- Calculate ideal body weight, body mass index, waist-to-hip ratio, and mid-arm muscle area and circumference.
- **Test vision using the Snellen chart.**

MENTAL STATUS EXAMINATION

- **In addition to data collected about the client's appearance during the general survey, observe:**
  - Level of consciousness
  - Posture and body movements
  - Facial expressions
  - Speech
  - Mood, feelings, and expressions
  - Thought processes and perceptions
- **Assess the client's cognitive abilities (the MMSE may be used):**
  - Orientation to person, time, and place
  - Concentration, ability to focus and follow directions
  - Recent memory of happenings today
  - Remote memory of the past
  - Recall of unrelated information in 5-, 10-, and 30-minute periods
  - Abstract reasoning (Explain a "Stitch in time saves nine.")
  - Judgment ("What one would do in case of . . . ?")
  - Visual perceptual and constructional ability (draw a clock or shapes of square, etc.)

Ask the client to empty the bladder (give the client a specimen cup if a urine sample is needed) and change into a gown. Ask him or her to sit on the examination table.

SKIN

- As you perform each part of the head-to-toe assessment, assess skin for color variations, texture, temperature, turgor, edema, and lesions.
- Teach the client skin self-examination.

HEAD AND FACE

- Inspect and palpate the head for size, shape, and configuration.
- Note consistency, distribution, and color of hair.
- Observe face for symmetry, facial features, expressions, and skin condition.
- Check function of cranial nerve (CN) VII: Have the client smile, frown, show teeth, blow out cheeks, raise eyebrows, and tightly close eyes.
- Evaluate function of CN V: Using the sharp and dull sides of a paper clip, test sensations of forehead, cheeks, and chin.
- Palpate the temporal arteries for elasticity and tenderness.
- As the client opens and closes the mouth, palpate the temporomandibular joint for tenderness, swelling, and crepitation.

EYES

- Determine function:
  - Test visual fields.
  - Assess corneal light reflex.
  - Perform cover and position tests.
- Inspect external eye:
  - Position and alignment of the eyeball in eye socket
  - Bulbar conjunctiva and sclera
  - Palpebral conjunctiva
  - Lacrimal apparatus
  - Cornea, lens, iris, and pupil

- Test pupillary reaction to light.
- Test accommodation of pupils.
- Assess corneal reflex (CN VII—facial).
- Use the ophthalmoscope to inspect:
  - Optic disc for shape, color, size, and physiologic cup
  - Retinal vessels for color and diameter and arteriovenous (AV) crossings
  - Retinal background for color and lesions
  - Fovea centralis (sharpest area of vision) and macula
  - Anterior chamber for clarity

EARS AND NOSE

- Inspect the auricle, tragus, and lobule for shape, position, lesions, discolorations, and discharge.
- Palpate the auricle and mastoid process for tenderness.
- Use the otoscope to inspect:
  - External auditory canal for color and cerumen (ear wax)
  - Tympanic membrane for color, shape, consistency, and landmarks
- Test hearing:
  - Whisper test
  - Weber's test for diminished hearing in one ear
  - Rinne test to compare bone and air conduction (tuning fork on mastoid; then in front of ear)
- Inspect the external nose for color, shape, and consistency. Palpate the external nose for tenderness.
- Check patency of airflow through nostrils (occlude one nostril at a time and ask client to sniff).
- Test CN I: Ask the client to close his or her eyes and smell for soap, coffee, or vanilla. (Occlude each nostril)

- Use an otoscope with a short wide tip to inspect internal nose for color and integrity of nasal mucosa, nasal septum, and inferior and middle turbinates.
- Transilluminate maxillary sinuses with a penlight to check for fluid or pus.

MOUTH AND THROAT

Put on gloves. Use a tongue depressor and penlight as needed.

- Inspect lips for consistency, color, and lesions.
- Inspect the teeth for number and condition.
- Check the gums and buccal mucosa for color, consistency, or lesions.
- Inspect the hard (anterior) and soft (posterior) palates for color and integrity.
- Ask the client to say "aah" and observe the rise of the uvula.
- Test CN X: Touch the soft palate to assess for gag reflex.
- Inspect the tonsils for color, size, lesions, and exudates.
- Inspect the tongue for color, moisture, size, and texture. Inspect the ventral surface of the tongue for frenulum, color, lesions, and Wharton ducts.
- Palpate the tongue for lesions.
- Test CN IX and CN X: Assess tongue strength by asking the client to press the tongue against the tongue blade.
- Assess CN VII and CN IX: Have the client close his or her eyes. Check taste by placing salt, sugar, and lemon on the tongue.

NECK

- Inspect the neck for appearance of lesions, masses, swelling, and symmetry.
- Test range of motion (ROM).

- Palpate the preauricular, postauricular, occipital, tonsillar, submandibular, and submental nodes.
- Palpate the trachea.
- Palpate the thyroid gland for size, irregularity, or masses.
- Auscultate an enlarged thyroid for bruits.
- Palpate carotid arteries and auscultate for bruits.

ARMS, HANDS, AND FINGERS

- Inspect the upper extremities for overall skin color, texture, moisture, masses, and lesions.
- Test function of CN XI (spinal) by shoulder shrug and turning head against resistance.
- Palpate arms for tenderness, swelling, and temperature.
- Assess epitrochlear lymph nodes.
- Test ROM of the elbows.
- Palpate the brachial pulse.
- Palpate ulnar and radial pulses.
- Test ROM of the wrist.
- Test ROM of the fingers.
- Inspect palms of hands and palpate for temperature.
- Use a reflex hammer to test biceps, triceps, and brachioradialis reflexes.
- Test rapid alternating movements of hands.
- Ask the client to close the eyes; test sensation:
  - Assess light touch, pain, and temperature sensation in scattered locations over hands and arms
  - Evaluate sensitivity of position of fingers.
  - Place a quarter or key in the client's hand to test stereognosis.
  - Assess graphesthesia by writing a number in the palm of the client's hand.
  - Assess two-point discrimination in the fingertips, forearm, and dorsal hands.

Ask client to continue sitting with arms at sides and stand behind client. Untie gown to expose posterior chest.

POSTERIOR AND LATERAL CHEST

- Inspect configuration and shape of scapulae and chest wall.
- Note use of accessory muscles when breathing and posture.
- Palpate for tenderness, sensation, crepitus, masses, lesions, and fremitus.
- Evaluate chest expansion at posterior intercostal spaces (comparing bilaterally).
- Percuss for tone at posterior intercostal spaces (comparing bilaterally).
- Determine diaphragmatic excursion.
- Auscultate for breath sounds, adventitious sounds, and voice sounds (bronchophony, egophony, and whispered pectoriloquy).
- Test for two-point discrimination on the client's back.
- Ask client to lean forward and exhale; use bell of stethoscope to listen over the apex and left sternal border of the heart.

Move to front of client and expose anterior chest. Allow client to maintain modesty.

ANTERIOR CHEST

- Inspect anteroposterior diameter of chest, slope of ribs, and color of chest.
- Note quality and pattern of respirations (rate, rhythm, and depth).
- Observe intercostal spaces for bulging or retractions and use of accessory muscles.
- Palpate for tenderness, sensation, masses, lesions, fremitus, and anterior chest expansion.
- Percuss for tone at apices above clavicles, then at intercostal spaces (comparing bilaterally).
- Auscultate for anterior breath sounds, adventitious sounds, and voice sounds.
- Pinch skin over sternum to assess mobility (ease to pinch) and turgor (return to original shape).

Ask client to fold gown to waist and sit with arms hanging freely.

BREASTS

Female Breasts

- Inspect size, symmetry, color, texture, superficial venous pattern, areolae, and nipples of both breasts.
- Inspect for retractions and dimpling of nipples: Have the client raise her arms overhead, press her hands on her hips, press her hands together in front of her, and lear forward.
- Palpate axillae for rashes, infection, and anterior, central, and posterior lymph nodes.

Male Breasts

- Inspect for swelling, nodules, and ulcerations.
- Palpate the breast tissue and axillae.

Assist client to supine position with the head elevated to 30° to 45°. Stand on client's right side.

NECK

Observe and evaluate jugular venous pressure.

Assist client to supine position (lower examination table.).

Complete examination of female breasts:

- Palpate breasts for masses and the nipples for discharge.
- Teach breast self-examination.

HEART

- Inspect and palpate for apical impulse.
- Palpate the apex, left sternal border, and base of the heart for any abnormal pulsations.

- Auscultate over aortic area, pulmonic area, Erb's point, tricuspid area, and mitral area (apex) for:
  - Heart rate and rhythm (with diaphragm of stethoscope). If irregular, auscultate for a pulse rate deficit.
  - S_1 and S_2 (with diaphragm of stethoscope)
  - Extra heart sounds, S_3 and S_4 (with diaphragm and bell of stethoscope)
  - Murmurs (using bell and diaphragm of the stethoscope)

Cover chest to lie on left side; use bell of stethoscope to listen to apex of the heart.

Ask the client to lie on left side; use bell and diaphragm of the stethoscope to listen to apex of the heart.

ABDOMEN

- Inspect for:
  - Overall skin color
  - Vascularity, striae, lesions, and rashes
  - Location, contour, and color of umbilicus
  - Symmetry and contour of abdomen
  - Aortic pulsations or peristaltic waves
- Auscultate for:
  - Bowel sounds (intensity, pitch, and frequency)
  - Vascular sounds and friction rubs (over spleen, liver, aorta, iliac artery, umbilicus, and femoral artery)
- Percuss for:
  - Tone over four quadrants
  - Liver location, size, and span
  - Spleen location and size

- Lightly palpate:
  – Abdominal reflex
  – Four quadrants to identify tenderness and muscular resistance
- Deeply palpate:
  – Four quadrants for masses
  – Aorta
  – Liver, spleen, and kidneys for enlargement or irregularities

Replace gown and position draping so lower extremities are exposed.

LEGS, FEET, AND TOES

- Inspect the lower extremities for overall skin coloration, texture, moisture, masses, lesions, and varicosities.
- Observe muscles of the legs and feet.
- Note hair distribution.
- Palpate joints of hips and test ROM. Palpate the femoral pulse.
- Palpate for:
  – Edema, skin temperature
  – Muscle size and tone of legs and feet
- Palpate knees including popliteal pulse.
- Palpate the ankles; assess dorsalis pedis and posterior tibial pulses. Test ROM.
- Assess capillary refill.
- Test
  – Sensation to dull and sharp sensations
  – Two-point discrimination (on thighs)
  – Patellar reflex, Achilles reflex, and plantar reflex
  – Position sense
  – Vibratory sensation on bony surface of big toe

- Perform heel-to-shin test.
- As warranted, perform special tests:
  - Position change for arterial insufficiency
  - Manual compression test
  - Trendelenburg test
  - Bulge knee test
  - Ballottement test
  - McMurray's test

Secure gown and assist client to standing position.

MUSCULOSKELETAL AND NEUROLOGIC EXAMINATION

Note: Parts of these systems have already been assessed throughout the physical examination.

- Check for spinal curvatures and scoliosis.
- Observe gait including base of support, weight-bearing stability, foot position, stride, arm swing, and posture.
- Observe as the client:
  - Walks heel to toe (tandem walk)
  - Hops on one leg, then the other
  - Performs Romberg's test
  - Performs finger-to-nose test

Perform the female and male genitalia examination last, moving from the less private to more private examination for client comfort.

GENITALIA

Female Genitalia

Have female client assume the lithotomy position. Apply gloves. Apply lubricant as appropriate.

- Inspect:
  - Distribution of pubic hair
  - Mons pubis, labia majora, and perineum for lesions, swelling, and excoriations
- Palpate:
  - Bartholin glands, urethra, and Skene glands
  - Labia minora, clitoris, urethral meatus, and vaginal opening for lesions, swelling, or discharge
- Inspect:
  - Size of vaginal opening and vaginal musculature
- Insert speculum and inspect:
  - Cervix for lesions and discharge
  - Vagina for color, consistency, and discharge
- Obtain cytologic smears and cultures.
- Perform bimanual examination; palpate:
  - Cervix for contour, consistency, mobility, and tenderness
  - Uterus for size, position, shape, and consistency
  - Ovaries for size and shape

Discard gloves and apply clean gloves and lubricant.

- Perform the rectovaginal examination; palpate rectovaginal septum for tenderness, consistency, and mobility.

Male Genitalia and Rectum

Sit on a stool. Have client stand and face you with gown raised. Apply gloves.

- Inspect the penis, including:
  - Base of penis and pubic hair for excoriation, erythema, and infestation
  - Skin and shaft of penis for rashes, lesions, lumps, or hardened or tender areas
  - Color, location, and integrity of foreskin in uncircumcised men
  - Glans for size, shape, lesions, or redness and location of urinary meatus
- Palpate for urethral discharge by gently squeezing glans.
- Inspect scrotum, including:
  - Size, shape, and position
  - Scrotal skin for color, integrity, lesions, or rashes
  - Posterior skin (by lifting scrotal sac)
- Palpate both testis and epididymis between thumb and first two fingers for size, shape, nodules, and tenderness. Palpate spermatic cord and vas deferens.
- Transilluminate scrotal contents for red glow, swelling, or masses. If a mass is found during inspection and palpation, have the client lie down and inspect and palpate for scrotal hernia.
- As client bears down, inspect for bulges in inguinal and femoral areas and palpate for femoral hernias.
- While client shifts weight to each corresponding side, palpate for inguinal hernia.
- Teach testicular self-examination.

Ask the client to remain standing and to bend over the exam table. Change gloves.

- Inspect:
  - Perianal area for lumps, ulcers, lesions, rashes, redness, fissures, or thickening of epithelium
  - Sacrococcygeal area for swelling, redness, dimpling, or hair

- While client bears down or performs Valsalva maneuver, inspect for bulges or lesions.
- Apply lubrication and use finger to palpate:
  - Anus
  - External sphincter for tenderness, nodules, and hardness
  - Rectum for tenderness, irregularities, nodules, and hardness
  - Peritoneal cavity
  - Prostate for size, shape, tenderness, and consistency
- Inspect stool for color and test feces for occult blood.

Developmental Information—Age 1 Month to 18 Years

Age	Physical Development	Language (Cognitive) Development (Based on PIAGET)	Psychosocial Development (Based on ERIKSON)	Nurse's Approach To Assessment
Overview of birth to 1 year		*Sensorimotor stage of development.*	*Developmental task: trust vs mistrust.* Learns to trust and to anticipate satisfaction. Sends cues to mother/caretaker. Begins understanding self as separate from others (body image).	Involve caretaker in assessment (eg, allow him or her to hold child in lap for parts of examination).

(continued)

Age	Physical Development	Language (Cognitive) Development (Based on PIAGET)	Psychosocial Development (Based on ERIKSON)	Nurse's Approach To Assessment
1–2 months	Lifts chin and chest off bed. Holds extremities in flexion and moves at random; weak neck muscles. Activity varies from quiet sleep to drowsiness to alert activity.	Can discriminate between various sensations and prefers certain ones. Follows moving objects with eyes.	Begins to bond with mother during alert periods.	Conserve infant's body heat. Assess while asleep or quiet. Place infant on table or in caretaker's arms. Give bottle if awake.
3–4 months	Head and back control developing. Holds rattle. Looks at own hands. Infant reflexes begin to disappear. Able to sit propped. Props self on forearm in prone position. Rolls from side to back and vice versa	Responds to parent. Social smile. Begins to vocalize; coos; babbles. Locates sounds by turning head, looking.	Learns to signal displeasure. Shows excitement with whole body. Begins to discriminate strangers. Squeals.	Speak softly to infant. Use brightly colored toys, bells, rattles to elicit necessary responses and to distract. Assess ears, mouth, nose last. Assess lungs and heart when quiet.

Age				
	and from back to abdomen. Takes objects to mouth. Drools with eruption of lower teeth.			
5–8 months	Begins to develop teeth. Birth weight doubled. Grasps objects. Sits unsupported.	Begins to imitate sounds, two-syllable words ("dada," "mama"). Responds to own name.	Increased fear of strangers. Definite likes/dislikes. Responds to "no."	Place on caretaker's lap (same as above).
9–12 months	Birth weight tripled. Anterior fontanelle nearly closed. Learns to pull in order to stand, creep, and crawl.	Says two-syllable words besides "dada," "mama." Understands simple commands. Imitates animal sounds.	Looks for hidden objects. Unceasing determination to move about. Clings to mother. Shows emotion. Plays peek-a-boo and pat-a-cake.	
1–3 years	Begins to walk and run well. Drinks from cup, feeds self. Develops fine motor control.	*Preoperational stage of development.* Has poor time sense. Increasing	*Developmental task: autonomy vs shame and doubt.* Estab-	Be flexible. Begin assessment with play period to establish rapport. Be

(continued)

Age	Physical Development	Language (Cognitive) Development (Based on PIAGET)	Psychosocial Development (Based on ERIKSON)	Nurse's Approach To Assessment
	Climbs. Begins self-toileting. Kneels without support. Steady growth in height/weight. Adult height will be approximately double the height at age 2. Dresses self by age 3.	verbal ability. Formulates sentences of 4 to 5 words by age 3. Talks to self and others. Has misconceptions about cause and effect. Interested in pictures. *Fears:* • Loss/separation from parents—peak • Dark • Machines/equipment • Intrusive procedures • Bedtime	lishes self-control, decision making, independence (autonomy). Extremely curious and prefers to do things by self. Demonstrates independence through negativism. Very egocentric; believes he or she controls the world. Attempts to please parents. Participates in parallel play; able to share some toys by age 3.	honest. Praise for cooperation. Begin slowly; speak to child. Involve caretaker/parent in holding on exam table. Let child hold security object. Allow child to play with stethoscope, tongue blade, flashlight before using on child if possible. Assess face, mouth, eyes, ears last. May need to restrain when lying prone. If resistant, save that part of the assessment for later.

Developmental Information—Age 1 Month to 18 Years

Age			
4–6 years	Growth slows. Locomotion skills increase and coordination improves. Tricycle/bicycle riding. Throws ball but has difficulty catching. Constantly active, increasing dexterity. Eruption of permanent teeth. Skips, hops, jumps rope.	Speaks to dolls and animals. Increasing attention span. Knows own sex by age 3. Preoperational stage of development continues. Language skills flourish. Generates many questions (eg, How, Why, What?) Simple problem solving. Uses fantasy to understand and problem solve. *Fears:* • Mutilation • Castration • Dark	Developmental tasks: *initiative vs guilt.* Attempts to establish self like his or her parents, but independent. Explores environment on own initiative. Boasts, brags, has feelings of indestructibility. Family is primary social group. Peers increasingly important. Assumes sex roles. Aggressive, very curious. Enjoys activities	Establish rapport through talking and play. Introduce self to child. Have parent present but direct conversation to child. Games such as "follow the leader" and "Simon says" can be used to elicit necessary behaviors. Explain each assessment in simple language. Ask for child's help and use flattery. Use pictures, models, or items he or she can see or touch. Reserve

(continued)

Age	Physical Development	Language (Cognitive) Development (Based on PIAGET)	Psychosocial Development (Based on ERIKSON)	Nurse's Approach To Assessment
		• Unknown • Inanimate • Unfamiliar objects Causality related to proximity of events. Enjoys mimicking and imitating adults.	such as sports, cooking, shopping. Cooperative play. Likes rules. May stretch the truth and tell large stories.	genital examination for last; drape accordingly.
6–11 years	Moves constantly. Physical play prevalent; sports, swimming, skating, etc. Increased smoothness of movement. Grows at rate of 2 in/7 lb a year. Eyes/hands well coordinated.	*Concrete operations stage of development.* Organized thought; memory concepts more complicated. Reads, reasons better. Focuses on concrete understanding.	*Developmental task: industry vs inferiority.* Learns to include values and skills of school, neighborhood, peers. Peer relationships important. Focuses more on reality, less on fantasy. Family is	Explain all procedures and impact on body. Encourage questioning and active participation in care. Be direct about explanation of procedures, based on what child will hear, see, smell, and feel. (In addition, explain

Age	Physical	Fears / Emotional	Cognitive	Psychosocial	Nursing Implications
		Fears: • Mutilation • Death • Immobility • Rejection • Failure		main base of security and identity. Sensitive to reactions of others. Seeks approval and recognition. Enthusiastic, noisy, imaginative, desires to explore. Likes to complete a task. Enjoys helping others.	body part involved, and use anatomical name and pictures to explain step by step.) Be honest. Reassure child that he or she is liked. Provide privacy. Involve parents, but give child choice as to whether parent will stay during exam. Reason and explain. Allow child some choice as to direction of assessment. May be able to proceed as if assessing adult. Praise cooperation.
12–18 years	Well developed. Rapid physical growth (early adolescence: maximum growth). Secondary sex characteristics.		*Formal operations stage of development.* Abstract reasoning, problem solving.	*Developmental task: identity vs role confusion.* Predominant values are those of peer group. Early	Respect privacy. Accept expression of feelings. Direct discussions of care and condition to child. Ask for child's

(*continued*)

Age	Physical Development	Language (Cognitive) Development (Based on PIAGET)	Psychosocial Development (Based on ERIKSON)	Nurse's Approach To Assessment
	(See Chapter 17, Genitourinary Assessment.)	Understanding of multiple cause-and-effect relationships. May plan for future career. *Fears:* • Mutilation • Disruption of body image • Rejection by peers	adolescence: outgoing and enthusiastic. Emotions are extreme, with mood swings. Seeking self-identity, sexual identity. Wants privacy and independence. Develops interests not shared with family. Concern with physical self. Explores adult roles.	opinions and encourage questions. Allow input into decisions. Be flexible with routines. Explain all procedures/treatments. Encourage continuance of peer relationships. Listen actively. Identify impact of illness on body image, future, and level of functioning. Correct misconceptions. Involve parent in assessment only if child requests presence.

Recommended Childhood and Adolescent Immunization Schedule

UNITED STATES · 2006

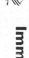

Vaccine ▼ Age ►	Birth	1 month	2 months	4 months	6 months	12 months	15 months	18 months	24 months	4-6 years	11-12 years	13-14 years	15 years	16-18 years
Hepatitis B¹	HepB	HepB		HepB¹		HepB					HepB Series			
Diphtheria, Tetanus, Pertussis²			DTaP	DTaP	DTaP		DTaP			DTaP	Tdap	Tdap		
Haemophilus influenzae type b³			Hib	Hib	Hib³	Hib								
Inactivated Poliovirus			IPV	IPV	IPV					IPV				
Measles, Mumps, Rubella⁴						MMR				MMR	MMR			
Varicella⁵						Varicella					Varicella			
Meningococcal⁶										MPSV4	MCV4	MCV4	MCV4	
Pneumococcal⁷			PCV	PCV	PCV	PCV			PCV		PPV			
Influenza⁸					Influenza (Yearly)					Influenza (Yearly)				
Hepatitis A⁹									HepA Series					

Vaccines within broken line are for selected populations

Legend: ▒ Range of recommended ages   ▒ Catch-up immunization   ▒ 11–12 year old assessment

This schedule indicates the recommended ages for routine administration of currently licensed childhood vaccines, as of December 1, 2005, for children through age 18 years. Any dose not administered at the recommended age should be administered at any subsequent visit when indicated and feasible. ▒ Indicates age groups that warrant special effort to administer those vaccines not previously administered. Additional vaccines may be licensed and recommended during the year. Licensed combination vaccines may be used whenever any components of the combination are indicated and other components of the vaccine are not contraindicated and if approved by the Food and Drug Administration for that dose of the series. Providers should consult the respective ACIP statement for detailed recommendations. Clinically significant adverse events that follow immunization should be reported to the Vaccine Adverse Event Reporting System (VAERS). Guidance about how to obtain and complete a VAERS form is available at www.vaers.hhs.gov or by telephone, 800-822-7967.

1. **Hepatitis B vaccine (HepB).** *AT BIRTH: All newborns* should receive monovalent HepB soon after birth and before hospital discharge. **Infants born to mothers who are HBsAg-positive** should receive HepB and 0.5 mL of hepatitis B immune globulin (HBIG) within 12 hours of birth. **Infants born to mothers whose HBsAg status is unknown** should receive HepB within 12 hours of birth. The mother should have blood drawn as soon as possible to determine her HBsAg status; if HBsAg-positive, the infant should receive HBIG as soon as possible (no later than age 1 week). **For infants born to HBsAg-negative mothers,** the birth dose can be delayed in rare circumstances but only if a physician's order to withhold the vaccine and a copy of the mother's original HBsAg-negative laboratory report are documented in the infant's medical record. *FOLLOWING THE BIRTH DOSE:* The HepB series should be completed with either monovalent HepB or a combination vaccine containing HepB. The second dose should be administered at age 1–2 months. The final dose should be administered at age ≥24 weeks. It is permissible to administer 4 doses of HepB (e.g., when combination vaccines are given after the birth dose); however, if monovalent HepB is used, a dose at age 6 months is not needed. **Infants born to HBsAg-positive mothers** should be tested for HBsAg and antibody to HBsAg after completion of the HepB series, at age 9–18 months (generally at the next well-child visit after completion of the vaccine series).

2. **Diphtheria and tetanus toxoids and acellular pertussis vaccine (DTaP).** The fourth dose of DTaP may be administered as early as age 12 months, provided 6 months have elapsed since the third dose and the child is unlikely to return at age 15–18 months. The final dose in the series should be given at age ≥4 years.

Tetanus and diphtheria toxoids and acellular pertussis vaccine (Tdap – adolescent preparation) is recommended at age 11–12 years for those who have completed the recommended childhood DTP/DTaP vaccination series and have not received a tetanus and diphtheria toxoid (Td) booster dose. Adolescents 13–18 years who missed the 11–12 year Td/Tdap booster dose should also: receive a single dose of Tdap if they have completed the recommended childhood DTP/DTaP vaccination series. Subsequent **tetanus and diphtheria toxoids (Td)** are recommended every 10 years.

3. **Haemophilus influenzae type b conjugate vaccine (Hib).** Three Hib conjugate vaccines are licensed for infant use. If PRP-OMP (PedvaxHIB® or ComVax® [Merck]) is administered at ages 2 and 4 months, a dose at age 6 months is not required. DTaP/Hib combination products should not be used for primary immunization in infants at ages 2, 4, or 6 months but can be used as boosters after any Hib vaccine. The final dose in the series should be administered at age ≥12 months.

4. **Measles, mumps, and rubella vaccine (MMR).** The second dose of MMR is recommended routinely at age 4–6 years but may be administered during any visit, provided at least 4 weeks have elapsed since the first dose and both doses are administered beginning at or after age 12 months. Those who have not previously received the second dose should complete the schedule by age 11–12 years.

5. **Varicella vaccine.** Varicella vaccine is recommended at any visit at or after age 12 months for susceptible children (i.e., those who lack a reliable history of chickenpox). Susceptible persons aged ≥13 years should receive 2 doses administered at least 4 weeks apart.

6. **Meningococcal vaccine (MCV4).** Meningococcal conjugate vaccine (MCV4) should be given to all children at the 11–12 year visit as well as to unvaccinated adolescents at high school entry (15 years of age). Other adolescents who wish to decrease their risk for meningococcal disease may also be vaccinated. All college freshmen living in dormitories should also be vaccinated, preferably with MCV4, although meningococcal polysaccharide vaccine (MPSV4) is an acceptable alternative. Vaccination against invasive meningococcal disease is recommended for children and adolescents aged ≥2 years with terminal complement deficiencies or anatomic or functional asplenia and certain other high risk groups (see *MMWR* 2005;54 [RR-7]:1–21); use MPSV4 for children aged 2–10 years and MCV4 for older children, although MPSV4 is an acceptable alternative.

7. **Pneumococcal vaccine.** The heptavalent **pneumococcal conjugate vaccine (PCV)** is recommended for all children aged 2–23 months and for certain children aged 24–59 months. The final dose in the series should be given at age ≥12 months. **Pneumococcal polysaccharide vaccine (PPV)** is recommended in addition to PCV for certain high-risk groups. See *MMWR* 2000; 49(RR-9):1–35.

8. **Influenza vaccine.** Influenza vaccine is recommended annually for children aged ≥6 months with certain risk factors (including, but not limited to, asthma, cardiac disease, sickle cell disease, human immunodeficiency virus [HIV], diabetes, and conditions that can compromise respiratory function or handling of respiratory secretions (including household members) in close contact with persons in groups at high risk (see *MMWR* 2005;54[RR8]:1–55). In addition, healthy children aged 6–23 months and close contacts of healthy children aged 0–5 months are recommended to receive influenza vaccine because children in this age group are at substantially increased risk for influenza-related hospitalizations. For healthy persons aged 5–49 years, the intranasally administered, live, attenuated influenza vaccine (LAIV) is an acceptable alternative to the intramuscular trivalent inactivated influenza vaccine (TIV). See *MMWR* 2005;54[RR-8]:1-55. Children receiving TIV should be administered a dosage appropriate for their age (0.25 mL if aged 6–35 months or 0.5 mL if aged ≥3 years). Children aged ≤8 years who are receiving influenza vaccine for the first time should receive 2 doses (separated by at least 4 weeks for TIV and at least 6 weeks for LAIV).

9. **Hepatitis A vaccine (HepA).** HepA is recommended for all children at 1 year of age (i.e., 12–23 months). The 2 doses in the series should be administered at least 6 months apart. States, counties, and communities with existing HepA vaccination programs for children 2–18 years of age are encouraged to maintain these programs. In these areas, new efforts focused on routine vaccination of 1-year-old children should enhance, not replace, ongoing programs directed at a broader population of children. HepA is also recommended for certain high-risk groups (see *MMWR* 1999; 48[RR-12]:1-37).

Advisory Committee on Immunization Practices www.cdc.gov/nip/acip • American Academy of Pediatrics www.aap.org • American Academy of Family Physicians www.aafp.org

The Childhood and Adolescent Immunization Schedule is approved by:

Recommended Immunization Schedule for Children and Adolescents Who Start Late or Who Are More Than 1 Month Behind

UNITED STATES • 2006

The tables below give catch-up schedules and minimum intervals between doses for children who have delayed immunizations. There is no need to restart a vaccine series regardless of the time that has elapsed between doses. Use the chart appropriate for the child's age.

CATCH-UP SCHEDULE FOR CHILDREN AGED 4 MONTHS THROUGH 6 YEARS

Vaccine	Minimum Age for Dose 1	Minimum Interval Between Doses			
		Dose 1 to Dose 2	Dose 2 to Dose 3	Dose 3 to Dose 4	Dose 4 to Dose 5
Diphtheria, Tetanus, Pertussis	6 wks	4 weeks	4 weeks	6 months	6 months[1]
Inactivated Poliovirus	6 wks	4 weeks	4 weeks	4 weeks[2]	
Hepatitis B[3]	Birth	4 weeks	8 weeks (and 16 weeks after first dose)		
Measles, Mumps, Rubella	12 mo	4 weeks[4]			
Varicella	12 mo				
Haemophilus influenzae type b[5]	6 wks	4 weeks if first dose given at age <12 months **8 weeks (as final dose)** if first dose given at age 12-14 months **No further doses needed** if first dose given at age ≥15 months	4 weeks[6] if current age <12 months **8 weeks (as final dose)**[6] if current age ≥12 months and second dose given at age <15 months **No further doses needed** if previous dose given at age ≥15 mo	**8 weeks (as final dose)** This dose only necessary for children aged 12 months-5 years who received 3 doses before age 12 months	
Pneumococcal[7]	6 wks	4 weeks if first dose given at age <12 months and current age <24 months **8 weeks (as final dose)** if first dose given at age ≥12 months or current age 24-59 months **No further doses needed** for healthy children if first dose given at age ≥24 months	4 weeks if current age <12 months **8 weeks (as final dose)** if current age ≥12 months **No further doses needed** for healthy children if previous dose given at age ≥24 months	**8 weeks (as final dose)** This dose only necessary for children aged 12 months-5 years who received 3 doses before age 12 months	

Recommended Childhood and Adolescent Immunization Schedule

CATCH-UP SCHEDULE FOR CHILDREN AGED 7 YEARS THROUGH 18 YEARS

Vaccine	Minimum Interval Between Doses		
	Dose 1 to Dose 2	Dose 2 to Dose 3	Dose 3 to Booster Dose
Tetanus, Diphtheria[1]	4 weeks	6 months	**6 months** if first dose given at age <12 months and current age <11 years, otherwise **5 years**
Inactivated Poliovirus[2]	4 weeks	4 weeks	IPV[2,5]
Hepatitis B	4 weeks	**8 weeks** (and 16 weeks after first dose)	
Measles, Mumps, Rubella	4 weeks		
Varicella[10]	4 weeks		

1. **DTaP.** The fifth dose is not necessary if the fourth dose was administered after the fourth birthday.

2. **IPV.** For children who received an all-IPV or all-oral poliovirus (OPV) series, a fourth dose is not necessary if third dose was administered at age ≥4 years. If both OPV and IPV were administered as part of a series, a total of 4 doses should be given, regardless of the child's current age.

3. **HepB.** Administer the 3-dose series to all children and adolescents <19 years of age if they were not previously vaccinated.

4. **MMR.** The second dose of MMR is recommended routinely at age 4-6 years but may be administered earlier if desired.

5. **Hib.** Vaccine is not generally recommended for children aged ≥5 years.

6. **Hib.** If current age <12 months and the first 2 doses were PRP-OMP (PedvaxHIB or ComVax [Merck]), the third (and final) dose should be administered at age 12-15 months or at least 8 weeks after the second dose.

7. **PCV.** Vaccine is not generally recommended for children aged ≥5 years.

8. **Td.** Adolescent tetanus, diphtheria, and pertussis vaccine (Tdap) may be substituted for any dose in a primary catch-up series or as a booster if age appropriate for Tdap. A five-year interval from the last Td dose is encouraged when Tdap is used as a booster dose. See ACIP recommendations for further information.

9. **IPV.** Vaccine is not generally recommended for persons aged ≥18 years.

10. **Varicella.** Administer the 2-dose series to all susceptible adolescents aged ≥13 years.

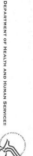

DEPARTMENT OF HEALTH AND HUMAN SERVICES®

CENTERS FOR DISEASE CONTROL AND PREVENTION

Report adverse reactions to vaccines through the federal Vaccine Adverse Event Reporting System. For information on reporting reactions following immunization, please visit www.vaers.hhs.gov or call the 24-hour national toll-free information line 800-822-7967. Report suspected cases of vaccine-preventable diseases to your state or local health department.

For additional information about vaccines, including precautions and contraindications for immunization and vaccine shortages, please visit the National Immunization Program Website at www.cdc.gov/nip or contact the **800-CDC-INFO (800-232-4636)** (in English, En Español – 24/7)

Recommended Adult Immunization Schedule, by Vaccine and Age Group
UNITED STATES, OCTOBER 2005–SEPTEMBER 2006

Vaccine ▼ Age group ▶	19–49 years	50–64 years	≥ 65 years
Tetanus, diphtheria (Td)*	1-dose booster every 10 yrs		
Measles, mumps, rubella (MMR)[2]*	1 or 2 doses	1 dose	
Varicella[3]*	2 doses (0, 4–8 wks)	2 doses (0, 4–8 wks)	
Influenza[4]*	1 dose annually	1 dose annually	
Pneumococcal (polysaccharide)[5,6]	1–2 doses		1 dose
Hepatitis A[7]*	2 doses (0, 6–12 mos, or 0, 6–18 mos)		
Hepatitis B[8]*	3 doses (0, 1–2, 4–6 mos)		
Meningococcal[9]	1 or more doses		

*– – – Vaccines below the broken line are for selected populations – – –

NOTE: These recommendations must be read along with the footnotes.

*Covered by the Vaccine Injury Compensation Program.

For all persons in this category who meet the age requirements and who lack evidence of immunity (e.g., lack documentation of vaccination or have no evidence of prior infection)

Recommended if some other risk factor is present (e.g., based on medical, occupational, lifestyle, or other indications)

This schedule indicates the recommended age groups and medical indications for which administration of currently licensed vaccines for persons aged ≥19 years. Licensed combination vaccines may be used whenever any components of the combination are indicated and when the vaccine's other components are not contraindicated. For detailed recommendations, consult the manufacturers' package inserts and the complete statements from the ACIP (www.cdc.gov/nip/publications/acip-list.htm).

Report all clinically significant postvaccination reactions to the Vaccine Adverse Event Reporting System (VAERS). Reporting forms and instructions on filing a VAERS report are available by telephone, 800-822-7967, or from the VAERS website at www.vaers.hhs.gov.

Information on how to file a Vaccine Injury Compensation Program claim is available at www.hrsa.gov/osp/vicp or by telephone, 800-338-2382. To file a claim for vaccine injury, contact the U.S. Court of Federal Claims, 717 Madison Place, N.W., Washington D.C. 20005, telephone 202-357-6400.

Additional information about the vaccines listed above and contraindications or vaccination is also available at www.cdc.gov/nip or from the CDC-INFO Contact Center at 800-CDC-INFO (232-4636) in English and Spanish, 24 hours a day, 7 days a week.

DEPARTMENT OF HEALTH AND HUMAN SERVICES
CENTERS FOR DISEASE CONTROL AND PREVENTION

CDC

Recommended Adult Immunization Schedule, by Vaccine and Medical and Other Indications
UNITED STATES, OCTOBER 2005–SEPTEMBER 2006

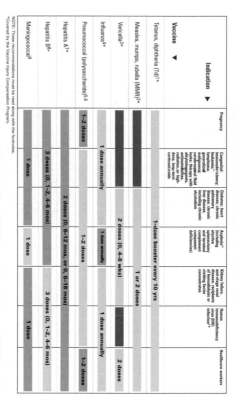

Vaccine ▼ / Indication ►	Pregnancy	Congenital immunodeficiency; leukemia; lymphoma; generalized malignancy; cerebrospinal fluid leaks; therapy with alkylating agents, antimetabolites, radiation, or high-dose, long-term corticosteroids	Diabetes; heart disease; chronic pulmonary disease; chronic liver disease, including chronic alcoholism	Asplenia[12] (including elective splenectomy and terminal complement component deficiencies)	Kidney failure, end-stage renal disease, recipients of hemodialysis or clotting factor concentrates	Human immunodeficiency virus (HIV) infection[4]	Healthcare workers
Tetanus, diphtheria (Td)[1]*	1-dose booster every 10 yrs						
Measles, mumps, rubella (MMR)[2]*			1 or 2 doses				
Varicella[3]*			2 doses (0, 4-8 wks)				
Influenza[4]*	1 dose annually		1 dose annually			1 dose annually	2 doses
Pneumococcal (polysaccharide)[5,6]	1-2 doses		1-2 doses			1-2 doses	
Hepatitis A[7]*			2 doses (0, 6-12 mos, or 0, 6-18 mos)				
Hepatitis B[8]*	3 doses (0, 1-2, 4-6 mos)				3 doses (0, 1-2, 4-6 mos)		
Meningococcal[9]	1 dose		1 dose			1 dose	

NOTE: These recommendations must be read along with the footnotes.

*Covered by the Vaccine Injury Compensation Program.

For all persons in this category who meet the age requirements and who lack evidence of immunity (e.g., lack documentation of vaccination or have no evidence of prior infection)

Recommended if some other risk factor is present (e.g., based on medical, occupational, lifestyle, or other indications)

Contraindicated

Approved by the Advisory Committee on Immunization Practices (ACIP),
the American College of Obstetricians and Gynecologists (ACOG), and the American Academy of Family Physicians (AAFP)

Footnotes

Recommended Adult Immunization Schedule, UNITED STATES, OCTOBER 2005–SEPTEMBER 2006

1. **Tetanus and Diphtheria (Td) vaccination.** Adults with uncertain histories of a complete primary vaccination series with diphtheria- and tetanus toxoid-containing vaccines should receive a primary series using combined Td toxoid. A primary series for adults is 3 doses; administer the first 2 doses at least 4 weeks apart and the third dose 6–12 months after the second. Administer 1 dose if the person received the primary series and if the last vaccination was received ≥10 years previously. Consult ACIP statement for recommendations for administering Td as prophylaxis in wound management (www.cdc.gov/nip/menu/preview/mmwrhtml/00041645.htm). The American College of Physicians Task Force on Adult Immunization supports a second option for Td use in adults: a single 10-booster at age 50 years for persons who have completed the full pediatric series, including the teenage/young adult booster. A newly licensed tetanus-diphtheria-acellular pertussis vaccine is available for adults. ACIP recommendations for its use will be published.

2. **Measles, Mumps, Rubella (MMR) vaccination.** *Measles component:* adults born before 1957 can be considered immune to measles. Adults born during or after 1957 should receive ≥1 dose of MMR unless they have a medical contraindication, documentation of ≥1 dose, history of measles based on healthcare provider diagnosis, or laboratory evidence of immunity. A second dose of MMR is recommended for adults who 1) were recently exposed to measles or in an outbreak setting; 2) were previously vaccinated with killed measles vaccine; 3) were vaccinated with an unknown type of measles vaccine during 1963–1967; 4) are students in postsecondary educational institutions; 5) work in a healthcare facility; or 6) plan to travel internationally. Withhold MMR or other measles-containing vaccines from HIV-infected persons with severe immunosuppression. *Mumps component:* 1 dose of MMR vaccine should be adequate for protection for those born during or after 1957 who lack a history of mumps based on healthcare provider diagnosis or who lack laboratory evidence of immunity. *Rubella component:* administer 1 dose of MMR vaccine to women whose rubella vaccination history is unreliable or who lack laboratory evidence of immunity. For women of child-bearing age, regardless of birth year, routinely determine rubella immunity and counsel women regarding congenital rubella syndrome. Do not vaccinate women who are pregnant or might become pregnant within 4 weeks of receiving the vaccine. Women who do not have evidence of immunity should receive MMR vaccine upon completion or termination of pregnancy and before discharge from the healthcare facility.

3. **Varicella vaccination.** Varicella vaccination is recommended for all adults without evidence of immunity to varicella. Special consideration should be given to those who 1) have close contact with persons at high risk for severe disease (healthcare workers and family contacts of immunocompromised persons) or 2) are at high risk for exposure or transmission (e.g., teachers of young children; child care employees; residents and staff members of institutional settings, including correctional institutions; college students; military personnel; adolescents and adults living in households with children; nonpregnant women of childbearing age; and international travelers). Evidence of immunity to varicella in adults includes any of the following: 1) documented age-appropriate vaccination with varicella vaccine (i.e., receipt of 1 dose before age 13 years or receipt of 2 doses [administered at least 4 weeks apart] at age ≥13 years); 2) born in the United States before 1966; 3) history of varicella disease based on healthcare provider diagnosis or self- or parental report of typical varicella disease for non–U.S.-born persons born before 1966 and all persons born during 1966–1997 (for a patient reporting a history of an atypical, mild case, or evidence of laboratory confirmation, if it was performed at the time of acute disease); 4) history of herpes zoster based on healthcare provider diagnosis; or 5) laboratory evidence of immunity. Do not vaccinate women who are pregnant or might become pregnant within 4 weeks of receiving the vaccine. Assess pregnant women for evidence of varicella immunity. Women who do not have evidence of immunity should receive dose 1 of varicella vaccine upon completion or termination of pregnancy and before discharge from the healthcare facility. Dose 2 should be given 4–8 weeks after dose 1.

4. **Influenza vaccination.** *Medical indications:* chronic disorders of the cardiovascular or pulmonary systems, including asthma; chronic metabolic diseases, including diabetes mellitus, renal dysfunction, hemoglobinopathies, or immunosuppression (including immunosuppression caused by medications or by HIV); any condition (e.g., cognitive dysfunction, spinal cord injury, seizure disorder or other neuromuscular disorder) that compromises respiratory function or the handling of respiratory secretions or that can increase the risk of aspiration; and pregnancy during the influenza season. No data exist on the risk for severe or complicated influenza disease among persons with asplenia; however, influenza is a risk factor for secondary bacterial infections that can cause severe disease among persons with asplenia. *Occupational indications:* healthcare workers and employees of long-term care and assisted living facilities. *Other indications:* residents of nursing homes and other long-term care and assisted living facilities; persons likely to transmit influenza to persons at high risk (i.e., in-home household contacts and caregivers of children birth through 23 months of age, or persons of all ages with high-risk conditions); and anyone who wishes to be vaccinated.

Footnotes

Recommended Adult Immunization Schedule, UNITED STATES, OCTOBER 2005–SEPTEMBER 2006

For healthy nonpregnant persons aged 5–49 years without high-risk condition who are not contacts of severely immunocompromised persons in special care units, intranasally administered influenza vaccine (FluMist®) may be administered in lieu of inactivated vaccine.

5. **Pneumococcal polysaccharide vaccination.** *Medical indications:* chronic disorders of the pulmonary system (excluding asthma), cardiovascular disease, diabetes mellitus, chronic liver disease, including liver disease as a result of alcohol abuse (e.g., cirrhosis); chronic renal failure or nephrotic syndrome; functional or anatomic asplenia (e.g., sickle cell disease or splenectomy [if elective splenectomy is planned, vaccinate at least 2 weeks before surgery]); immunosuppressive conditions (e.g., congenital immunodeficiency, HIV infection [vaccinate as close to diagnosis as possible when CD4 cell counts are highest], leukemia, lymphoma, multiple myeloma, Hodgkin disease, generalized malignancy, organ or bone marrow transplantation), chemotherapy with alkylating agents, antimetabolites, or high-dose, long-term corticosteroids; and cochlear implants. *Other indications:* Alaska Natives and certain American Indian populations; residents of nursing homes and other long-term care facilities.

6. **Revaccination with pneumococcal polysaccharide vaccine.** One-time revaccination after 5 years for persons with chronic renal failure or nephrotic syndrome; functional or anatomic asplenia (e.g., sickle cell disease or splenectomy); immunosuppressive conditions (e.g., congenital immunodeficiency, HIV infection, leukemia, lymphoma, multiple myeloma, Hodgkin disease, generalized malignancy, organ or bone marrow transplantation); or chemotherapy with alkylating agents, antimetabolites, or high-dose, long-term corticosteroids. For persons aged ≥65 years, one-time revaccination if they were vaccinated ≥5 years previously and were aged <65 years at the time of primary vaccination.

7. **Hepatitis A vaccination.** *Medical indications:* persons with clotting factor disorders or chronic liver disease. *Behavioral indications:* men who have sex with men or users of illegal drugs. *Occupational indications:* persons working with hepatitis A virus (HAV)-infected primates or with HAV in a research laboratory setting. *Other indications:* persons traveling to or working in countries that have high or intermediate endemicity of hepatitis A (for a list of countries, visit www.cdc.gov/travel/diseases.htm#hepa) as well as any person wishing to obtain immunity. Current vaccines should be given in a 2-dose series at either 0 and 6–12 months, or 0 and 6–18 months. If the combined hepatitis A and hepatitis B vaccine is used, administer 3 doses at 0, 1, and 6 months.

8. **Hepatitis B vaccination.** *Medical indications:* hemodialysis patients (use special formulation [40 µg/mL] or two 20-µg/mL doses) or patients who receive clotting factor concentrates. *Occupational indications:* healthcare workers and public-safety workers who have exposure to blood in the workplace, and persons in training in schools of medicine, dentistry, nursing, laboratory technology, and other allied health professions. *Behavioral indications:* injection-drug users; persons with more than one sex partner in the previous 6 months; persons with a recently acquired sexually transmitted disease (STD); and men who have sex with men. *Other indications:* household contacts and sex partners of persons with chronic hepatitis B virus (HBV) infection; clients and staff of institutions for the developmentally disabled; all clients of STD clinics; inmates of correctional facilities; and international travelers who will be in countries with high or intermediate prevalence of chronic HBV infection for >6 months (for list of countries, visit www.cdc.gov/travel/diseases.htm#hepa).

9. **Meningococcal vaccination.** *Medical indications:* adults with anatomic or functional asplenia, or terminal complement component deficiencies. *Other indications:* first-year college students living in dormitories; microbiologists who are routinely exposed to isolates of *Neisseria meningitidis*; military recruits; and persons who travel to or reside in countries in which meningococcal disease is hyperendemic or epidemic (e.g., the "meningitis belt" of sub-Saharan Africa during the dry season [December–June], particularly if contact with the local populations will be prolonged. Vaccination is required for all government of Saudi Arabia for all travelers to Mecca during the annual Hajj. Meningococcal conjugate vaccine is preferred for adults meeting any of the above indications who are aged ≤55 years, although meningococcal polysaccharide vaccine (MPSV4) is an acceptable alternative. Revaccination after 5 years may be indicated for adults previously vaccinated with MPSV4 who remain at high risk for infection (e.g., persons residing in areas in which disease is epidemic).

10. **Selected conditions for which *Haemophilus influenzae* type b (Hib) vaccine may be used.** *Haemophilus influenzae* type b conjugate vaccines are licensed for children aged 6 weeks–71 months. No efficacy data are available on which to base a recommendation concerning use of Hib vaccine for older children and adults with the chronic conditions associated with an increased risk for Hib disease. However, studies suggest good immunogenicity in patients who have sickle cell disease, leukemia, or HIV infection; or have had splenectomies; administering vaccine to these patients is not contraindicated.

Approved by the Advisory Committee on Immunization Practices (ACIP), the American College of Obstetricians and Gynecologists (ACOG), and the American Academy of Family Physicians (AAFP)

Psychosocial Development

YOUNG ADULT DEVELOPMENTAL TASK: INTIMACY VS ISOLATION

Behavior to Assess:

Accepts self: physically, cognitively, and emotionally
Establishes independence from parental home
Expresses love responsibly, emotionally, and sexually
Establishes an intimate bond with another human being
Finds a social friendship group
Becomes involved as part of a community
Establishes a philosophy of living and life
Begins a profession or a life's work that provides a means of contribution
Learns to solve problems of life that accompany independence from parental home

MATURE ADULT DEVELOPMENTAL TASK: GENERATIVITY VS STAGNATION

Behavior to Assess:

Establishes/maintains healthful life patterns
Discovers self as a life-mate for another person
Derives satisfaction from contributing to growth and development of others
Establishes an abiding intimacy
Helps children grow and mature

Maintains a stable home

Finds pleasure in an established work or profession

Takes pride in self and family accomplishments and contributions

Contributes to the community to support its growth and development

Adjusts to physical changes of aging

Develops deep, sustained friendships

Integrates leisure with work life

Develops a philosophy of life that includes an understanding of mortality

Prepares for eventual retirement

Supports aging parents/relatives

AGING ADULT DEVELOPMENTAL TASK: EGO INTEGRITY VS DESPAIR

Behavior to Assess:

Adjusts to changing physical self

Recognizes changes present as a result of aging, in relationships and activities

Maintains relationships with children, grandchildren, other relatives

Continues interests outside self and home

Completes transition from retirement at work to satisfying alternative activities

Establishes relationships with others his or her own age

Adjusts to deaths of relatives, spouse, and friends

Maintains maximum level of physical functioning through diet, exercise, and personal care

Finds meaning in past life and faces inevitable mortality of self and significant others

Integrates philosophical or religious values into understanding of self to promote comfort

Reviews accomplishments and recognizes meaningful contributions he or she has made to community and relatives

Height–Weight–Head Circumference Charts for Children

Published May 30, 2000 (modified 10/16/00).
SOURCE: Developed by the National Center for Health Statistics in collaboration with the National Center for Chronic Disease Prevention and Health Promotion (2000). http://www.cdc.gov/growthcharts

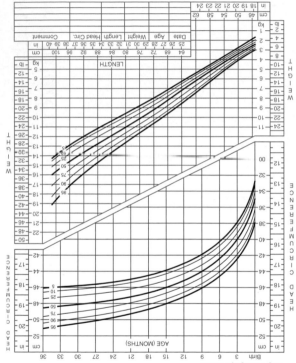

Birth to 36 months: Girls
Head circumference-for-age and
Weight-for-length percentiles

Height-Weight-Head Circumference Charts for Children

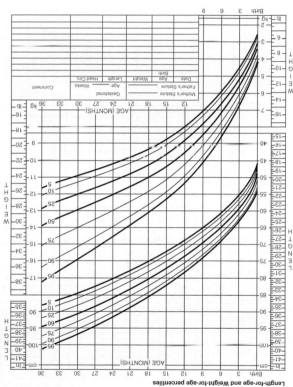

Birth to 36 months: Girls
Length-for-age and Weight-for-age percentiles

2 to 20 years: Girls
Stature-for-age and Weight-for-age percentiles

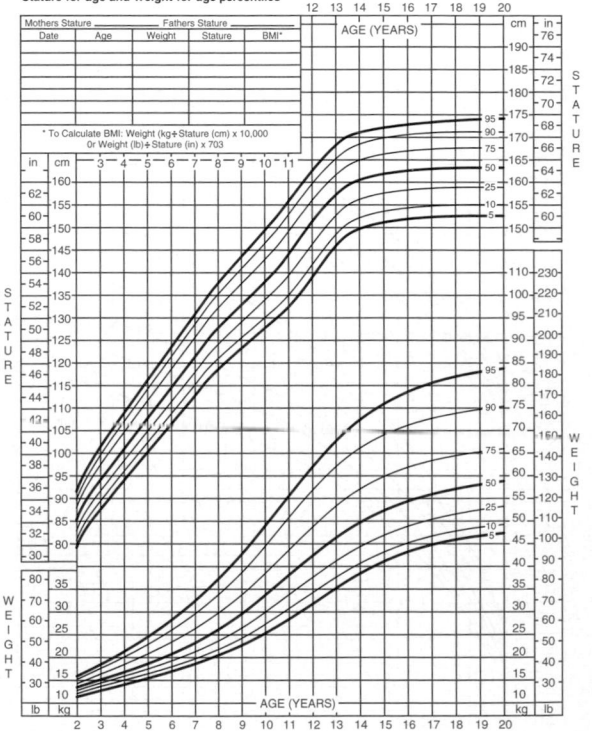

Height-Weight-Head Circumference Charts for Children

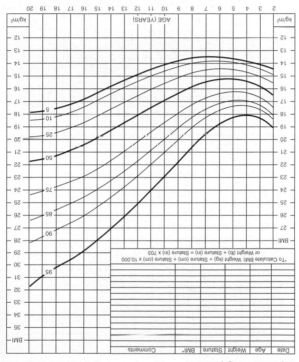

2 to 20 years: Girls
Body mass index-for-age percentiles

Date	Age	Weight	Stature	BMI*	Comments

*To Calculate BMI: Weight (kg) ÷ Stature (cm) ÷ Stature (cm) x 10,000
or Weight (lb) ÷ Stature (in) ÷ Stature (in) x 703

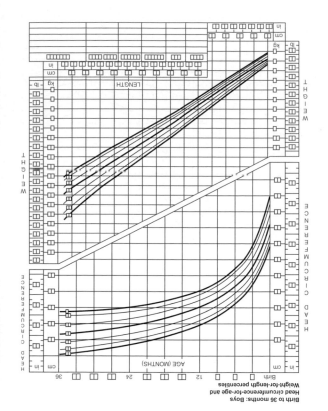

Birth to 36 months: Boys
Head circumference-for-age and
Weight-for-length percentiles

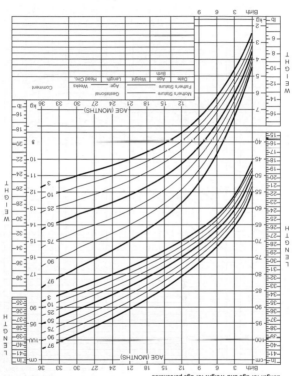

Length-for-age and Weight-for-age percentiles
Birth to 36 months: Boys

2 to 20 years: Boys
Body mass index-for-age percentiles

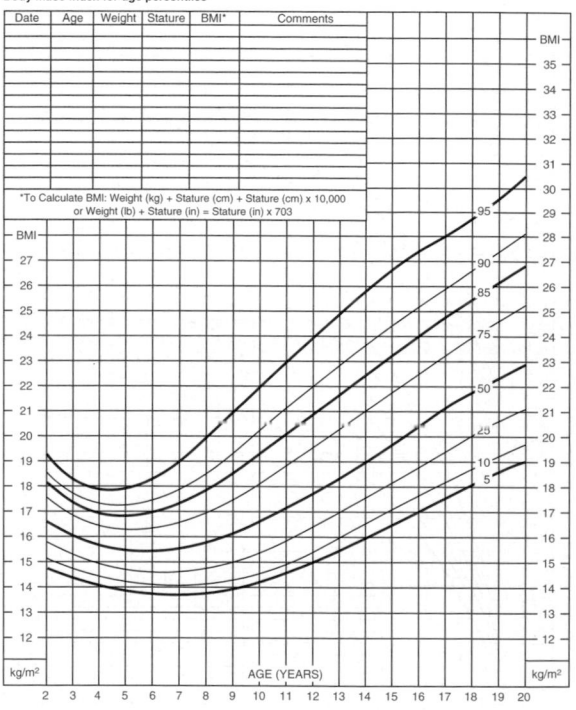

2 to 20 years: Boys
Stature-for-age and Weight-for-age percentiles

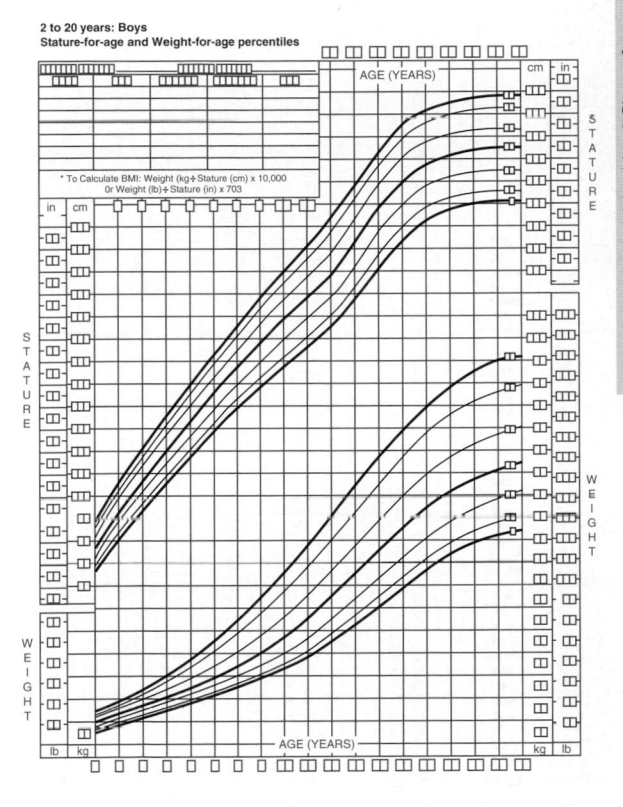

* To Calculate BMI: Weight (kg ÷ Stature (cm) x 10,000
Or Weight (lb) ÷ Stature (in) x 703

AGE (YEARS)

How to Examine Your Own Skin

You can systematically and regularly assess your skin for abnormalities by using the following recommended procedure for skin assessment from the American Cancer Society.

Face the mirror:

1. Check your face, ears, neck, chest, and belly.

2. Check both sides of your arms, the tops and palms of your hands, and your nail beds.

Sit down:

3. Check the front of your thighs, shins, tops of your feet, in between your toes, toenail beds, and bottoms of your feet.

How to Examine Your Own Skin

Stand up:

You will need a hand mirror for the backs of your thighs.

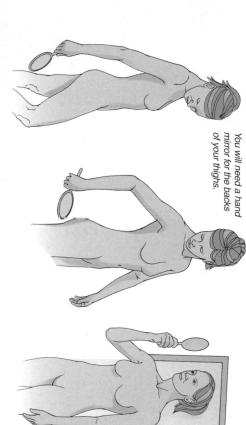

4. Now look at the back of your feet, your calves, and the backs of your thighs—first one leg, then the other.

5. Use the hand mirror to check the buttocks, genital area, lower back, upper back, and the back of the neck.

It may be helpful to look at your back in a wall mirror by using hand mirror.

Get familiar with your own skin and pattern of moles, freckles and birth marks. Be alert to changes in the number, size, shape or color of any of these. The best way to do this is to examine your skin. It may also be helpful to have someone who can check the skin on your back.

The best time to do this simple monthly exam is right after a bath or shower. Mark the date on your calendar. Use a full-length mirror and hand mirror so you can check any moles, blemishes, or birthmarks from the top of your head to your toes; note anything new, e.g., a change in shape, size, or color, or a sore that does not heal.

If you perform the exam regularly, you will know what is normal for you and can feel confident. Remember the warning signs and check with your health care professional or dermatologist if you find something new or different.

Courtesy of the American Cancer Society.

How to Examine Your Own Skin

Breast Self-Examination (BSE)

- Lie down and place your right arm behind your head. The exam is done while lying down, and not standing up, because when lying down the breast tissue spreads evenly over the chest wall and it is as thin as possible, making it much easier to feel all the breast tissue.

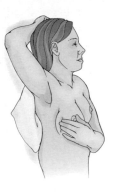

- Use the finger pads of the three middle fingers on your left hand to feel for lumps in the right breast. Use overlapping dime-sized circular motions of the finger pads to feel the breast tissue.

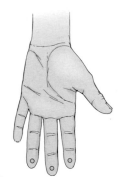

Source: American Cancer Society.

- Use three different levels of pressure to feel all the breast tissue. Light pressure is needed to feel the tissue closest to the skin; medium pressure to feel a little deeper; and firm pressure to feel the tissue closest to the chest and ribs. A firm ridge in the lower curve of each breast is normal. If you're not sure how hard to press, talk with your doctor or nurse. Use each pressure level to feel the breast tissue before moving on to the next spot.

- Move around the breast in an up and down pattern starting at an imaginary line drawn straight down your side from the underarm and moving across the breast to the middle of the chest bone (sternum or breastbone). Be sure to check the entire breast area going down until you feel only ribs and up to the neck or collar bone (clavicle).

There is some evidence to suggest that the up and down pattern (sometimes called the vertical pattern) is the most effective pattern for covering the entire breast and not missing any breast tissue.

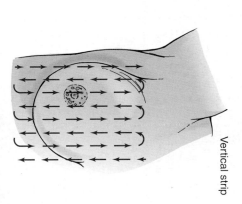

Vertical strip

Breast Self-Examination (BSE)

- Repeat the exam on your left breast, using the finger pads of the right hand. While standing in front of a mirror with your hands pressing firmly down on your hips, look at your breasts for any changes of size, shape, contour, or dimpling. (The pressing down on the hips position contracts the chest wall muscles and enhances any breast changes.)

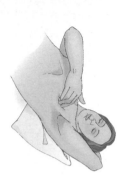

- Examine each underarm while sitting up or standing and with your arm only slightly raised so you can easily feel in this area. Raising your arm straight up tightens the tissue in this area and makes it very difficult to examine.

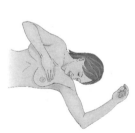

This procedure for doing breast self-exam represents changes in previous procedure recommendations. These changes represent an extensive review of the medical literature and input from an expert advisory group. There is evidence that the woman's position (lying down), area felt, pattern of coverage of the breast, and use of different amounts of pressure increase the sensitivity of BSE as measured with silicon models, and for clinical breast examination (CBE) using patient models with known small noncancerous lumps in their breasts.

Remember, if you find any changes, see your doctor right away.

Testicular Self-Examination

Testicular self-examination (TSE) is to be performed once a month; it is neither difficult nor time consuming. A convenient time is often after a warm bath or shower when the scrotum is more relaxed.

1. Stand in front of a mirror and check for scrotal swelling.
2. Use both hands to palpate the testis; the normal testicle is smooth and uniform in consistency.
3. With the index and middle fingers under the testis and the thumb on top, roll the testis gently in a horizontal plane between the thumb and fingers (*A*).
4. Feel for any evidence of a small lump or abnormality.
5. Follow the same procedure and palpate upward along the testis (*B*).
6. Locate the epididymis (*C*), a cordlike structure on the top and back of the testicle that stores and transports sperm. It is normal
7. Repeat the examination for the other testis. It is normal to find that one testis is larger than the other.
8. If you find any evidence of a small, pealike lump, consult your physician. It may be due to an infection or a tumor growth.

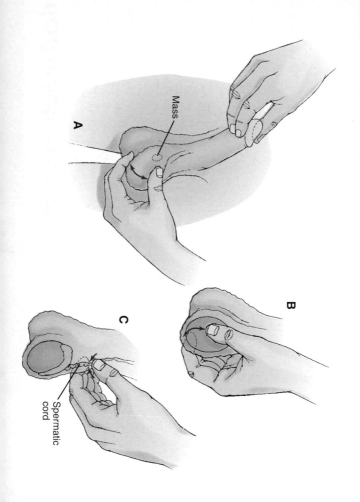

Classification and Management of Blood Pressure for Adults*

BP Classification	SBP* (mm Hg)	DBP* (mm Hg)	Lifestyle Modification	Initial Drug Therapy	
				Without Compelling Indications	With Compelling Indications (See Table 4–3)
Normal	<120	and <80	Encourage		
Prehypertension	120–139	or 80–89	Yes	No antihypertensive drug indicated.	Drug(s) for compelling indications.†
Stage 1 Hypertension	140–159	or 90–99	Yes	Thiazide-type diuretics for most. May consider ACEI, ARB, BB, CCB, or combination.	Drug(s) for compelling indications.† Other antihypertensive drugs (diuretics, ACEI, ARB, BB, CCB) as needed.
Stage 2 Hypertension	≥160	or ≥100	Yes	Two-drug combination for most† (usually thiazide-type diuretic and ACEI or ARB or BB or CCB).	

DBP, diastolic blood pressure; SBP, systolic blood pressure.

Drug abbreviations: ACEI, angiotensin converting enzyme inhibitor; ARB, angiotensin receptor blocker; BB, beta-blocker; CCB, calcium channel blocker.

*Treatment determined by highest BP category.

†Initial combined therapy should be used cautiously in those at risk for orthostatic hypotension.

‡Treat patients with chronic kidney disease or diabetes to BP goal of <130/80 mm Hg.

From the Seventh Report of the Joint National Committee on Prevention, Detection, Evaluation, and Treatment of High Blood Pressure. (2003). *JAMA,* 289 (19), 2560–2572.

Sample Adult Nursing Health History and Physical Assessment

HEALTH HISTORY

A. Client Profile

S.L. is a 72-year-old white female, born on a small farm in southern Missouri. Appears younger than stated age. English speaking, with a German ethnic origin. High school graduate and presently retired from restraint work. Lives in a one-bedroom apartment on first floor. Drives own car. Seeks health care in local community hospital 4 miles from home. Major reason for seeking health care is for routine check-up—has not had one for 8 years. Understands that she has adult-onset diabetes mellitus (type 2), which is controlled with 1800-calorie diet and moderate amount of exercise. Also has "mild rheumatoid arthritic" pains in right hip and finger joints in early mornings; relieved with exercise, warm baths, and ASA.

Treatments/medications:

1. Prescribed: none
2. OTC
   a. ASA gr at H.S. for "arthritis aches." Takes about 2x per month. Denies nausea, abdominal pains or evidence of bleeding while taking
   b. Mylanta at H.S. for "gas pains."
   c. Ducolax suppository 3x/week for past 4 years.
   d. Multivitamin 1 qd, for past 4 years.

Past illnesses/hospitalizations:

1. Appendectomy age 18.
2. Left arm fracture age 20.
3. Cholecystectomy age 56, performed for complaint of gas pains after eating fatty foods. Satisfied with care received at local hospital.

Allergies:

Denies food, drug, and environmental allergies.

B. Developmental History

Developmental Level: Integrity vs Despair

Describes childhood as a very happy time for her. Becomes excited and smiles as she relates stories of her childhood on the farm. States she was an average child and ran and played like all the others. Companions were brothers and sisters. Has been married for 55 years. Describes relationship with husband as close and sharing. Owned and operated a restaurant for 30 years with husband and was a waitress at another restaurant after they retired from their own. Lived in a large house until 1988. Currently lives in a one-bedroom apartment. Active in church and society. Volunteers at community functions. She and her husband are active in their church. States she enjoys being retired and lives a "comfortable" life. Does not voice financial concerns. Has begun to write will and distribute personal heirlooms to son and grandchildren. States she is not afraid of death and wishes to have the "business part taken care of" in order to enjoy the rest of her life together with her husband.

C. Health Perception–Health Management Pattern

1. Client's rating of health:
   Scale: 10-best; 1-worst
   5 years ago: 10
   Now: 8

5 years from now: 6

Sees health deterioration as normal aging process and states, "I feel really good when I look at a lot of people my age with all their problems and the medicine they take."

2. Health does not interfere with self-care or other desired activities of daily living. Unaware of signs, symptoms, and Tx of hyperglycemia and hypoglycemia. Denies use of alcohol, tobacco, and drugs.

3. Client seeks health care only in emergencies. Last medical exam September 1996. Keeps active and feels well. Feels lifestyle and faith "keep her going." Does not check own blood sugar or do breast self-exams.

D. Nutritional-Metabolic Pattern

States she is on a "no concentrated sweet" meal pattern as follows: Eats breakfast of whole wheat toast, one boiled egg, orange juice, and decaf. coffee at 7 AM. Eats lunch at noon. Today had tuna, lettuce salad, apple, and milk. Eats light supper around 6 PM. Typical dinner includes small serving broiled meat, green vegetables, piece of fruit, and glass of milk. Tries not to snack but will have fruit if she feels the urge. Drinks two 8-oz glasses of water a day. Drinks decaf. coffee—no tea or colas. Voices no dislikes or food intolerances.

Wears dentures. Last dental exam October 1996. Denies problems with proper fit, eating, chewing, swallowing, sore throat, sore tongue, or colds. Complains of "canker sore" if she eats strawberries. Denies n/v, abdominal pain, or excessive gas. Complains of dyspepsia approx. 2x/month, relieved by Mylanta. Does not associate this with time she takes ASA.

Describes skin and scalp as dry. Uses lotions frequently. Denies easy bruising, pruritus, or nonhealing sores. Nails are hard and brittle. Hair is fine and soft.

Current weight: 120 lb; height: 5'4"

Previous weight: 150 lb 10 years ago. Desires to maintain current weight.

Weight fluctuates ± 5 lb/month. Client states, "I've always had to watch what I eat because I gain so easily." Denies intolerance to heat or cold, or voice changes.

E. Elimination Pattern

Bowel habits: Soft, formed, med, brown bowel movement (BM) every third day after Dulcolax suppository. States she becomes constipated without use of laxative. Denies mucous, bloody, or tarry stools. States discomfort with BMs starting in September 1996. When having to strain with BVs felt "some kind of mass" prolapsing from rectum. Consulted her doctor, who explained to her "it was a piece of my colon slipping out." No surgical treatment or exercises prescribed. Gently reinserts tissue when this happens.

Bladder habits: Voids 4–5x/day, clear yellow urine Denies current problems with cysturia, hematuria, polyuria, hesitancy, incontinence, or nocturia. Complaint of urgency during the colder months with no increase in frequency. Had polyuria and polydipsia prior to diagnosis of diabetes type 2. Developed UTI at age 60, at which time she sought medical advice and was diagnosed with type 2 diabetes mellitus.

F. Activity-Exercise Pattern

1. ADLs on an average day: Arises at 6 A.M. Eats breakfast and does housekeeping. In early afternoon goes to the community center to eat lunch, quilt, and visit. Goes home around 2 P.M. Walks about four blocks with a friend every day. Cleans own house daily for one 2-hour period (includes dusting, vacuuming, washing). Denies palpitations, chest pain, SOB, fatigue, wheezing, claudication, cramps, stiffness, or joint pain or swelling with activity. Walking relieves ache in hips and makes her feel good. After walking, returns home and relaxes with crafts and visiting with husband. During evenings attends church-related activities. Expresses satisfaction with activity and believes she functions above the level of the average person her age.

2. Hygiene: Showers and washes hair every day.

3. Occupational activities: Retired from being a cook and waitress. Volunteers to cook for church group. Occasionally has lower back pains when carrying large amounts of food or when carrying large trays.

G. Sexuality–Reproduction Pattern

Menstrual history: Age of menarche: approx. 12 years; age of menopause: 50 years. States, "going through my change of life wasn't difficult for me physically or emotionally." Described menstrual period as regular, lasting 4 days with moderate flow. Denies postmenopausal spotting at this time.

Obstetric history: Gravida 1, Para 1. No complications with pregnancy or childbirth.

Contraception: Never used any form.

Sexual activities: Sexually active. States, "My husband and I have good relations." Denies pain, discomfort, or postcoital bleeding.

Special problems: Denies history of any sexually transmitted diseases. Denies problem with vaginal itching. Last Pap smear: negative in 1988.

H. Sleep–Rest Pattern

Goes to bed at 10 PM. Denies difficulty falling asleep or sleeping. Feels well rested when she arises at 6 AM. Never used sleep medications. Denies orthopnea and nocturnal dyspnea. Enjoys reading 1 to 2 pages of Bible history each evening.

I. Sensory–Perceptual Pattern

1. *Vision:* Has worn glasses "all of my life." Cannot recall age at which they were prescribed. Prescription change from bifocals to trifocals August 1996. Complains of blurred vision without glasses. Denies diplopia, itching, excessive tearing, discharge, redness, or trauma to eyes.
2. *Hearing:* Believes she is "a little slow to grasp, and I think it may be because of my hearing." Does not wear hearing aid. Cannot recall last hearing test. Denies tinnitus, pain, discharge, or trauma to ears. Does not ask for questions to be repeated when asked at normal voice tone and level.
3. *Smell:* Denies difficulty with smell, pain, postnasal drip, sneezing, or frequent nosebleeds.
4. *Touch:* States "occasionally my feet feel numb"; subsides on own.
5. *Taste:* No difficulty tasting foods.

J. Cognitive Pattern

Speech clear without slur or stutter. Follows verbal cues. Expresses ideas and feelings clearly and concisely. States she has had a gradual loss of memory over past 5 to 6 years. Believes long-term memory is better than short term. She can recall past weekly events but has trouble recalling dates, times, and places of events. Learns best by writing information down and then reviewing it. Makes major decisions jointly with husband after prayer.

K. Role–Relationship Pattern

Client has been married 55 years. Describes relationship as the best part of her life right now. Only son lives in Minnesota, and they visit one to two times a year. Is very fond of three grandchildren. Expresses desire to visit more often but states, "He has his own life and family now." Communicates once a month by phone. Explains her relationship with other members of the church and community groups as friendly and "familylike." Lives with husband in first-floor apartment. Has casual relationship with apartment neighbors—friendly but distant. Was the oldest of five children. See family genogram.

L. Self-Perception–Self-Concept Pattern

Describes self as a normal person. Talkative, outgoing, and likes to be around people but hates noisy environments. Happy with the person she has become and states, "I can definitely live with myself." States a weakness is that she worries about "little things" more now than she used

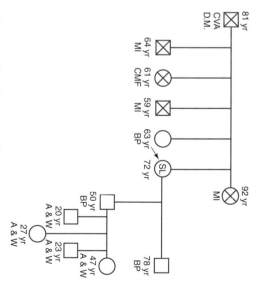

to and tends to be irritated more easily. Cannot place specific onset of these feelings. Feels good about self-control of diabetes.

M. Coping–Stress Tolerance Pattern

States husband's high blood pressure has never been a source of stress to her. Shares confidences with husband and with a few close friends. Most stressful time in life was losing two brothers and a sister, all in 1994. States with the support of husband and church she handled it "better than most people would have." States she prays and eats when under stress. Cannot identify any major stresses that have occurred in the last year.

N. Value–Belief Pattern

Religious preference is Lutheran. Values relationship with husband, family, and God. Enjoys helping others in the church and community. Believes God is loving, supportive, and forgiving. Places God as first priority in life. States prayer is extremely important to her and practices it daily. States this personalizes her relationship with God. Has been Lutheran all her life and states she and her husband share in church activities together.

PHYSICAL ASSESSMENT

A. General Physical Survey

Ht: 5′4″, Wt: 120 lb, Radial pulse: 71, Resp: 16, BP: R arm—120/72, L arm—120/70, Temp: 98.6°F. Client alert and cooperative. Sitting comfortably on table with arms crossed and shoulders slightly slouched forward. Smiling with mild anxiety. Dress is neat and clean. Walks steadily with posture slightly stooped.

B. Skin, Hair, and Nail Assessment

1. *Skin:* Pale pink, warm and dry to touch. Skinfold returns to place after 1 second when lifted over clavicle. Tan "age spots" on posterior hands bilaterally in clusters of four to five and evenly distributed over lower extremities. A 3-cm

nodule with 2-mm macule in center noted in right axilla; indurated, nontender, and nonmobile. No evidence of vascular or purpuric lesions. No edema.

2. *Hair:* Chin length, gray, straight, clean, styled, medium-textured, evenly distributed on head. No scalp lesions or flaking. Fine blend hair evenly distributed over arms bilaterally and sparsely on legs bilaterally. No hair noted on axilla or on chest, back, or face.

3. *Nails:* Fingernails medium length, and thickness, clear. Splinter hemorrhages noted on right thumb near fingertip in midline. No clubbing or Beau lines.

C. Head and Neck Assessment

Head symmetrically rounded, neck nontender with full ROM. Neck symmetrical without masses, scars, pulsations. Lymph nodes nonpalpable. Trachea in midline. Thyroid norpalpable. Carotid arteries equally strong without bruits. Identifies light and deep touch to various parts of face.

CN V: Identifies light touch and sharp touch to forehead, cheek, and chin. Bilateral corneal reflex intact. Masseter muscles contract equally and bilaterally. Jaw jerk + 1.

CN VII: Identifies sugar and salt on anterior two thirds of tongue. Smiles, frowns, shows teeth, blows cheeks, and raises eyebrows as instructed.

D. Eye Assessment

Eyes 2 cm apart without protrusion. Eyebrows sparse with equal distribution. No scaliness noted. Lids pink without ptosis, edema, or lesions, and freely closeable bilaterally. Lacrimal apparatus nonedematous. Sclera white without increased vascularity or lesions noted. Palpebral and bulbar conjunctiva slightly reddened without lesions noted. Irises uniformly blue. PERRLA. EOMs intact bilaterally. Peripheral vision equal to examiner's.

Visual acuity: With glasses off vision is blurred at 14″ away, but can identify number of fingers held up. With glasses on reads newspaper print at 14″.

Funduscopic exam: Red reflex present bilaterally. Optic disc round with well-defined margins. Physiologic cup occupies disc. Arterioles smaller than venules. No A-V nicking, no hemorrhages, or exudates noted. Macula not seen. (CNs II, III, IV, and VI intact.)

E. Ear Assessment

Auricle without deformity, lumps, or lesions. Right auricle with tag at top of pinna. Auricles and mastoid processes non-tender. Bilateral auditory canals contain moderate amount dark-brown cerumen. Tympanic membrane difficult to view due to wax.

Whisper test: Client identifies one out of two words in four attempts. Weber test: No lateralization of sound to either ear. Rinne test: AC is greater than BC both ears (CN VIII).

F. Nose and Sinuses Assessment

External structure without deformity, asymmetry, or inflammation. Nares patent. Turbinates and middle meatus pale pink, without swelling, exudate, lesions, or bleeding. Nasal septum midline without bleeding, perforation, or deviation. Frontal and maxillary sinuses nontender. Identifies smells of coffee and soap (CN I).

G. Mouth and Pharynx Assessment

Lips moist with peach lipstick. No lesions or ulcerations. Buccal mucosa pink and moist without discoloration or increased pigmentation. No ulcers or nodules. Upper and lower dentures secure. Gums pink and moist without inflammation, bleeding, or discoloration. Hard and soft palates smooth without lesions or masses. No lesions, discolorations, or ulcerations on floor of mouth, oral mucosa, or gums. Gag reflex intact, and client identifies sugar and salt on posterior tongue. Uvula in midline and elevates on phonation. (CNs IX and X intact.) Tonsils present without exudate, edema, ulcers, or enlargement.

H. Cardiac Assessment

No pulsations visible. No heaves, lifts, or vibrations. PMI: 5th ICS to LMCL. Clear, brief heart sounds throughout. Physiologic S_2. No gallops, murmurs, or rubs. AP = 72/min and regular.

I. Peripheral Vascular System Assessment

Arms: Equal in size and symmetry bilaterally; pale pink; warm and dry to touch without edema, bruising, or lesions noted. Radial pulses equal in rate and amplitude, and strong. Allen test: Right equal 2-second refill, left equal 2-second refill. Brachial pulses strong, equal, and even. Epitrochlear nodes nonpalpable.

Legs: Legs large in size and bilaterally symmetrical. Skin intact, pale pink; warm and dry to touch without edema, bruising, lesions, or increased vascularity. Superficial inguinal, horizontal, and vertical lymph nodes nonpalpable. Femoral pulses strong and equal without bruits. Popliteal pulse nonpalpable with client supine or prone. Dorsalis pedis and posterior tibial pulses strong and equal. No edema palpable. Homans negative bilaterally. No retrograde filling noted when client stands. Toenails thick and yellowed. Special maneuver for arterial insufficiency: feet regain color after 4 seconds and veins refilled in 5 seconds.

J. Thorax and Lung Assessment

Skin pale pink without scars, pulsations, or lesions. No hair noted. Thorax expands evenly bilaterally without retractions or bulging. Slope of ribs = $40°$. No use of auxiliary respiratory muscles and no nasal flaring. Mild kyphosis. Respirations even, unlabored, and regular (16/min). No cough noted. No tenderness, crepitus, or masses. Tactile fremitus decreases below T5 bilaterally posteriorly, and 4th ICS anteriorly bilaterally. Thorax resonance throughout. Diaphragmatic excursion: Left—on inspiration diaphragm descends to T11, and on expiration diaphragm ascends to T9. Right—on inspiration diaphragm descends to T12, and on expiration diaphragm ascends to T9. Vesicular breath sounds heard in all lung fields. No rales, rhonchi, friction rubs, or abnormal whispered pectoriloquy, bronchophony, or egophony noted.

K. Breast Assessment

Breasts moderate in size, round, and symmetrical bilaterally. Skin pale pink with light-brown areola. No dimpling or retraction. Free movement in all positions. Engorged vein noted running across UOQ to areola in right breast. Nipples inverted bilaterally. No discharge expressed. No thickening or tenderness noted. A 2-cm, hard, immobile round mass noted in left breast in LUOQ. Client denies ever noticing this. Nontender to palpation. Lymph nodes nonpalpable. Client does not know how to do breast self-exam.

L. Abdominal Assessment

Abdomen rounded, symmetrical without masses, lesions, pulsations, or peristalsis noted. Abdomen free of hair, bruising, and increased vascularity. Healed with appendectomy scar. Umbilicus in midline, without herniation, swelling, or discoloration. Bowel sounds low pitched and gurgling at 22/minute × four quads. Aortic, renal, and iliac arteries auscultated without bruit. No venous hums or friction rubs auscultated over liver or spleen. Tympany percussed over all four quads. An 8-cm liver span percussed in RMCL. Area of dullness percussed at 9th ICS in left postaxillary line. No tenderness or masses noted with light and deep palpation in all four quadrants. Liver and spleen nonpalpable.

M. Genitourinary–Reproductive Assessment

No bulging or masses in inguinal area. A 1-cm nodule palpated in right groin. Labia pink with decreased elasticity and vaginal secretions. No bulging of vaginal wall, purulent foul drainage, or lesions. Skene's gland not visible. Anal area pink with small amount of hair. Rectal mucosa bulges with straining.

N. Musculoskeletal Assessment

Posture slightly stooped with mild kyphosis. Gait steady, smooth, and coordinated with even base. Limited ROM of lateral flexion and extension of spine. Paravertebrals equal in size and strength. Shrugs shoulders and moves head to right and left against resistance (CN XI intact); upper extremities and lower extremities have full ROM. Muscles moderately firm bilaterally. No deviations, inflammations, or bony deformities. Small callus on left heel. Moves upper and lower extremities freely against gravity and against resistance. Rheumatoid nodule noted on dorsal surface of left hand.

O. Neurologic Assessment

Mental status: Pleasant and friendly. Appropriately dressed for weather with matching colors and patterns. Clothes neat and clean. Facial expressions symmetrical and correlate with mood and topic discussed. Speech clear and appropriate. Oriented to person, place. Follows through with train of thought. Carefully chooses words to convey feelings and ideas.

time, and events. Remains attentive and able to focus on exam during entire interaction. Short-term memory intact, long-term memory before 1992 unclear—especially cannot recall dates and sequencing of events. General information questions answered correctly 100% of the time. Vocabulary suitable to educational level. Explains proverb accurately. Gives semiabstract answers and enjoys joking. Is able to identify similarities 5 seconds after asked. Answers to judgment questions in realistic manner.

Cranial nerves: I–XII intact (integrated throughout exam).

Cerebellar and motor function: Alternates finger to nose with eyes closed; occasionally tends to hit opposite side of nose. Rapidly opposes fingers to thumb bilaterally, without difficulty. Alternates pronation and supination of hands rapidly without difficulty. Heel to shin intact bilaterally. Romberg: minimal swaying. Tandem walk: steady. No involuntary movements noted.

Sensory status: Superficial light- and deep-touch sensation intact on arms, legs, neck, chest, and back. Position sense of toes and fingers intact bilaterally. Identifies point localization correctly. Identifies coin placed in hand and number written on palm of hand correctly.

Two-Point Discrimination (in mm)	Right	Left
Fingertips	6	6
Dorsal hand	15	15
Chest	45	49
Forearm	39	35
Back	45	45
Upper arm	40	45

Reflexes	Right	Left
Biceps	2+	2+
Triceps	2+	2+
Patellar	3+	3+
Achilles	2+	2+
Abdominal	1+	1+
Babinski	neg	neg

Motor status: Muscle tone firm at rest, abdominal muscles slightly relaxed. Muscle size adequate for age. No fasciculations or involuntary movements noted. Muscle strength moderately strong and equal bilaterally.

Client's Strengths

- Positive attitude and outlook in life
- Motivation to comply with prescribed diet
- Strong support systems: husband and spiritual beliefs
- No physical limitations

Nursing Diagnoses

- Risk for Ineffective Health Maintenance related to lack of knowledge concerning importance of regular medical checkups, re: lesion in UOQ of left breast not seen by physician, no Pap smear, and no follow-up with diabetes

- Acute right hip pain
- Constipation related to lack of bowel routine and laxative overuse
- Knowledge Deficit: Signs, symptoms, and treatment of hyperglycemia/hypoglycemia
- Knowledge Deficit: Management and causes of constipation
- Knowledge Deficit: self breast exam technique
- Knowledge Deficit: Importance of self-blood glucose monitoring

Collaborative Problems

- Potential complication: Hyperglycemia, hypoglycemia
- Potential complication: Hypertension

Assessment of Family Functional Health Patterns

The nurse obtains data about the family's functional health patterns by interviewing the family as a group or by interviewing one or two family members who are reliable historians and seem knowledgeable about their family's health patterns. If data reveal a particular problem identified with an individual family member, the nurse can then focus attention or obtaining more data from that individual.

I. FAMILY PROFILE

The purpose of the family profile is to obtain biographical family data (age, sex, and current health status of each family member). A genogram may be used to illustrate this information.

II. HEALTH PERCEPTION–HEALTH MANAGEMENT PATTERN

Subjective Data

- Describe your family's general health during the past few years.
- Has your family been able to participate in its usual activities (work, school, sports)?
- Describe what your family does to try to stay healthy (diet, exercise, etc).
- From whom does your family seek health care? When?
- Describe how your family members check their health status (eg, eye exams, dental exams, breast exams, testicular exams, medical checkups).

- Describe any behaviors in your family that are considered unhealthy.
- Who cares for family members who are or who become ill?
- How would you know if a family member were ill?

Objective Data

1. Observe the appearance of family members.
2. Observe the home (hazards and safety devices, storage facilities, cooking facilities).

III. NUTRITIONAL–METABOLIC PATTERN

Subjective Data

- Describe typical breakfast, lunch, supper, and snacks that you eat as a family.
- What type of drinks do you usually have during the day and at night?
- How would you describe your family's appetite in general?
- How often does your family seek dental care? Are there any dental problems in your family?
- Does anyone in your family have skin rashes or problems with sores healing? Explain.
- Who usually prepares the family meals? Who shops for groceries?

Objective Data

1. Observe kitchen appliances, availability of food, and types of foods kept in the home, if possible.
2. Observe preparation of a family meal, if possible.
3. Observe family members for obvious signs of malnutrition or obesity.

IV. ELIMINATION PATTERN

Subjective Data

- How often do family members have bowel movements? Urinate?
- Are laxatives used in your family? Explain.
- Are there problems with disposing of waste or garbage?
- Describe any recycling you do.
- Does your family have pets (indoor or outdoor)? How are their wastes disposed?
- Do you have problems with insects in your home? Explain.

Objective Data

1. Observe bathroom facilities.
2. Inspect home for insects.
3. Observe garbage and waste disposal.

V. ACTIVITY-EXERCISE PATTERN

Subjective Data

- Describe how your family exercises. Frequency?
- How does your family relax?
- What does your family do for enjoyment?
- Describe a typical day of activities in your family (work, school, play, games, meals, hobbies, house cleaning, yard work, cooking, exercise).

Objective Data

1. Observe the pace of family activities.
2. Observe any exercise equipment kept in home.

VI. SLEEP–REST PATTERN

Subjective Data

- When does your family generally go to bed and awaken? Do family members go to bed and arise at different times? Explain.
- Does your family seem to get enough time to sleep? To rest and relax?
- Do any family members work at night? How does this affect other family members?

Objective Data

1. Observe sleeping areas.
2. Observe temperament and energy level of family members.

VII. SENSORY–PERCEPTUAL PATTERN

Subjective Data

- Are there any hearing or visual problems that affect your family members?
- Are there any deficits in a family member's ability to taste and smell that affect how food is prepared for the family?
- Does pain seem to be a family problem? Explain. How is this managed?
- What is the usual form of pain relief used by family members?

Objective Data

1. Observe any visual or hearing aids used by family members.
2. Observe medications kept on hand to relieve pain.

VIII. COGNITIVE PATTERN

Subjective Data

- Who makes the major family decisions? How?
- Describe the highest educational level of all family members.
- Does your family understand any illnesses and treatments that affect any of your family members?
- How does your family enjoy learning (eg, reading, watching television, attending classes)?
- Are there any problems with memory in the family? Explain.

Objective Data

1. Observe language spoken by all family members.
2. Observe use of words (vocabulary level), and ability to grasp ideas and express self.
3. Are family decisions present or future oriented? Observe family decision-making strategies.
4. Observe school attended by children.

IX. SELF-PERCEPTION–SELF-CONCEPT PATTERN

Subjective Data

- Describe the general mood of your family (eg, sad, happy, eager, depressed, anxious, relaxed).
- Do you consider yourselves to be a close family? How do you spend time together? Is this time satisfying?

- Do family members share any common goals? Explain.
- What does the family enjoy doing most together?
- How does your family deal with disagreements?
- How do your family members express their affection, feelings, and/or concerns? Are they allowed to do so freely? Explain.
- Does your family seem to discuss problems that affect individual members?
- How does your family deal with change?

Objective Data

1. Observe family discussions.
2. Observe mood and temperament of family.
3. Observe how family members deal with conflict.
4. How do family members show concern and consideration for each other's needs and desires?

X. ROLE–RELATIONSHIP PATTERN

Subjective Data

- Describe how your family members support each other, show affection, and express concerns.
- Describe any problems with relationships between family members.
- Describe your family resources (financial, community support systems, family support systems).
- How active is your family in your neighborhood and/or community?
- Explain family responsibilities for various household chores (washing, cooking, driving, lawn maintenance, etc).
- Explain how discipline is used in your family. How are family members rewarded? Describe any aggression and/or violence that occurs in your family.

Objective Data

1. Observe family interaction patterns (verbal and nonverbal).
2. Explore which family members take responsibility for managing and leading family activities.
3. Observe living space and ownership of rooms by family members.

XI. SEXUALITY-REPRODUCTIVE PATTERN

Subjective Data

If appropriate: Are sexual partners within home satisfied with sexual relationship and activities? Describe any problems.

- Are contraceptives used?
- Is family planning used? How?
- Are parents comfortable answering questions and explaining topics related to sexuality to their children?

XII. COPING–STRESS TOLERANCE PATTERN

Subjective Data

- What major changes have occurred in your family during the past year (eg, divorce, marriage, family members leaving home, new members coming into home, death, illness, births, accidents, change in finances and/or occupation)?
- How does your family *cope* with major stressors (eg, exercise, discussion, prayer, drugs, alcohol, violence)?
- Who in the family copes best with stressors?
- Who has the most difficult time coping with stress?
- Who outside the family (eg, friends, church, support groups) seems to help your family most during difficult times?

Objective Data

1. Observe effect and pace of family interactions.

XIII. VALUE–BELIEF PATTERN

Subjective Data

- What does your family consider to be most important in life?
- What does your family want from life?
- What rules does your family hold most important?
- Is religion important in the family? What religion are family members? What religious practices are important to the family? Is a relationship with God important to the family?
- What does your family look forward to in the future?
- From where do the family's hope and strength come?

Objective Data

1. Observe family rituals and/or traditions.
2. Observe pictures and other articles (religious or other) in home.
3. Listen to general topics discussed in home by family members.
4. Observe the type of television programs viewed by family members and the type of music to which family members listen.

Nursing Diagnoses (Wellness, Risk, and Actual) Grouped According to Functional Health Patterns

I. HEALTH PERCEPTION-HEALTH MANAGEMENT PATTERN

Wellness Diagnoses

Health-Seeking Behaviors
Effective Therapeutic Regimen Management

Risk Diagnoses

Risk for Falls
Risk for Injury
Risk for Suffocation
Risk for Poisoning
Risk for Trauma
Risk for Perioperative Positioning Injury
Risk for Altered Development
Risk for Altered Growth

Actual Diagnoses

Adult Failure to Thrive
Energy Field Disturbance
Delayed Growth and Development
Delayed Surgical Recovery
Ineffective Health Maintenance
Ineffective Therapeutic Regimen:
    Management Individual
Ineffective Therapeutic Regimen Management: Family
Ineffective Therapeutic Regimen Management:
    Community
Noncompliance
Sedentary Lifestyle

2. NUTRITIONAL-METABOLIC PATTERN

Wellness Diagnoses

Effective Breast-feeding
Readiness for Enhanced Nutritional Metabolic Pattern
Readiness Enhanced Skin Integrity

Risk Diagnoses

Risk for Imbalanced Body Temperature
 Hypothermia
 Hyperthermia
Risk for Infection
Risk for Imbalanced Nutrition: More than body
 requirements
Risk for Imbalanced Nutrition: Less than body
 requirements
Risk for Aspiration
Risk for Imbalanced Fluid Volume
Risk for Constipation
Risk for Delayed Surgical Recovery
Risk for Impaired Skin Integrity
Risk for Latex Allergy

Actual Diagnoses

Decreased Adaptive Capacity: Intracranial
Ineffective Thermoregulation
Fluid Volume Deficit

Fluid Volume Excess
Imbalanced Nutrition: Less Than Body Requirements
Imbalanced Nutrition: More Than Body
 Requirements
Ineffective Breast-feeding
Interrupted Breast-feeding
Ineffective Infant Feeding Pattern
Impaired Swallowing
Ineffective Protection
Impaired Tissue Integrity
Altered Oral Mucous Membrane
Latex Allergy
Impaired Skin Integrity
Dentition Impaired

3. ELIMINATION PATTERN

Wellness Diagnoses

Readiness for Enhanced Bowel
 Elimination Pattern
Readiness for Enhanced Urinary
 Elimination Pattern

Risk Diagnoses

Risk for constipation
Risk for Impaired Urinary Elimination
Risk for Urge Urinary Incontinence

Actual Diagnoses

Altered Bowel Elimination
  Constipation
  Perceived Constipation
  Diarrhea
  Bowel Incontinence
Altered Urinary Elimination
  Urinary Retention
  Total Urinary Incontinence
  Functional Urinary Incontinence
  Reflex Urinary Incontinence
  Urge Urinary Incontinence
  Stress Urinary Incontinence

4. ACTIVITY–EXERCISE PATTERN

Wellness Diagnoses

Readiness for Enhanced:
  Cardiac Output
  Diversional Activity Pattern
  Activity–Exercise Pattern
  Home Maintenance Management
  Self-care Activities
  Tissue Perfusion
  Breathing Pattern
  Organized Infant Behavior

Risk Diagnoses

Risk for Disuse Syndrome
Risk for Perioperative Positioning Injury
Risk for Disorganized Infant Behavior
Risk for Peripheral Neurovascular Dysfunction
Risk for Altered Respiratory Function

Actual Diagnoses

Impaired Gas Exchange
Activity Intolerance
Ineffective Airway Clearance
Ineffective Breathing Pattern
Decreased Cardiac Output
Decreased Adaptive Capacity: Intracranial
Disuse Syndrome
Diversional Activity Deficit
Impaired Home Maintenance
Impaired Physical Mobility
Dysfunctional Ventilatory Weaning Response
Inability to Sustain Spontaneous Ventilation
Self-Care Deficit: (specify type: Feeding,
  Bathing/Hygiene, Dressing/Grooming, Toileting)
Ineffective Tissue Perfusion: (specify type: Cerebral,
  Cardiopulmonary, Renal, Gastrointestinal,
  Peripheral)

Disorganized Infant Behavior
Impaired Walking
Impaired Wheelchair Mobility
Impaired Wheelchair Transfer Ability
Impaired Bed Mobility
Sedentary Lifestyle
Wandering

5. SEXUALITY–REPRODUCTIVE PATTERN

Wellness Diagnosis

Readiness for Enhanced Sexuality Patterns

Risk Diagnoses

Risk for Ineffective Sexuality Pattern
Risk for Falls

Actual Diagnoses

Sexual Dysfunction
Ineffective Sexuality Patterns

6. SLEEP–REST PATTERN

Wellness Diagnosis

Readiness for Enhanced Sleep

Risk Diagnoses

Risk for Disturbed Sleep Pattern
Risk for Sleep Deprivation

Actual Diagnoses

Disturbed Sleep Pattern
Sleep Deprivation

7. SENSORY–PERCEPTUAL PATTERN

Wellness Diagnosis

Readiness for Enhanced Comfort Level

Risk Diagnoses

Risk for Pain (acute, chronic)
Risk for Aspiration
Risk for Autonomic Dysreflexia

Actual Diagnoses

Acute Pain
Chronic Pain
Dysreflexia
Disturbed Sensory–Perception (specify Visual,
Auditory, Kinesthetic, Gustatory, Tactile,
Olfactory)

Nausea
Unilateral Neglect

8. COGNITIVE PATTERN

Wellness Diagnosis

Readiness for Enhanced Cognition

Risk Diagnosis

Risk for Disturbed Thought Processes

Actual Diagnoses

Acute Confusion
Chronic Confusion
Decisional Conflict (Specify)
Impaired Environmental Interpretation Syndrome
Knowledge Deficit (Specify)
Disturbed Thought Processes
Impaired Memory

9. ROLE–RELATIONSHIP PATTERN

Wellness Diagnoses

Readiness for Enhanced
Relationships

Parenting
Role Performance
Communication
Social Interaction
Caregiver Role
Grieving

Risk Diagnoses

Risk for Dysfunctional Grieving
Risk for Loneliness
Risk for Impaired Parent/Infant/Child Attachment

Actual Diagnoses

Impaired Verbal Communication
Dysfunctional Family Processes
Dysfunctional Family Processes: Alcoholism
Interrupted Family Processes
Anticipatory Grieving
Dysfunctional Grieving
Impaired Parenting
Parental Role Conflict
Ineffective Role Performance
Impaired Social Interaction
Social Isolation
Caregiver Role Strain

10. SELF-PERCEPTION-SELF-CONCEPT PATTERN

Wellness Diagnoses

Readiness for Enhanced Self-Perception
Readiness for Enhanced Self-Concept

Risk Diagnoses

Risk for Hopelessness
Risk for Body Image Disturbance
Risk for Situational Low Self-Esteem

Actual Diagnoses

Anxiety
Fatigue
Fear
Hopelessness
Powerlessness
Disturbed Personal Identity
Disturbed Body Image
Disturbed Self-Esteem
Chronic Low Self-Esteem
Situational Low Self-Esteem
Death Anxiety

11. COPING-STRESS TOLERANCE PATTERN

Wellness Diagnoses

Readiness for Enhanced Individual Coping
Readiness for Enhanced Family Coping
Readiness for Enhanced Community Coping

Risk Diagnoses

Risk for Ineffective Coping (Individual, Family, or Community)
Risk for Self-Abuse
Risk for Self-Mutilation
Risk for Suicide
Risk for Violence: Self Directed or Other Directed
Risk for Spiritual Distress
Risk for Post-Trauma Syndrome
Risk for Relocation Syndrome

Actual Diagnoses

Impaired Adjustment
Caregiver Role Strain
Disabled Family Coping
Disturbed Energy Field

Ineffective Individual Coping
Defensive Coping
Ineffective Denial
Ineffective Family Coping: Disabling
Compromised Family Coping
Ineffective Community Coping
Posttrauma Response
Rape–Trauma Syndrome
Relocation Stress Syndrome
Self-Mutilation
Chronic Sorrow

12. VALUE–BELIEF PATTERN

Wellness Diagnosis

Readiness for Enhanced Spiritual Well-Being

Risk Diagnosis

Risk for Spiritual Distress
Risk for Impaired Religiosity

Actual Diagnoses

Impaired Religiosity
Spiritual Distress
Death Anxiety

NANDA diagnoses are used with permission from North American Nursing Diagnosis Association (2004-6) Nursing Diagnoses: Definitions and Classification. Philadelphia: NANDA International.

Functional Health Patterns identified by M. Gordon (1982) Nursing Diagnosis: Process & Application. New York: McGraw Hill.

Collaborative Problems*

Potential Complication: Cardiac/Vascular

PC: Decreased cardiac output
PC: Dysrhythmias
PC: Pulmonary edema
PC: Deep vein thrombosis
PC: Hypovolemia
PC: Compartmental syndrome
PC: Pulmonary embolism

Potential Complication: Metabolic/Immune/Hematopoietic

PC: Hypoglycemia/hyperglycemia
PC: Negative nitrogen balance
PC: Electrolyte imbalances
PC: Sepsis
PC: Acidosis (metabolic, respiratory)
PC: Alkalosis (metabolic, respiratory)
PC: Allergic reaction
PC: Thrombocytopenia
PC: Opportunistic infections

Potential Complication: Gastrointestinal/Hepatic/Biliary

PC: Paralytic ileus
PC: Hepatic dysfunction
PC: Hyperbilirubinemia
PC: GI bleeding

Potential Complication: Neurologic/Sensory

PC: Increased intracranial pressure
PC: Seizures
PC: Neuroleptic malignant syndrome
PC: Alcohol withdrawal
PC: Increased intraocular pressure

Potential Complication: Renal/Urinary

PC: Acute urinary retention
PC: Renal insufficiency
PC: Renal calculi

Potential Complication: Muscular/Skeletal

PC: Joint dislocation

Potential Complication: Respiratory

PC: Hypoxemia
PC: Atelectasis/pneumonia
PC: Tracheobronchial constriction
PC: Pneumothorax

Potential Complication: Reproductive

PC: Fetal distress
PC: Postpartum hemorrhage
PC: Pregnancy-associated hypertension
PC: Prenatal bleeding
PC: Preterm labor

Potential Complication: Medication Therapy Adverse Effects

PC: Adrenocorticosteroid therapy adverse effects
PC: Antianxiety therapy adverse effects
PC: Antiarrhythmic therapy adverse effects
PC: Anticoagulant therapy adverse effects
PC: Anticonvulsant therapy adverse effects
PC: Antidepressant therapy adverse effects
PC: Antihypertensive therapy adverse effects
PC: Beta-adrenergic blocker therapy adverse effects
PC: Calcium channel blocker therapy adverse effects
PC: Angiotensin-converting enzyme therapy adverse effects
PC: Antineoplastic therapy adverse effects
PC: Antipsychotic therapy adverse effects

(Carpenito, L. J. (2004). *Nursing diagnosis: Application to clinical practice* (10th ed). Philadelphia: Lippincott Williams & Wilkins.)
*Frequently used collaborative problems are represented on this list. Other situations not listed here could qualify as collaborative problems.

Spanish Translation for Nursing Health History and Physical Examination

BIOGRAPHICAL DATA

English	Spanish
What is your name?	¿Cómo se llama Ud.?
	¿Cómo te llamas? (for child)
How old are you?	¿Cuántos años tiene?
Where do you live?	¿Dónde vive Ud.?
Are you allergic to anything?	¿Tiene Ud. alérgias a algún medicamento?
Do you have any handicaps?	¿Tiene minusvalía?
	¿Incapacidad física?
Do you have any illnesses that you know of?	¿Padece Ud. de una enfermedad?
	¿Más de una?
Have you had any past surgeries?	¿Ha sido operado?

FUNCTIONAL HEALTH PATTERN HISTORY

Health Perception/Health Management Pattern

English	Spanish
Rate your health on a scale of 1 to 10 (1 being poor, 10 being good).	Estime su salud en una escala de uno a diez (cuando uno significa malo y diez bueno).
Describe your current health.	Describa cómo está su salud.
When was your last tetanus shot?	¿Ha tenido inyección de tétano? ¿Cuándo fue la última?
Do you use drugs? If yes, explain.	¿Toma Ud. medicamentos? ¿drogas? Si 'sí,' ¿cuales son?
Do you use alcohol? If yes, explain.	¿Toma alcohol? Si 'sí,' ¿de qué clase y cuánto toma?
Do you use caffeine? If yes, explain.	¿Toma cafeína? ¿En qué forma y cuánto por día?

Nutritional/Metabolic Pattern

English	Spanish
What do you eat for breakfast? For lunch? For supper? For snacks?	¿Qué come por el desayuno? ¿por el almuerzo? ¿por la cena? ¿bocaditos? ¿tapas?
Describe the condition of your: • Skin • Hair • Nails	Por favor, describa la condición • de la piel • del pelo • de las uñas
Have you recently gained or lost weight? How much?	¿Ha experimentado un bajo o aumento de peso?

Elimination Pattern

English	Spanish
Describe your bowel pattern. How often? Color and consistency?	¿Cuándo hizo la deposición/defecación/evacuación la última vez? (¿Cuándo fue al baño la última vez?) ¿Puede describir el patrón de la defecación? ¿Cuántas veces a la semana? ¿Color? ¿Textura?
Describe your urinary pattern. How often? Color?	Puede describir el color de la orina? ¿Cuántas veces al día orina? (hace pi pi)
Do you need to urinate at night?	¿Hay que orinar de noche?
Is there a sense of urgency?	¿Hay un sentido de urgencia?

Activity/Exercise Pattern

English	Spanish
What activities do you do in a normal day?	Describa un día normal. ¿Cuáles actividades hace?
What do you do to relax?	¿Qué hace para descansar?
Do you physically exercise? Explain.	¿Hace ejercicio? Descríbalo, por favor.

Spanish Translation for Nursing Health History and
Physical Examination

Sexual/Reproduction Pattern

English	Spanish
How old were you when you started menstruating? Or when you stopped menstruating?	¿Cuántos años tenía cuando comenzó la menstruación? (a menstruar) ¿Cuándo paró la menstruación?
How many times have you been pregnant?	¿Cuántos embarazos ha tenido?
How many children do you have?	¿Cuántos niños/hijos tiene?
Do you do anything to prevent pregnancy?	¿Hace algo por evitar el embarazo?
Do you have any sexually transmitted diseases?	¿Padece de enfermedades transmitidos por el sexo?

Sleep/Rest Pattern

English	Spanish
What time do you go to bed at night?	¿A qué hora se aqueste?
How long do you sleep each night?	¿Cuántas horas se duerme de noche?
Does anything wake you?	¿Hay algo que lo despierte?
What helps you fall asleep?	¿Qué le ayuda dormir?
Do you take naps? How often?	¿Toma siestas? ¿Con frecuencia?

Sensory/Perceptual Pattern

English	Spanish
When was your last eye exam?	¿Cuándo fué el último examen de los ojos?
Do you have any problems:	¿Padece de problemas de
• Seeing?	• la vista?
• Hearing?	• oir? escuchar?
• Smelling?	• oler?
• Tasting?	• saber?
• Feeling?	• sentir sensaciones?
Do you have any pain now? Show me on this picture.	¿Tiene dolor ahora? ¿En dónde le duele? Muéstramelo en este dibujo.
• What causes it?	• ¿Qué cree que causa el dolor?
• What relieves it?	• ¿Qué reduce o quita el dolor?
• When does it occur?	• ¿Cuándo ocurre el dolor?
• How often?	• ¿y la frecuencia del dolor?
• How long does it last?	• ¿Cuánto tiempo dura el dolor?
• Show me on this scale how bad it hurts (use facial scale)	• Muéstreme lo malo que es el dolor en esta escala.

Cognitive Pattern

English	Spanish
What did your doctor tell you?	¿Qué es lo que le dijo el medico?
Do you have questions about your illness? Or treatments?	¿Quiere preguntar algo sobre la enfermedad? ¿sobre los tratamientos?

Role/Relationship Pattern

English	Spanish
Who do you live with?	¿Con quién vive Ud. ?
Are you married?	¿Está Ud. casado? casada (fem.)
Does your family get along well?	¿La familia se acuerdan/se portan bien?
What is your role in your family?	¿Qué es el papel que hace en la familia?

Self-Perception/Self-Concept Pattern

English	Spanish
What are your strengths?	¿Cuáles son las fuerzas que tiene en cuanto a la salud?
What are your weaknesses?	¿Cuáles son las debilidades?

Coping/Stress Tolerance Pattern

English	Spanish
What is stressful in your life?	¿Cuáles son los estreses de su vida?
What or who helps you most when you have a problem?	Cuándo hay un problema, ¿quién lo ayuda mas?

Value/Belief Pattern

English	Spanish
What is very important to you in life?	¿Qué mas le importa en la vida?
What religion are you?	¿A qué religion corresponde?
Are there certain foods you cannot have?	¿Hay comidas o ingredients que no puede comer?
Do you want a priest or hospital chaplain to visit you?	¿Quiere que el padre el capillán del hospital le hace una visita?

PHRASES TO USE TO HELP THE CLIENT THROUGH THE PHYSICAL ASSESSMENT

English	Spanish
Please	Por favor
Take off all your clothes and put on this gown.	Saque toda la ropa y ponga esta bata.
Urinate in this cup.	Orina (hace pi pi) en esta taza.
Lie down.	Acuéstese, por favor.
Stand up.	Póngase en pie, por favor.
Sit up.	Siéntese.
Get up and sit again.	Levántese y siéntese de nuevo.
Roll over to your right.	Gírese a la derecha.
Roll over to your left.	Gírese a la izquierda.
Take a deep breath.	Respira profundo.
Hold it.	Manténgalo.
Breathe out.	Respira de nuevo.
Cough.	Tosa.
Bend your leg.	Doble la pierna.
Bend your arm.	Doble el brazo.
Look up.	Mire para arriba.
Look down.	Mire para abajo.
Look to your right.	Mire al lado derecho.
Look to your left.	Mire al lado izquierdo.

Spanish Translation for Nursing Health History and Physical Examination

References and Bibliography

Allal, A., Nicoucar, K., Mach, N., & Dulguerov, P. (2003). Quality of life in patients with oropharynx carcinomas: Assessment after accelerated radiotherapy with or without chemotherapy versus radical surgery and postoperative radiotherapy. *Head & Neck, 25*(10), 833–841.

American Academy of Ophthalmology. (2005). *Comprehensive adult eye evaluation, preferred practice patterns.* San Francisco. www.aao.org

American Academy of Ophthalmology. (2006). Policy statement: Frequency of ocular examinations. San Francisco: Author.

American Academy of Ophthalmology. (2002). Pediatric eye evaluations (preferred practice pattern). San Francisco: Author.

American Academy of Pediatrics. (1997). Policy statement: Breast feeding and the use of human milk. *Pediatrics, 100*(6), 1035–1039.

American Academy of Pediatrics. (2000). Task force on infant sleep position and sudden infant death syndrome. *Pediatrics, 105*(3), 650–656.

American Cancer Society. (2006). *Cancer facts and figures.* Atlanta: Author.

American College of Obstetricians and Gynecologists. (2005). ACOG committee opinion number 315, September 2005. Obesity in pregnancy. *Obstetrics and Gynecology, 106*(3), 671–675.

American Dental Association. (2001). *Taking care of teeth and gums.* Chicago: Author.

American Dental Association. (2001). *Gum disease: Are you at risk.* Chicago: Author.

American Dental Association. (2002). *Your child's teeth.* Chicago: Author.

American Heart Association. (2000). *Dietary guidelines for healthy American adults.* AHA Scientific Position. Retrieved March 11, 2004, from http://www.americanheart.org

American Heart Association. (2004). *Tips for exercise success: Getting started on an exercise program.* Retrieved March 16, 2004, from http://www.americanheart.org

American Medical Association. (1992). *Diagnostic and treatment guidelines on elder abuse.* The Hartford Institute for Geriatric Nursing, New York: New York University.

American Nurses Association. (1998). *Culturally competent assessment for family violence.* Washington D.C.: Author.

Andrews, M., & Boyle, J. (2002). *Transcultural concepts in nursing care* (2nd ed.). Philadelphia: Lippincott Williams & Wilkins.

Apgar, V. (1953). A proposal for a new method of evaluation of the newborn infant. *Current Researchers in Anesthesia and Analgesia*, July–August, 1953, p. 260.

Atbasogcaronlu, E., Ozguven, H., & Olmez, S. (2003). Dissociation between inattentiveness during mental status testing and social inattentiveness in the scale for the assessment of negative symptoms attention subscale. *Psychopathology, 36*(5), 263–268.

Ballard, J. L., Khoury, J. C., Wedig, K., Wang, L., Eilers-Walsman, B. L., & Lipp, R. (1991). New Ballard Score: Expanded to include extremely premature infants. *Journal of Pediatrics, 19*(3), 417–423.

Bickley, L. S. (2003). *Bates' guide to physical examination and history taking* (8th ed.). Philadelphia: Lippincott Williams & Wilkins.

Bowles, K., & Cater, J. (2003). Screening for risk of rehospitalization from home care: Use of the outcomes assessment information set and the probability of readmission instrument. *Research in Nursing & Health, 26*(2), 118–128.

Brink, T., Yesavage, J. A., Lum, O., Heersema, P., Adey, M., & Rose, T. (1982). Screening tests for geriatric depression. *Clinical Gerontologist, 1*(1), 37–44.

Campbell, J. C. (2003). Danger Assessment. In Humphreys, J. & Campbell, J. C. (2004). *Family violence and nursing practice*. Philadelphia: Lippincott, Williams & Wilkins.

Campbell, J., & Humphreys, J. (1993). *Nursing care of survivors of family violence*. St. Louis: Mosby.

Campinha-Bacote, J. (2003). *The process of cultural competence in the delivery of healthcare services* (4th ed.). Cincinnati, OH: Transcultural C.A.R.E. Associates.

Carpenito-Moyet, L. J. (2006). *Nursing diagnosis: Application to clinical practice* (10th ed.). Philadelphia: Lippincott Williams & Wilkins.

Carrier-Kohlman, V., Lindsey, A. M., & West, C. M. (2003). *Pathophysiologic phenomena in nursing: Human response to illness* (3rd ed., pp. 235–254). St. Louis: Saunders.

Centers for Disease Control and Prevention. (2006) Stroke Facts and Statistics. Division for Heart Disease and Stroke Prevention, National Center for Chronic Disease Prevention and Health Promotion. Retrieved November 2006 from http://www.cdc.gov/Stroke/stroke_facts.htm#facts.

Child Abuse Prevention and Treatment Act, Public Law 104-235, §111; 42 U.S.C. 510g (2003).

Criddle, L., Bonnono, C., & Fisher, S. (2003). Standardizing stroke assessment using the National Institute of Health stroke scale. *Journal of Emergency Nursing, 29*(6), 541–548.

Daniel, W. A., Jr. (1985). Growth at adolescence clinical correlations. *Seminars in Adolescent Medicine, 1*(1), 15–24.

Datner, E., & Ferroggiaro, A. (1999). Violence during pregnancy. *Emergency Medical Clinics of North America, 17*(3), 645.

Dennis, C. (2003). The breastfeeding self-efficacy scale: Psychometric assessment of the short form. *Journal of Obstetric, Gynecologic and Neonatal Nursing, 32*(6), 734–744.

DePaula, T., Lagana, K., & González-Ramirez, L. (1996). Mexican Americans. In J. Lipton, S. Dribble, & P. Minarik (Eds.), *Culture and nursing care: A pocket guide*. San Francisco: UCSF Press.

Dion, L., Malouin, F., McFayden, B., & Richards, C. (2003). Assessing mobility and locomotor coordination after stroke with the rise-to-walk task. *Neurorehabilitation & Neural Repair, 17*(2), 83–92.

Dudek, S. G. (1997). *Nutrition handbook for nursing practice* (3rd ed.). Philadelphia: Lippincott-Raven Publishers.

Elder Mistreatment: Abuse, neglect and exploitation in an aging America. Retrieved May 20, 2006 from http://www.nap.edu/books/0309084342/ html/238.html

Erikson, E. (1963). *Childhood and society* (2nd ed.). New York: W. W. Norton.

Family Violence Prevention Fund. (1999). *Preventing domestic violence: Clinical guidelines on routine screening*. San Francisco: Author. www.fvpf.org.

Ferraro, M., Demaio, J., Krol, J., Trudell, C., Rannekleiv, K., & Edelstein, L. (2002). Assessing the motor status score: A scale for the evaluation of upper limb motor outcomes in patients with stroke. *Neurorehabilitation & Neural Repair, 16*(3), 283–289.

Gallagher, L. P., & Kreidler, M. C. (1987). *Nursing and health: Maximizing human potential throughout the life cycle*. Norwalk, CT: Appleton & Lange.

Giger, J., & Davidhizar, R. (2003). *Transcultural nursing: Assessment and intervention*. St. Louis: Mosby.

Gillum, K. (1996). Epidemiology of hypertension in African American women. *American Heart Journal, 13,* 385–395.

Gordon, M. (2002). *Manual of nursing diagnosis* (10th ed.). St. Louis: Mosby-Year Book.

Hawkins, D. F. (1993). Inequality, culture, and interpersonal violence. *Health Affairs* (Winter).

Hegar, A. H., Emans, S. J., & Muram, D. (2000). *Evaluation of the sexually abused child: A medical textbook and photographic atlas*. New York: Oxford University Press.

Houston, A., & Cowley, S. (2002). An empowerment approach to needs assessment in health visiting practice. *Journal of Clinical Nursing, 11*(5), 640–650.

Howard, G., Howard, V. J., Kapholi, C., Oli, M. K., & Huston, S. (2001). Decline in U.S. stroke mortality: An analysis of temporal patterns of sex, race, and geographic region. *Stroke, 32*(10), 2213–2220.

Humphreys, J., & Campbell, J. C. (2004). *Family violence and nursing practice*. Philadelphia: Lippincott Williams & Wilkins.

Jacobson, N., Gift, A., & Jacox, A. (1990). Advances in physical assessment. *Nursing Clinics of North America, 25*(4), 743–833.

Kelley, J., Avant, K., & Frisch, N. (1995). A trifocal model of nursing diagnosis: Wellness reinforced. *Nursing Diagnosis, 6*(3), 123–128.

Lamberg, L. (2000). Domestic violence: What to ask, what to do. *Journal of the American Medical Association, 284*(5), 554.

Leininger, M., & McFarland, M. (2002). *Transcultural nursing: Concepts, theories, research and practice.* New York: McGraw-Hill.

Lipson, J., Dibble, S., & Minarik, C. (1996). *Culture and nursing care: A pocket guide.* San Francisco: UCSF Nursing Press.

Manuszak, M., & Ross, J. (2003). Identification and management of vascular risk: Beyond low density lipoprotein cholesterol. *Official Journal of the American Association of the Occupational Health Nurse, 51*(12), 221–234.

Marshall, W. A., & Tanner, J. M. (1969). Summary of sequence of sexual development: Boys/girls. *Archives of Disease in Childhood, 44,* 291.

Matucci-Cerinic, M., D'Angelo, S., Denton, C., Vlachoyiannopoulos, P., & Silver, R. (2003). Assessment of lung involvement. *Clinical and Experimental Rheumatology, 21*(3), S19.

Messager, S., Hann, C., Goddard, P., Dettmar, P., & Maillard, J. (2003). Assessment of skin viability: Is it necessary to use different methodologies. *Skin Research and Technology, 9*(1), 321–330.

Metropolitan Life Insurance Company. (2000). Height and weight table. *Statistical Bulletin.*

Miller, B. (2002). Breast cancer risk assessment in patients seen in a gynecological oncology clinic. *International Journal of Gynecological Cancer, 12*(4), 389–393.

Murray, R. B., & Zentner, J. P. (1993). *Nursing assessment and health promotion strategies through the life span* (5th ed.). Norwalk, CT: Appleton & Lange.

National Center on Elder Abuse. (1998). National elder abuse incidence study. Final report. Washington, DC: Author.

National Institutes of Health. (2003). National high blood pressure education program: The 7th report of the Joint National Committee on Prevention, Detection, Evaluation and Treatment of High Blood Pressure. Bethesda, MD.

Nettina, S. (2001). *The Lippincott manual of nursing practice* (7th ed.). Philadelphia: Lippincott Williams & Wilkins.

Nogami, A. (2002). Idiopathic left ventricle tachycardia: assessment and treatment. *Cardiac Electrophysiology Review, 6*(2), 448–457.

North American Nursing Diagnosis Association. *Nursing diagnoses: Definitions and classification (2003–2004).* Philadelphia: Author.

North American Nursing Diagnosis Association International. (2005–2006). *Nursing diagnoses: Definition & classification 2005–2006.* Philadelphia: Author.

Nursing Network on Violence Against Women International. (2004). *Assessment tools.* Retrieved November 2005 from www.nnvawi.org.

Olaleye, D., Perkins, B., & Bril, V. (2002). Evaluation of three screening tests and a risk assessment model for diagnosis of peripheral neuropathy in the diabetes clinic. *Journal of the Peripheral Nervous System, 7*(2), 137.

Overfield, T. (1995). *Biological variation in health and illness: Race, age, and sex differences.* Menlo Park, CA: Addison-Wesley.

Pablo, A., Izaga, M., & Alday, L. (2003). Assessment of nutritional status on hospital admission nutritional scores. *European Journal of Clinical Nutrition, 57*(7), 824–831.

Palou, A., Serra, F., & Pico, C. (2003). General aspects on the assessment of functional foods in the European union. *European Journal of Clinical Nutrition, 57*(S1), S12–S17.

Peddle, N., Wang, C. T., Diaz, J., & Reid, R. (2002). Current trends in child abuse prevention and fatalities—the 2000 fifty state survey. Retrieved November 2005 from www.preventchildabuse.org/learn_more/research_ docs/2000_50_survey.pdf

Peterson, A., Hryshko-Mullen, A., & Cortex, Y. (2003). Assessment and diagnosis of nicotine dependence in mental health settings. *American Journal on Addictions, 12*(3), 192–197.

Piaget, J. (1967). *Six psychological studies:* New York: Vintage Books.

Pillitteri, A. (2003). *Maternal and child health nursing: Care of the childbearing and childrearing family* (4th ed.). Philadelphia: Lippincott Williams & Wilkins.

Ponzer, S., Skoog, A,, & Bergstrom, G. (2003). The short musculoskeletal function assessment questionnaire (SMFA). *Acta Orthopaedica Scandinavica, 74*(6), 756–763.

Price, S. A., & Wilson, L. M. (1997). *Pathophysiology, clinical concepts of disease process* (5th ed., pp. 819–848). St. Louis: Mosby-Year Book.

Purnell, L. & Paulanka, B. (2003). *Transcultural health care: A culturally competent approach* (2nd ed.). Philadelphia: F. A. Davis.

Rankin, E. A., & Mitchel, M. L. (2000). Creating a pain management educational module for hospice nurses: Integrating the new JCAHO standards and the AHCPR pain management guidelines. *Journal of Hospice and Palliative Nursing, 2*(3), 91–100.

Regan, J. M., & Peng, P. (2000). Neurophysiology of cancer pain. *Cancer Control, 7*(2), 111–119.

Rice, E. M. (1989). Geriatric assessment. *Advancing Clinical Care* (May–June), 8–15.

Sanchez-Muniz, F., Carbajal, A., Rodenas, S., Mendez, M., Raposo, R., & Ruiz, T. (2003). Nutritional assessment, health markers and lipoprotein profile in postmenopausal women belonging to a closed community. *European Journal of Clinical Nutrition, 57*(S1), S26–530.

Schiffman, R., Walt, J., Jacobson, G., Doyle, J., Lebovics, G., & Sumner, W. (2003). Utility assessment among patients with dry eye disease. *Ophthalmology, 110*(7), 1412–1420.

Schmermund, A., Mohlenkamp, S., Stang, A., Gronemeyer, D., Seibel, R., & Hirch, H. (2002). Assessment of clinically silent atherosclerotic disease and established and novel risk factors for predicting myocardial infarction and cardiac death in healthy middle-aged subjects. *American Heart Journal, 144*(2), 212–218.

Schwartz, J., & Vinson, R. (2003). Self-assessment examination of the American academy of dermatology. *Journal of the American Academy of Dermatology, 49*(5), 971.

Shimada, M., Hayat, J., Meguro, K., OO, T., Jafri, S., & Yamadori, A. (2003). Correlation between functional assessment staging and "basic age" by the Binet scale supports the retrogenesis model of Alzheimer's disease: A preliminary study. *Psychogeriatrics, 3*(2). 82–87.

Spector, R. E. (2003). *Cultural diversity in health and illness* (6th ed.). Upper Saddle River, NJ: Prentice-Hall.

Stark, E. (2001). Heath intervention with battered women: From crisis intervention to complex social prevention. In C. M. Renzetti, J. L. Edleson, & R. K. Bergen (Eds.), *Sourcebook on violence against women* (pp. 345–370). Thousand Oaks, CA: Sage Publications.

Symon, A., MacDonald, A., & Ruta, D. (2002). Postnatal quality of life assessment; introducing the mother-generated index. *Birth 29*(1), 40–46.

Synder, L., Wallerstedt, D., Lahl, L., Nehrebecky, M., Soballe, P., & Klein, P. (2003). Development of breast cancer education and risk assessment program. *Oncology Nursing Forum, 30*(5), 803–811.

Takata, G., Chan, L., Morphew, T., Mangione-Smith, R., Morton, S., & Shkelle, P. (2003). Evidence of assessment of the accuracy of methods of diagnosing middle ear effusion in children with otitis media with effusion. *Pediatrics, 11*(2), 1379–1388.

Tanner, J. M. (1962). *Growth at adolescence* (2nd ed.). Oxford: Blackwell Scientific Publications.

Teasdale, G., & Jennett, B. (1974). Assessment of coma and impaired consciousness: A practical scale. *Lancet, 2,* 81–83.

U.S. Department of Agriculture, U.S. Department of Health and Human Services. (2005). *Nutrition and your health: Dietary guidelines for Americans* (6th ed.). Washington, DC: Author.

United States Department of Health and Human Services. (2004). Bone health and osteoporosis: A report of the Surgeon General. Retrieved November 2006 from http://www.surgeongeneral.gov/library/bonehealth/content.html.

Wall, P. D., & Melzack, R. (1994). *Textbook of pain* (3rd ed., pp. 523–540). London: Longman Group U.K. Limited.

Washington State Department of Health. (2004). Domestic violence and pregnancy: Guidelines for screening and referral. Publication #950-143, pp. 2–28. Olympia, WA: Author.

Weeks, S. K., McGarin, P. E., Michaels, T. K. & Pennius, B. W. J. H. (2003). Comparing various short-form geriatric depression scales leads to the GDS-5/15. *Journal of Nursing Scholarship 35*(2), 133–137.

Index

Page numbers followed by a *f* indicate a figure; page numbers followed by a *t* indicate a table; page numbers followed by a *b* indicate a box.